Cognitive Therapy
with Chronic Pain Patients

Carrie Winterowd, PhD, is an Associate Professor of Counseling Psychology and Counseling in the School of Applied Health and Educational Psychology at Oklahoma State University. She has been working with chronic pain patients in her private practice for the past 10 years. Dr. Winterowd received her PhD in Counseling Psychology at The University of Kansas in 1993. She was a post-doctoral fellow at the Center for Cognitive Therapy at the University of Pennsylvania. She is a licensed psychologist (Health Service Psychologist) in the state of Oklahoma and is a Founding Fellow of the Academy of Cognitive Therapy (ACT). Much of her current research is focused in the area of health psychology. She is a member of the Association for the Advancement of Behavior Therapy (AABT), the American Psychological Association (APA), the International Association for Cognitive Psychotherapy (IACP), the International Association for the Study of Pain (IASP), and the American Pain Society (APS).

Aaron T. Beck, MD, University Professor of Psychiatry, University of Pennsylvania, is a graduate of Brown University (1942) and Yale Medical School (1946). The recipient of numerous awards and honorary degrees, he is the only psychiatrist to receive research awards from the American Psychological Association and the American Psychiatric Association. The author or coauthor of over 400 articles, he has recently published a new book, *Prisoners of Hate: The Cognitive Basis of Anger, Hostility and Violence.* He is President of The Beck Institute of Cognitive Therapy.

Daniel M. Gruener, MD, completed his psychiatric training at Jefferson Medical College in 1991 and served as Chief Resident in Psychiatry during his last year of training. Dr. Gruener is board-certified in both Psychiatry and Pain Medicine. He has been on the volunteer teaching faculty of Jefferson Medical College since 1992. Dr. Gruener has divided his time, both academically and clinically, between the fields of Psychiatry and Pain Medicine. He has been active in both clinical and administrative work in Psychiatry and has served as President of the Medical Staff of Friends Hospital in Philadelphia, as well as two years as the Medical Director of Inpatient Services. Dr. Gruener has spent time doing clinical research, teaching, clinical practice and writing related to Pain Medicine and Psychiatry. He has lectured at numerous conferences, continuing medical education programs and similar venues across the United States and remains a highly requested lecturer. Active in many causes related to Pain Medicine, he currently serves as President of the Greater Philadelphia Pain Society, a branch of the American Pain Society, and just completed editing, *A Guidebook for Managing Pain in the Hospital,* with the Society. Active in clinical practice, Dr. Gruener was named one of the "Top Docs" for 2002 in *Philadelphia Magazine.* He is President of the Northeast Neuroscience Institute, a medical education company devoted to the advancement of research and education in both Psychiatry and Pain Medicine. He continues to serve a patient population via a private group practice in Abington, Pennsylvania.

Cognitive Therapy
with Chronic Pain Patients

Carrie Winterowd, PhD
Aaron T. Beck, MD
Daniel Gruener, MD

 Springer Publishing Company

Springer Publishing Company, Inc.
536 Broadway
New York, NY 10012-3955

Acquisitions Editor: Sheri W. Sussman
Production Editor: Sara Yoo
Cover design by Joanne Honigman
Cover artwork by Karla Winterowd

01   02   03   04   05   /   5   4   3   2   1

Library of Congress Cataloging-in-Publication Data

Winterowd, Carrie.
    Cognitive therapy with chronic pain patients / Carrie Winterowd,
Aaron T. Beck, Daniel Gruener.
        p. ; cm.
    Includes bibliographical references and index.
    ISBN 0-8261-4595-7
    1. Chronic pain—Treatment.   2. Cognitive therapy.
I. Beck, Aaron T.   II. Gruener, Daniel.   III. Title.
    [DNLM: 1. Pain—psychology.   2. Pain—therapy.   3. Chronic
Disease—psychology.   4. Chronic Disease—therapy.   5. Cognitive
Therapy.   WL 704 W788c 2003]
RB127. W565 2003
616'.0472—dc22

                                                        2003059044

Printed in the United States of America by Maple-Vail Book
Manufacturing Group.

Dedications

I would like to dedicate this book to my husband, Phil, and
my children, Austin and Kayla.
Thank you for your love and support.

— *Carrie Winterowd, PhD*

To Phyllis.

— *Aaron T. Beck, MD*

To my wife Karen, and my children, Jennifer and Laura
for their love, talent and patience.

— *Daniel Gruener, MD*

Contents

Part V Assertiveness

Part VI Pharmacotherapy

Part VII Preparing for the End of Therapy and Beyond

Preface

Although other articles and books have been written on cognitive-behavioral therapy applications to chronic pain, this is the first treatment manual available for readers interested in applying Aaron T. Beck's cognitive therapy approach with chronic pain patients. Cognitive therapy has been highly effective with a number of patient concerns and has a strong research base to confirm its efficacy. Cognitive therapy with chronic pain patients is unique in that it emphasizes a strong theoretical foundation that guides intervention strategies. Patients learn how to identify, evaluate, and modify their negative, unrealistic appraisals of their pain and its impact on their lives within the context of a supportive, collaborative therapeutic relationship. Rather than substituting positive thoughts for negative thoughts, patients are taught to evaluate the *accuracy* of their thoughts, beliefs, and images related to their pain prior to developing alternative, more realistic thoughts. Patients are taught to become their own "scientists" or "investigators" on themselves and their pain. They learn to view their thoughts and beliefs as hypotheses or hunches to test out and then collect evidence to confirm or disconfirm them. Behavioral experiments and journaling are typical homework assignments developed between therapists and patients to evaluate negative thoughts and intense emotions related to pain. This evaluation process is one of the key ingredients in cognitive therapy that distinguishes it from other cognitive-behavioral approaches.

One of the advantages of using the cognitive therapy approach with the chronic pain population is its active and structured therapeutic focus. Most individuals can be treated within a short time frame. By teaching patients the basic skills they need to cope with their pain and other psychosocial events, chronic pain patients will become more independent, more compliant with medical treatment, as well as more hopeful and realistic in coping with their pain and their lives. The key skills that chronic pain patients can learn in cognitive therapy include how to (1) identify, evaluate, and modify their negative, unrealistic appraisals of their pain, themselves, their world, and their future and (2) develop problem-solving skills in order to make decisions, accomplish tasks, and set realistic goals. In learning and applying these skills, chronic pain patients may experience less pain, less emotional distress, improved coping skills, and better relationships with others, including medical professionals, people at work, family, and friends.

It is hoped that this treatment manual provides psychologists, psychiatrists, social workers, counselors, and other health care professionals with the "how to's" of cognitive therapy with chronic pain patients. Many of the ideas and case examples presented have been based on clinical experience. Please note that the names and identities of actual patients have been changed to ensure their anonymity. Some case examples represent an integration of several patient cases. Throughout this manual, clients who have chronic pain will be referred to as patients. This does not mean that we view them as "sick" or "ill," but rather, it reflects the medical and psychosocial nature of their problems, and it is often used by a variety of health care professionals who work with this population. In addition, the term "therapist," will be used denote the health care professionals (e.g. psychiatrists, psychologists, counselors, social workers, physicians) who provide psychotherapy services to clients/patients.

This treatment manual offers improvements to and new knowledge on cognitive therapy with chronic pain patients compared with existing books on cognitive-behavioral approaches to chronic pain in the following ways. First, this book describes Beck's cognitive therapy approach to patients with chronic pain. Second, it provides an easy-to-follow structured approach, with case examples and therapist–patient dialogues to demonstrate the cognitive therapy approach. Third, cognitive therapy emphasizes a collaborative relationship with other professionals involved in chronic pain patients' care; this manual illustrates ways to improve collaborative efforts between professionals and patients. Fourth, many books and manuals on cognitive-behavioral approaches to chronic pain assume that mental health professionals work in multidisciplinary chronic pain treatment centers or programs, which may not be the case. Although some patients are seen in chronic pain clinics, there are a number of towns and cities that do not have such specialty clinics. Therefore, this book is primarily geared toward professionals who may see chronic pain patients as part of their practice in hospital settings, community mental health centers, university counseling centers, and private practice settings. Those professionals who work in pain specialty clinics may also find this book to be of assistance to them.

The book has seven main sections. The first section, Chapters 1, 2, 3 and 4 provides an overview of pain, assessment, and treatment considerations for patients with chronic, noncancer pain. Chapter 1 explains some of the theories of pain as well as the treatment approaches to pain management. Chapter 2 introduces readers to the cognitive conceptualization of chronic pain. Chapter 3 explains the usual course and structure of cognitive therapy with chronic pain patients. Intake interviewing strategies and the assessment process are highlighted in chapter 4.

The second section of the book provides information on behavioral interventions in therapy. Pain monitoring, and activity monitoring, scheduling, and pacing are covered in chapter 5, while relaxation training and distraction techniques are covered in chapter 6. These behavioral approaches help patients cope better with their pain.

In the third section of this book, readers will learn cognitive interventions to help chronic pain patients identify, evaluate, and modify (1) automatic thoughts about pain (in chapters 7, 8, and 9), (2) imagery related to pain (in chapter 10), and (3) intermediate and core beliefs about pain (in chapters 11 and 12).

In the fourth section of this book, therapists will learn how to address psychosocial stressors associated with chronic pain in therapy, including medical care problems (chapter 13), family, friends, and lifestyle issues (chapter 14), and occupational, financial, and legal difficulties (chapter 15). Therapists will learn how to intervene with patients experiencing stressors in these areas.

In the fifth section of this book, assertiveness training interventions will be illustrated as a way to promote chronic pain patients' self-efficacy in obtaining quality care and social support (chapter 16). Pharmacotherapy issues for chronic pain patients will be addressed in the sixth section of this book as well as potential substance-related problems for this population (chapter 17). Relapse prevention, is the topic of the last section of this book. As therapy is brought to a close, it is important for therapists to discuss with patients what was accomplished in therapy, to reinforce positive treatment outcomes, and reduce the likelihood of relapse when therapy ends.

Cognitive therapy is an active, directive, time-limited approach with an emphasis on identifying, evaluating, and modifying patients' negative thoughts and beliefs about their pain, themselves, their world, and their future. Skill development in problem-solving approaches is also highlighted. Cognitive therapy has been effective with a variety of patients because of its emphasis on (1) setting specific, measurable goals with patients, (2) developing a collaborative (team) approach to resolving problems, (3) educating patients about the cognitive model (so that someday they too can become their own cognitive therapist), (4) incorporating structure within and between sessions to guide the psychotherapy process, and (5) encouraging patients to learn from their experiences in session by providing them with regular homework assignments to help them practice necessary coping skills.

Interestingly, patients with chronic pain are being referred more often to psychotherapists because of the potential difficulties in coping with pain and significant psychosocial stressors. Cognitive therapists can assist physicians and specialists in evaluating and treating the psychological aspects of patients' medical conditions in hopes of reducing their pain levels, increasing their level of functioning, and improving medical compliance with treatment recommendations. Cognitive therapy can provide an important service to these individuals in evaluating what it means to have chronic pain, how to cope with these painful experiences, and how to gain more support from friends, family, physicians, and attorneys. It is for these reasons that this treatment manual has been developed to serve clinicians who may work with chronic pain patients.

Acknowledgments

We would like to thank a number of people who have helped us with different aspects of this book including its development and production. Special thanks go to Sheri W. Sussman, Editorial Director at Springer Publishing. We are very grateful to Sheri and her staff at Springer for their unwavering support and encouragement in the development and production of this manuscript. We are indebted to Barbara Marinelli for her assistance to Drs. Beck and Winterowd, particularly in coordinating phone contacts and other communications. Jessica Handelsman and Kimberly Ling served as copyeditors on earlier drafts of our manuscript and we are very grateful for their feedback.

Carrie Winterowd, PhD and Aaron T. Beck, MD

Special thanks to Trevor Richardson who served as my graduate assistant last year and helped me stay organized. I would also like to thank Dr. Robert Tromley, Benita Big Foot, Anita Warrior, Syd Church, and Jenny Sheader-Wood for reviewing earlier drafts of the manuscript. Laura Densmore, Debbie Holman, Stephanie Porterfield, Jenny Sheader-Wood, and Ginger Welch assisted me with library research and article reviews. Although much of their work was not included in this book due to space issues, their work served as an important foundation for the writing of this book.

Dr. Ed Heck introduced me to cognitive therapy when I was a graduate student at the University of Kansas. His passion and enthusiasm for this subject provided the impetus for me to become a cognitive therapist.

I am grateful to the folks at the Center for Cognitive Therapy, especially Dr. Aaron T. Beck and Dr. Michael Natale, who provided me with a unique postdoctoral training experience to specialize in cognitive therapy with chronic pain patients. I also want to thank the clients I have worked with during the course of my career as a psychologist. They inspired me to write this book. Drs. Maureen Sullivan, Trish Long, Margaret Johnson, Donald Boswell, and Ms. Alison Chakraborty have provided unwavering personal support and encouragement along the way. Thanks to all of my friends and colleagues for believing in me. Last, I would like to acknowledge my husband, Phil, my children, Austin and Kayla, my parents, K.B. and Carol, my sister, Karla, and my lifelong friend, Debbie, for their love and support during the journey of writing my first book.

Carrie Winterowd, PhD

I would like to thank my friend and colleague, Dr. Stephen Lande for his ongoing assistance in this and many other projects. A special thanks to my patients for teaching me so much about medicine. Finally, I would like to thank my parents for allowing me to pursue this path.

Daniel Gruener, MD

PART I

OVERVIEW OF PAIN, ASSESSMENT, AND TREATMENT CONSIDERATIONS

1

Theories of Pain and Treatment Approaches to Pain Management

Everyone has been in pain at some point in his or her life. However, unrelieved chronic pain is perhaps one of the most challenging problems faced by health care consumers as well as health care practitioners and providers. It is a problem of enormous magnitude in society, yet there is overwhelming evidence that it is inadequately treated. Nearly 75% of people dying from cancer have unrelieved pain (Brescia, Portenoy, & Ryan, 1992). If we fail to treat people with terminal illnesses, how can we expect people with noncancer pain to obtain proper treatment and relief? It is estimated that from 75 million to 80 million people in the United States suffer from some sort of chronic pain, at an annual cost of $65 billion to $70 billion (Tollison, 1993). Approximately 80% of all physician visits in the United States involve pain complaints (Stucky, Gold, & Zhang, 2001). Chronic back pain is probably the most frequently identified pain condition in the chronic pain population. Health care professionals (ie., physicians, nurses, psychiatrists, psychologists, counselors, social workers) are likely to work with patients who have chronic pain and will need an understanding of the etiology and treatment of pain.

WHAT IS PAIN?

Pain has been defined as "an unpleasant sensory and emotional experience associated with actual or potential tissue damage or described in terms of such damage" (Merskey & Bogduk, 1994, p. 210). This definition of pain, adopted by the International Association for the Study of Pain, emphasizes the mind–body connection in terms of the pain experience. This means that the sensory experience of pain cannot be separated from the emotional experience. Turk, Meichenbaum, and Genest (1993) described pain as a subjective experience involving our senses, our emotions, our thoughts, and our actions or behaviors. If pain truly has a subjective component, then perhaps the best definition of pain is what patients tell us it is.

SUBTYPES OF PAIN

Pain can be *cancer* or *noncancer related*. This manual is geared toward working with patients who have chronic noncancer pain. However, many of the techniques described in this book can be used with patients who have cancer-related chronic pain.

Pain can also be acute or chronic. In the past, chronic pain was defined as pain that lasted more than 6 months and acute pain as pain that lasted less than 6 months. The main flaw in these definitions is the arbitrary designation of time course for pain. *Chronic pain* is now defined as pain that persists beyond the time one would expect normal healing to occur, and *acute pain* is defined as pain that lasts within a specified time frame for a given condition (Bonica, 1990). For example, a person breaks his right arm. We expect the arm to heal in 6 weeks, assuming it is a simple fracture. Three months later, the same person continues to complain of pain, especially a burning sensation in his right arm. At that point, we would classify this pain as chronic.

Acute pain serves a useful function in signaling potential injury or damage to muscles, tissues, or nerves. For example, if a person experiences a sharp pain in the right lower quadrant of her abdomen, this pain may signal an illness such as appendicitis. Without the pain, the appendix might have burst, leading to sepsis and possibly death.

Chronic pain serves no useful purpose. It is a result of persistent tissue injury and ongoing activation of pain receptors that may lead to pharmacological, physiological, and anatomical changes in the central nervous system, where pain information is processed. Unlike acute pain, chronic pain no longer warns the patient of bodily harm.

Chronic pain typically has more than one etiology. Pain may be caused by a number of different factors, including injuries, diseases/pathology, and medical procedures (Turk et al., 1993). Most patients who have presented with chronic pain have consulted with a number of health care practitioners, have received a variety of diagnoses or potentially no diagnoses at all, and have undergone multiple failed treatments. Chronic pain patients often suffer from anxiety and depression, either as part of the pain's underlying etiology or as a result of continuing refractory pain (Payne, 1998).

Pain is further subdivided by its underlying cause. *Nociceptive pain* (i.e., musculoskeletal) is the type of pain that results from an injury, sending a signal via specialized pain receptors in the spinal cord to the brain. There are no permanent changes or alterations to the central nervous system. Examples of nociceptive pain (also known as nonneuropathic pain) are bone fractures, arthritis, burns, lacerations, and injury to internal organs.

To illustrate nociceptive pain, imagine a patient who has broken a bone. Specialized pain receptors called nociceptors are activated in the patient and send an electrical signal up the spinal cord to the brain. The signal is processed as pain. This is rather simple and straightforward. The patient's bone heals within several weeks; the painful signal ceases to be sent to the brain, and the painful sensation stops (no permanent central nervous system changes).

Contrast this with the next subtype of pain, *neuropathic pain.* Neuropathic pain is pain due to damage or dysfunction of nerves. After a neuropathic injury, there are changes and alterations in the central nervous system (including the brain and spinal cord) or the peripheral nervous system (i.e., peripheral nerves leading to the spinal cord), becoming permanent in nature over time. For example, a person injures her back in a car accident and herniates a disc. That person undergoes a laminectomy procedure, during which damaged disc material is removed. Unbeknownst to the neurosurgeon, there may be nerve root damage caused by the accident and the surgery itself, leading to a neuropathic pain syndrome. A year later, the patient complains of a severe burning sensation in her right leg, a neuropathic pain condition known as radicular pain, which is extremely common but unfortunately missed by some physicians. Without an understanding of neuropathic pain, the neurosurgeon might schedule a magnetic resonance imaging (MRI) test for the patient, find that the surgery was successful and that the spine is stable, pronounce the patient healed, and assume that the patient's pain is psychogenic in nature.

It is estimated that two million Americans suffer from neuropathic pain (Bennett, 1994). Neuropathic pain has been called "the silent disease," although not because patients are silent about it. In fact, they complain about it a great deal. Most neuropathic pain goes undetected by health care providers, often because they have not been trained adequately in the diagnosis and treatment of neuropathic pain. Some examples of neuropathic pain are diabetic neuropathy, postherpetic neuralgia, complex regional pain syndrome (formerly known as reflex sympathetic dystrophy), and neuropathy related to acquired immunodeficiency syndrome (AIDS).

Patients with neuropathic pain often present with sensory changes such as allodynia (i.e., pain due to a stimulus that does not normally provoke pain, (e.g., light touch), hyperalgesia (i.e., an increased response to a stimulus that is normally painful, e.g., a pinprick), and hyperpathia (i.e., a syndrome characterized by an abnormally painful reaction to a stimulus, especially a repetitive stimulus, e.g., a repetitive pinprick, as well as lowered pain threshold). These symptoms are the result of changes occurring in the central or peripheral nervous system (Woolf & Mannion, 1999). For example, patients with neuropathic pain in its most advanced form report that wind blowing on their skin is exquisitely painful. It is not unusual to see these patients in hospital beds where the affected extremity (e.g., leg or arm) is outside the sheet because the pressure of a thin hospital sheet causes intense pain in that extremity.

Another type of pain is *mixed pain.* This occurs when a patient has elements of both nociceptive and neuropathic pain. For example, a person has a low back injury. He herniates a disc in his back, which is a mechanical nociceptive problem; the disc in his back compresses nerve roots, causing a neuropathic problem. Thus, this patient has both nociceptive and neuropathic pain. If the physician does not understand the etiology and treatment of neuropathic pain and treats only the nociceptive component, the patient is receiving inadequate treatment.

The next type of pain is *idiopathic or unspecified pain.* Idiopathic pain is undiagnosed pain, which may, in fact, be neuropathic in nature.

The last category of pain is *psychogenic pain.* Psychogenic pain refers to a process whereby pain is purely psychological in nature and no true physical pathology exists. Psychogenic pain is extremely rare. What often happens is that the physician does not do an adequate assessment of pain and, therefore, fails to come up with the physiological mechanism to explain why a person is suffering from pain. (For example, complex pain syndromes may be inaccurately diagnosed as psychogenic in origin.) Some patients are referred to mental health professionals because the pain is believed to be psychogenic in nature. Based on clinical experiences, many patients referred with so-called psychogenic pain turned out to have a physiological basis for their pain. However, psychogenic overlay is quite common to pain patients, which means that psychological factors can influence the experience of pain.

MODELS OF PAIN PERCEPTION

Our understanding of pain has evolved greatly since the concept of pain being regulated by neural pathway gates between the brain and the site of pain (e.g., gate control theory). We now conceptualize pain perception as follows. Pain is detected by nociceptive receptors located in the periphery (i.e., peripheral nerves), deep tissues (e.g., muscles and tendons), and viscera (i.e., internal organs). The two types of nociceptive fibers, A-delta and C fibers, project to the dorsal horn (bottom) of the spinal cord (see Figure 1.1). That pain signal, which is essentially an electric signal, gets relayed to the dorsal horn of the spinal cord. The signal then travels up the spinal cord via ascending pathways and terminates in an area of the brain called the thalamus, where that signal is processed (see Figure 1.2). From the thalamus, the signal is relayed to several areas of the brain, primarily the somatosensory cortex of the cerebral cortex, where memories and thoughts are processed, and the limbic system, where emotions are processed. The brain has an effect on that pain signal; the brain actually modulates it and changes it. At each point along the pathway, the signal may be modulated by intrinsic neurons or by descending input from higher centers, for example, the cerebral cortex. Damage at any point along the pathway from the peripheral nervous system to the cerebral cortex can lead to neuropathic pain (Hyman & Cassen, 1996).

FIGURE 1.1 Neuroanatomy of Pain Pathways: Dorsal Horn of Spinal Cord

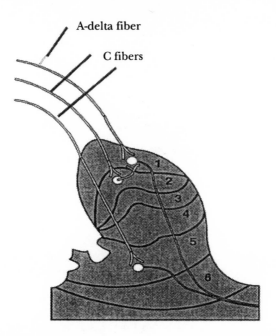

From "Pain," by R. Payne and D. Dale, 1996, *Scientific American Medicine, 3.* Copyright 1996 Richard Payne. Reprinted with permission.

FIGURE 1.2 Neuroanatomy of Pain Pathways: View of the Brain

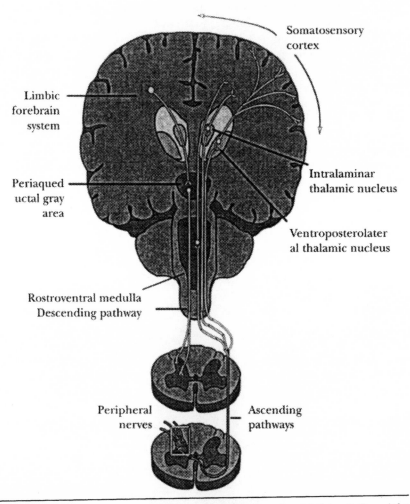

From "Pain," by R. Payne and D. Dale, 1996, *Scientific American Medicine, 3,* Copyright 1996 Richard Payne. Reprinted with permission.

Neuropathic pain is different etiologically from nociceptive pain. It is important to understand the difference between nociceptive and neuropathic pain given that the treatment pathways are quite different (this will be discussed in chapter 17). How does pain know to become neuropathic as opposed to nociceptive? Normal neuronal function depends on an actively maintained equilibrium between neurons and their environment. Any disruption in this equilibrium can initiate profound changes in sensory function and can lead to neuropathic pain.

There are two types of neurotransmitters (substances crucial to nerve transmission) in the brain: the excitatory neurotransmitters that increase the rate of neuronal firing (i.e., glutamate) and the inhibitory neurotransmitters that reduce neuronal firing (i.e., gabaaminobutyric acid, or GABA). Glutamate and GABA are normally in homeostasis; in other words, they balance each other out. However, glutamate becomes hyperactivated in response to a neuropathic injury.

For example, a person has a neuropathic injury, and type C fibers become activated. This leads to an increase in glutamate levels. Receptors become uncoupled (i.e., the N-methyl-D-aspartate [NMDA] receptor and the alpha-amino-3-hydroxy-5-melthyl-4-isoxazolepropion, acid [AMPA] receptor). Opening these receptors leads to an influx of cations (electrolytes) such as sodium, potassium, and calcium. This rise of intracellular cations leads to a cascade of events. Cell membranes destabilize; neurons gradually depolarize, and their responses become increasingly amplified. This process has been referred to as the "wind up phenomenon" (Ollat & Cesaro, 1995). In other words, the entire nervous system is being wound up. Nerves are firing more rapidly in response to a stimulus and eventually fire spontaneously without a stimulus. As a result of the hyperactivation of the nervous system, patients become more easily sensitized to pain than before.

Suppose a person is lightly tapped 20 times on his left hand while at the same time his right hand is hit extremely hard. The nerves in the person's right hand become hyperpolarized (excited). Next, both arms are tapped with equal pressure. The person feels more pressure or pain in his right hand because the nerves in the right arm have been supersensitized as compared with the left. Suppose the person's right arm is hit so hard that nerve damage results. It is possible that the person will experience neuropathic pain in the right arm spontaneously without any stimulus.

Another way of conceptualizing this process is called the "kindling model" (Ollat & Cesaro, 1995). Suppose a person is starting a fire in a fireplace or at a campsite. This person cannot take two big logs, light a match under these logs, and expect them to ignite. The match will burn down, and the person will merely burn her hand. Instead, little pieces of wood, twigs, and paper, referred to as kindling, must be gathered and placed underneath the large logs. Next, the kindling is lit with a match. The kindling essentially alters the chemical composition of the wood in the larger logs, making them more sensitive to the heat source, and ultimately a raging fire results. This is a simple way of conceptualizing the evolution of neuropathic pain. As the regular firing of the pain message occurs, this process of firing alters the central nervous system, making it more sensitive to future pain signals, resulting in more frequent, nonfunctional pain.

The kindling model is also an explanation of how seizures in the brain evolve. We now believe that it may explain the pathogenesis of a variety of neuropsychiatric conditions such as bipolar disorder, anxiety states, withdrawal states related to substance abuse, and even migraine headaches.

This model also explains why pain and psychiatric conditions often occur comorbidly and may have overlapping features. In other words, psychiatric conditions are also the result of hyperactivation of the nervous system, as mentioned above. When two or more medical or psychological conditions occur at the same time (comorbidity), they may share common features, which may relate to the similar underlying causes of these disorders. For example, it is very common for people suffering from chronic pain to experience symptoms such as depression, anxiety, and sleep disorders. This comorbidity explains why we use common medications and treatment pathways to treat a variety of neuropsychiatric complaints such as pain, insomnia, anxiety, and depression (Kanazi, Johnson, & Dworkin, 2000).

PSYCHOLOGICAL ASPECTS OF PAIN

When the pain signal is processed in the brain, certain thoughts or memories may be activated in the somatosensory cortex, and certain emotions may be activated in the limbic system. Thus, when a person experiences a pain sensation, he or she will have some emotional response(s) to it and will experience certain thoughts and/or images during or immediately following the pain.

For example, a chronic pain patient with herniated discs in his lower back bent down to pick up the newspaper on the ground. He experienced an intense, stabbing sensation in his lower back. He felt very frustrated and thought, "Why is this happening to me? I can't even pick up a newspaper without experiencing pain. I shouldn't have to deal with this." At the same time, he also felt hopeless and thought, "I'll never be able to live a normal life again." The emotions he experienced were frustration and hopelessness. His cognitions were negative in nature, focusing on his physical limitations and his life in general.

Similarly, thoughts and emotions that are activated in the brain may modulate the pain signal. In other words, patients' thoughts, memories, and emotions can influence the experience of pain physiologically in the central and peripheral nervous systems.

Suppose a 45-year-old man has a father who died of a heart attack at the age of 45. Imagine that man is having lunch in a Mexican restaurant and is eating spicy food. He begins to experience chest discomfort. Although this discomfort is merely heartburn, his memory of his father's death (including his thoughts and feelings about it) actually modulates the pain sensation, sending it back down the spinal cord to the nerves that innervate the chest wall, and that man experiences the pain as being more severe than it really is.

Conversely, suppose a woman trips and sprains her ankle very badly. The sprain leads to severe pain. She then gets good news. She won the lottery. Her positive emotions are experienced in the limbic system of the brain. This area of the brain modulates the pain and sends it back down to the ankle, and the pain is not experienced as intensely as it would be were her mood not elevated. This serves as a physiologic explanation for the mind–body connection.

Another example of how our emotional states and our thoughts mediate our pain perception is the classic story of the marathon runner who trips in the middle of a race and sprains an ankle. Despite the potentially devastating pain, the person actually experiences no pain and, in fact, finishes the race and does not feel pain until he crosses the finish line. This is because his excitement about the race, including his optimistic thoughts, coupled with the aerobic exercise involved in this activity, causes an increase in endogenous opioids in the brain, which include endorphins and enkephalins. These are naturally occurring morphine-like substances circulating in the brain that increase in response to positive emotional states and aerobic exercise. It is believed that psychological treatment such as cognitive therapy may actually help increase these endogenous opioids in patients' brains by changing thought processes and emotional states and thus reducing pain perceptions without using large amounts of medications.

PAIN VERSUS SUFFERING

Pain and suffering are not necessarily the same. People can experience pain without suffering. For example, some patients have a high tolerance of pain. They may cope with pain as well as its consequences fairly well. As a result, these people do not typically seek out counseling or psychotherapy services.

Other patients do not tolerate pain very well. They experience physical suffering. When patients engage in negative, catastrophic thinking about their pain, they are experiencing cognitive suffering. For example, pain is often viewed as a sign that something is wrong. Having chronic pain can lead to a heightened sense of danger as well as a variety of distressing emotions because of the duration and intensity of the pain (emotional suffering). There are also a number of personal, social, and environmental consequences to having chronic pain that may be very difficult for patients to deal with, for example, physical limitations, life role changes (e.g., work, finances, and leisure), relationship issues, and legal problems. This is known as psychosocial suffering.

Chronic pain patients tend to experience a great deal of emotional suffering as a result of the long-term nature of their pain as well as the limited effects of medical interventions on their physical well-being. It is estimated that the incidence of psychological problems in the chronic pain population ranges from 30% to 100% (Turk, Rudy, & Steig, 1987). Research indicates that chronic pain patients experience greater psychological distress and psychosocial problems compared with people who have acute pain or no pain (Erdal & Zautra, 1995; Trief, Elliott, Stein, & Frederickson, 1987). In fact, the incidence of depression in chronic pain patients tends to be higher than that for the general population (Magni, Caldieron, Rigatti-Luchini, & Merskey, 1990; for reviews, see Banks & Kerns, 1996; Gupta, 1986; Romano & Turner, 1985; Sullivan, Reesor, Mikail, & Fisher, 1992). In addition to depression (major depressive disorder, dysthymia; Miller, 1993), chronic pain patients can develop significant problems related to anxiety (i.e., generalized anxiety disorder, panic disorder, hypochondriasis, and post-traumatic stress disorder; e.g., Gaskin, Greener, Robinson, & Geisser, 1992; Miller, 1993), and anger (Feldman, Downey, & Schaffer-Neitz, 1999; Gaskin et al., 1992; Summers, Rapoff, Varghese, Porter, & Palmer, 1991). In fact, chronic pain patients tend to suppress their anger more than others (e.g., Braha & Catchlove, 1986–1987; Pilowsky & Spence, 1976). These emotional states are directly related to the severity of pain experienced. Patients who report higher pain severity are more likely to be depressed (e.g., Brown, Nicassio, & Wallston, 1989; Feldman et al., 1999), anxious (al Absi & Rokke, 1991; Arntz, Dreessen, & De Jong, 1994), and angry (e.g., Feldman et al., 1999; Gaskin et al., 1992; Summers et al., 1991) than patients who report less pain.

A significant percentage of chronic pain patients are diagnosed with at least one personality disorder (31% to 51%; Weisberg & Keefe, 1999). Given the incidence of psychological distress and personality disorders in the chronic pain population, these patients can be difficult to work with (Maras, 2003).

Fatigue and irritability are common symptoms in chronic pain patients. Other emotions can negatively affect pain, including resentment, hopelessness, helplessness, and despair (e.g., Miller, 1993). However, substance use problems are relatively rare in chronic pain patients. The risk of substance abuse in chronic pain patients is comparable to the general population. In most cases, these substance problems predated patients' chronic pain diagnoses.

Why are chronic pain patients at risk for these emotional problems? Cognitive therapists would argue that these patients develop emotional difficulties as a result of negative, unrealistic thoughts and beliefs about their pain and its consequences, in addition to preexisting problems. Initially, most chronic pain patients are hopeful about their medical problems and maintain faith in the medical profession to resolve their pain. This is often the case with acute pain. People try to make sense of their pain; they may interpret it in a negative way. As pain continues beyond reasonable medical expectations for healing, patients may interpret their pain as uncontrollable and unfixable. These thoughts may also begin to generalize to other aspects of their lives. Patients may experience depression, anxiety, and anger when they focus on their pain and on their physical limitations and think their pain is uncontrollable: "I can't control my pain. If I am not in control of my body, I won't be functional at all. Something bad is going to happen to me. It is going to be a catastrophe." They may also blame themselves for having pain: "Why me? Bad things only happen to bad people, right? So I must have done something bad."

Experiencing unrelieved pain over time as well as the impact or consequences of having pain in their lives can be very distressing. Physical limitations may affect patients' range of motion, general pace, and the ability to engage in previously enjoyed tasks and activities, including work. As a result, they may have negative thoughts about their abilities to do things. Other potential difficulties include job loss or job reassignments, financial hardship, declining productivity, and strained family relationships. Patients are more vulnerable to depression, anxiety, and anger, as well as thoughts of inadequacy and worthlessness if they cannot return to work. When the pain continues despite medical interventions, patients may perceive themselves as having less control over various facets of their lives. Therefore, patients may view themselves as more vulnerable to illness or harm over time.

Emotionally distressed patients tend to focus on negative events and stressors in their life, including their pain. Unfortunately, this tends to exacerbate their experience of pain. As a result, a stress–pain cycle can develop. Negative thoughts and emotional distress can lead to increased muscle tension, which can in turn increase pain levels, resulting in further distress. A cycle occurs, with pain causing distress and distress causing more pain.

ROLE OF BELIEFS, ATTITUDES, AND BEHAVIORS

Beliefs and attitudes are very important in managing physical illnesses and conditions such as chronic pain. Having a realistic and hopeful attitude is one important aspect of pain management. In fact, pain beliefs and pain self-efficacy (i.e., believing in one's ability to cope with pain) have been related to psychological adjustment, physical functioning and pain levels (e.g., Jensen, Romano, Turner, Good, & Wald, 1999; Kaivanto, Estlander, Moneta, & Vanharanta, 1995; Lackner, Carosella, & Feuerstein, 1996; Stroud, Thorn, Jensen, & Boothby, 2000), as well as treatment outcomes (e.g., Tota-Faucette, Gil, Williams, Keefe, & Goli, 1993; Waldrop, Lightsey, Ethington, Woemmel, & Coke, 2001). Catastrophizing thoughts about pain has been associated with pain, psychological distress, and perceived disability (e.g., Severeijns, Vlaeyen, van den Hout, & Weber, 2001).

How people act or behave can also influence their physical health. Chronic pain and the physical limitations related to it can lead to a number of potentially troublesome behaviors, including inactivity, social withdrawal and isolation, overeating, complaining, and frequent office visits to physicians. Therefore, another aspect of pain management is behavioral (or action-oriented) in nature.

Cognitive therapy addresses these aspects of pain management: the importance of realistic, healthy beliefs, attitudes, and behaviors in reducing the emotional and physical suffering associated with pain. Cognitive therapy is a specific theory of psychotherapy originally developed by the second author. This type of therapy teaches patients skills in cognitive coping (e.g., distraction, self-talk, and imagery), cognitive restructuring (i.e., identifying, evaluating, and modifying negative, unrealistic thoughts, images, and beliefs), problem solving, and relaxation training. Patients learn to view pain as a dynamic, multifaceted experience involving sensory perceptions, thinking patterns, affective responses, and behaviors, given their environmental contexts (e.g., level of support and cultural/societal attitudes toward pain). Thoughts, feelings, behaviors, and physiological sensations of pain are all interrelated. According to the cognitive model of chronic pain, negative, unrealistic thoughts, images, and beliefs can have a significant and negative impact on the experience of pain sensations, moods (e.g., hopeless, depression, anxiety, and anger), behaviors (e.g., isolation, and disturbed sleep), and other adverse physiological sensations. Therefore, the primary target for change is patients' negative, unrealistic cognitions about pain, the consequences of having pain, and other life stresses. Therapists also help patients identify behaviors that exacerbate pain and stress and teach them new coping strategies as well as adaptive, healthy behaviors. Emotional and sensory experiences of patients are also highly valued and are explored in cognitive therapy. In fact, changes in emotional or sensory states (e.g., pain) serve as cues to exploring the thoughts and images that are associated with emotional distress or painful sensations.

Cognitive therapists help chronic pain patients by providing them with a supportive, yet structured, therapeutic environment in which to discuss their experiences of pain and how it is affecting their lives. Therapy is geared toward identifying any emotional, cognitive, behavioral, physiological, and/or environmental (e.g., family, social, cultural, and societal) difficulties that might be influencing patients' experiences of pain. Although therapy goals vary for each patient, depending on the presenting problems, the ultimate goals are to teach these patients how to cope better with their pain and their moods and to enhance their functioning in various life roles. For many patients, being able to talk about their concerns or issues in therapy with professionals who are empathic and supportive (while at the same time active and problem-oriented) is very different from the type of treatment they may receive from other health care professionals.

Cognitive therapy is usually recommended when (1) patients' pain condition becomes chronic in nature; (2) the pain itself becomes unmanageable; (3) the pain affects patients' psychological functioning, or when emotional distress exacerbates pain; (4) patients are having difficulty coping with their medical treatment (e.g., becoming fearful of seeing their doctor or undergoing medical testing); and (5) patients experience significant psychosocial stressors, for example, strained relationships with family members or friends, physical limitations (e.g., inability to perform tasks and activities), loss of employment, and financial difficulties, among others. Long-term pain can have rippling effects for patients and can affect their relationships with others and their life roles.

Cognitive therapy can be conducted in groups, which is a highly efficient modality of treatment. Chronic pain groups are particularly common in pain clinics. Group therapy provides opportunities for support and validation as well as for helping others. Many patients also benefit from individual cognitive therapy sessions, because these sessions can be individually tailored to the particular needs of each patient to increase the likelihood of successful treatment outcomes (Spence, 1998). Individual therapy provides the opportunity for more attention to individual concerns. Some patients may benefit from a combination of individual and group cognitive therapy intervention. This manual was written from an individual therapy perspective, but it can be adapted for cognitive therapy groups.

There may be cases when cognitive therapy is not recommended for certain patients. For example, patients who have severe cognitive impairments may have difficulty remembering information learned in therapy, including cognitive restructuring techniques. These patients may benefit from behavioral interventions or supportive therapies instead.

Cognitive therapy may need to be adapted for patients who are more concrete and less abstract in their thinking compared with the average patient. However, this does not necessarily mean that cognitive therapy is contraindicated for these patients. They may prefer the behavioral strategies, such as relaxation and activity scheduling or pacing, or educational interventions (e.g., learning the types of cognitive errors), instead of other cognitive strategies.

Therapists should also keep in mind that some patients might be better suited to other therapies if they are really not interested in the cognitive-behavioral approach. Some patients may desire other types of therapy based on their particular needs. It is therefore important for therapists to educate their patients about the type of therapy they provide before therapy starts.

Cognitive therapy may not be recommended for patients who are highly psychotic at the time of initiating therapy. In such cases, inpatient hospitalization would be recommended. After patients have been on a course of antipsychotic medication and have been stabilized, then cognitive therapy could be recommended. In fact, cognitive therapy has been used successfully with patients who have schizophrenia and other psychotic disorders (Rector & Beck, 2001).

In summary, cognitive therapy with chronic pain patients may be contraindicated for patients who have severe cognitive deficits, lack interest in or motivation for cognitive therapy, or are highly psychotic at the time of starting therapy.

Cognitive therapy serves as an important component in a holistic team approach to treating patients with chronic pain. Patients receive services from a variety of health care professionals for pain management. In the next section, we offer an overview of the pain treatment approaches patients might receive as well as the professional groups that provide these services. These are the professional groups with whom mental health professionals typically communicate about their patients' progress.

APPROACHES TO PAIN TREATMENT

Pain treatment used to be dichotomized into medical and psychological treatments similar to the mind–body dualism theory. In other words, chronic pain patients were initially treated by physicians or chiropractors. When medical treatments failed to diagnose or alleviate the pain, patients were referred to mental health professionals to treat the pain as a psychiatric or psychological condition.

Today, most health care professionals, including medical and mental health professionals, embrace the mind–body connection because pain typically has a biological as well as a psychological basis. Although medical intervention is a given with chronic pain patients, many chronic pain patients benefit from an interdisciplinary approach that includes medical care, physical and/or occupational therapy, and psychiatric and psychotherapy/counseling services and interventions in order to help them manage their physical and emotional suffering.

As a therapist begins providing psychotherapy services for a chronic pain patient, it is important to obtain a clear understanding of the concurrent pain treatments that the patient is undergoing. Types of concurrent pain treatments besides psychotherapy can include:

- medical care
- chiropractic care
- physical therapy
- occupational therapy
- recreational therapy
- massage therapy and myelotherapy
- weight management/nutrition therapy

The medical approach is usually the first avenue sought out by chronic pain patients. They are often under the medical care of one or more physicians, such as a pain specialist, a neurologist, an orthopedic surgeon, and a primary care physician. They are primarily focused on the diagnosis and treatment of patients' chronic pain conditions. Physicians typically use conservative, traditional methods of treatment, including physical examinations, range of motion assessments (i.e., patients' ability to move different muscles and parts of the body), laboratory testing for diagnostic purposes (e.g., x-rays, MRIs, electrocardiograms [EKGs], computerized axial tomography [CAT] scans, and myelograms), medication for pain management, injection therapies, and surgical interventions. They also provide referrals to other professionals for specific treatments or therapies.

Chiropractors treat acute and chronic pain conditions by physically manipulating the spine and the bones in the body to correctly adjust or align them. They may also provide targeted massage to specific muscle groups. Treatments can occur once a week or more often, depending on the condition. Chiropractors may offer recommendations on dietary concerns and herbal remedies for patients with chronic pain. However, they do not prescribe pain medication. Some patients may prefer to work with a chiropractor rather than a medical doctor or doctor of osteopathy. Other patients may seek chiropractic services after they have exhausted all possible forms of traditional medical intervention (laboratory testing, examinations, medication, and surgery).

Physical therapy (also known as physiotherapy) is a very common treatment recommended for patients with acute or chronic pain. Physical therapists (PTs) provide a variety of services including the physical treatment of joint and muscle groups (the physical therapist moves the joint or muscle group to strengthen it), the use of massage for specific muscle groups, the development of exercise programs to strengthen joints or muscle groups, the implementation of electrical stimulation treatments (e.g., transcutaneous electrical nerve stimulations [TENS unit]), and the use of cold (e.g., ice) and heat treatments for specific pain locations in the body.

Another pain approach that may be recommended by clinicians is occupational therapy. Occupational therapists (OTs) help patients learn how to physically manage the daily activities and functions of living, such as cooking meals, eating, drinking, and using appliances, as well as learning appropriate postures, such as sitting and getting in and out of bed correctly. OTs help patients learn how to use utensils, equipment, and appliances independent of others and in ways that facilitate their physical recovery. Depending on the pain condition, patients may have a limited range of motion for certain muscle groups that could affect their ability to handle day-to-day activities. Patients may not be able to do some activities until their condition improves. OTs work with physicians to determine those activities patients can master as well as those activities they cannot perform at the present time.

Recreational therapy is another approach to pain treatment and rehabilitation. Recreational therapists (RTs) use leisure and recreational activities (e.g., art and sports) to help patients cope with their pain. They build patients' repertoire of leisure and creative activities as part of a holistic approach to enhance their well-being and functioning. Some RTs may teach patients relaxation techniques.

Massage therapy may also be recommended as a form of pain treatment for acute and chronic conditions. Massage therapists work the muscles of the body to increase circulation to as well as remove toxins from specific muscle groups. Many massage therapists incorporate background music to set the tone for deep muscle relaxation and massage. There are different forms of massage, including Swedish, deep tissue, manual lymph drainage, neuromuscular therapy, and sports massage.

Myelotherapists are trained to do pressure point therapy to help relax the muscle impulses. Patients are taught how to put pressure on different points of their body to induce relaxation of muscle groups.

Chronic pain patients may also be referred to a dietitian or nutritionist for assistance in developing a healthy, well-balanced diet. Extra weight can cause additional strain and tension to muscles, ligaments, and nerves that are trying to heal. Many candidates for surgery (e.g., back) need to be at an optimal weight before surgery can be scheduled. If patients are overweight or obese, a healthy, low-fat diet can be incorporated to help them lose the weight needed to help reduce pain levels, to prepare for surgery, and to increase their energy and activity levels.

Surgery may be recommended for some patients to correct muscle tissue or neurologic damage immediately following an injury or the diagnosis of a condition. Patients may be referred to an orthopedic surgeon (for muscle tissue damage or pathology) or a neurosurgeon (for nerve damage or pathology) for such services. Surgery may be performed for a number of different acute and chronic pain conditions such as joint (e.g., knee, ankle, elbow, and temporomandibular), back and neck (e.g., disc fusions), and upper and lower extremity problems, as well as neuropathy.

Psychotherapy services offer another important approach to pain treatment. The use of behavioral and cognitive-behavioral psychotherapies in medical settings has often been referred to as behavioral medicine. In the field of behavioral medicine, people's behaviors and thinking processes are viewed as important factors that influence pain and emotions. It is felt that changing behaviors and developing more realistic, helpful thoughts will optimize overall well-being. Behavioral and cognitive-behavioral interventions have been recognized as effective in treating pain, for example, relaxation training, hypnosis, cognitive restructuring, and biofeedback (Ruksznis, 1996). Although it is rare for patients to become pain free, cognitive therapy teaches patients how to cope with their pain and its effects on their lives. More medical professionals are realizing the contributions of a biopsychosocial approach to treating pain compared with biomedical interventions alone, and many of them are recommending cognitive-behavioral therapy for their patients. Why? Because the cognitive-behavioral approach has been identified as a commonly accepted form of psychotherapy for patients with chronic pain, given its efficacy and its regular use in medical settings. It has been used with a variety of chronic pain patients including arthritis patients, back pain patients, patients with carpal tunnel syndrome (Feverstein et al., 1999), patients with complex regional pain syndromes (Stanton-Hicks et al., 1998), headache patients, myofascial pain patients, upper extremity pain patients (Spence, 1998), and patients with multiple pain problems.

EFFICACY OF BEHAVIORAL, COGNITIVE-BEHAVIORAL, AND COGNITIVE THERAPIES WITH CHRONIC PAIN PATIENTS

There are two major behavioral medicine approaches to pain management in the research literature: behavioral and cognitive-behavioral therapies (Turner & Clancy, 1988). Cognitive therapy best fits into the cognitive-behavioral approach in this research. In behavioral and cognitive-behavioral therapies, patients identify and change behaviors that are unhealthy or self-defeating, by incorporating techniques such as modeling (learning by observing), relaxation training and/or biofeedback, desensitization (graded exposure to feared stimuli, based on classical conditioning), operant conditioning (e.g., changing reinforcement contingencies to modify pain responses, rewarding activity, time-based medication intake, and ignoring pain behaviors), and assertiveness and social skills training (e.g., Cardona, 1994; Linton, 1979). The main feature that distinguishes cognitive-behavioral therapy from behavioral therapy is the additional emphasis on patients' thoughts and beliefs related to their pain and current life situation.

BEHAVIORAL THERAPIES

During the 1970s and 1980s, many pain researchers explored the effectiveness of behavioral therapies with chronic pain patients. In general, behavioral approaches to pain management have been effective in reducing pain levels, the use of pain medication, and psychological distress as well as improving physical functioning (e.g., range of motion, walking time, activity levels, and sleep) in a variety of chronic pain patient populations such as arthritis patients (e.g., see Bradley, Young, Anderson, McDaniel, Turner, & Agudelo, 1984, for a review), back pain patients (e.g., Fordyce, Brockway, Bergman, & Spengler, 1986), headache patients (e.g., Appelbaum, 1991; Larsson & Melin, 1989; Lisspers & Ost, 1990), myofascial pain patients (e.g., Banks, Jacobs, Gevirtz, & Hubbard, 1998), and patients with nonspecific pain (e.g., Dahl & Faellstroem, 1989) either by itself (i.e., no comparison group) or compared with control conditions or other treatment conditions (e.g., traditional medical treatment, physical therapy, and exercise). Some behavioral approaches were equally effective in treating pain compared with medical treatments (e.g., medication therapy) for chronic pain patients (e.g., Holroyd et al., 1988). Many behavioral therapy programs for pain management combine behavioral techniques in treating pain, for example, relaxation and biofeedback (e.g., Achterberg, McGraw, & Lawlis, 1981), and progressive muscle relaxation and breathing/imagery (e.g., Varni, 1981; Varni & Gilbert, 1982; Varni, Gilbert, & Dietrich, 1981). Some components of behavioral therapy programs have been compared, for example, biofeedback versus progressive muscle relaxation and imagery (Spence, Sharp, Newton-John, & Champion, 1995) and time-contingent versus behavior-contingent interventions (Fordyce et al., 1986). Time-contingent interventions (i.e., receive medications and participate in activities and exercises on fixed time intervals) appear to be more effective than behavior-contingent interventions (using pain levels to determine medications taken and activity level/exercise participation; e.g., Fordyce et al., 1986). In addition, behavioral interventions (e.g., relaxation) combined with instructions to practice appear to have added benefit compared with behavioral interventions alone (e.g., Appelbaum, 1991; Keel, Bodoky, Gerhard, & Muller, 1998).

COGNITIVE-BEHAVIORAL TREATMENTS

Over the past 15 to 20 years, more attention has been given to cognitive-behavioral approaches to pain management in the research literature than to behavioral treatments (Grant & Haverkamp, 1995). In fact, many clinics now incorporate a cognitive-behavioral approach to treating pain. A number of studies demonstrate the efficacy of cognitive-behavioral approaches to chronic pain in reducing pain levels, the use of pain medications, negative thoughts, and the extent of physical disability as well as enhancing pain control, psychological adjustment (e.g., moods, pain behaviors, coping, and self-efficacy), physical functioning and health status (e.g., range of motion and activity level), and psychosocial functioning with a variety of chronic pain patients. These include arthritis patients (e.g., see reviews by Blanchard, 1992; Keefe & Van Horn, 1993; Parker, Iverson, Smarr, & Stucky-Ropp, 1993; see also James, Thom, & Williams, 1993; Nicholson & Blanchard, 1993), back pain patients (e.g., Basler, Jakle, & Kroner-Herwig, 1997; Engstrom, 1983; Linton, Bradley, Jensen, Spangfort, & Sundell,1989; Nicholas, Wilson, & Goyen, 1992), patients with chronic whiplash associated disorders (Söderlund & Lindberg, 2001), patients with irritable bowel syndrome (e.g., Greene and Blanchard, 1994; Schwarz, Taylor, Scharff, & Blanchard, 1990; Toner et al., 1998; Vollmer & Blanchard, 1998), knee pain patients (e.g., Keefe et al., 1990), patients with mixed or miscellaneous pain (e.g., Pearce & Erskine, 1993; Ross & Berger, 1996; Williams et al., 1996), noncardiac chest pain patients (van Peski-Oosterbabaan et al., 1999), upper extremity pain patients (e.g., tendonitis, bursitis, rotator cuff syndrome, and carpal tunnel syndrome; see review by Spence, 1998), and acute pain patients at risk for chronicity (Linton & Andersson, 2000). In most of these studies, cognitive behavioral therapy was compared with waiting list controls, placebo medication conditions, and other treatment conditions (e.g., medical interventions alone, physical therapy alone, psychoeducation, and support groups). However, some studies have found that cognitive-behavioral therapy is just as effective as other psychotherapies with chronic pain patients (e.g., Pilowsky, Spence, Rounsefell, Forsten, & Soda, 1995). Cognitive-behavioral therapy is also effective (compared to control conditions) in treating secondary issues related to chronic pain (e.g., insomnia, Currie, Wilson, Pontefract, & deLaplante, 2000).

COMPARISON OF BEHAVIORAL AND COGNITIVE-BEHAVIORAL APPROACHES TO PAIN MANAGEMENT

There is firm evidence in the research literature that both cognitive-behavioral and behavioral treatments are superior to no treatment control conditions on a variety of outcomes (e.g., pain, cognitive coping, pain behaviors, psychological adjustment, and psychosocial functioning). These effects are maintained at follow-up for a variety of chronic pain patients (see meta-analysis studies by Morley, Eccleston, & Williams, 1999; see also a review by McCracken & Turk, 2002). In addition, multidisciplinary pain treatment programs that incorporated cognitive-behavioral therapy and behavioral therapy approaches were significantly more successful than unimodal treatment or no-treatment controls (see meta-analysis studies by Cutler et al., 1994; Flor, Fydrich, & Turk, 1992). Cognitive-behavioral therapy has been shown to be just as effective as (e.g., see Attanasio, Andrasik, & Blanchard, 1987; Newton-John, Spence, & Schotte, 1995), and in some cases, more effective than behavioral therapy with chronic pain patients (e.g., Kerns, Turk, Holzman, & Rudy, 1986; Kole-Snijders et al., 1999; Reese, 1983; Turner, 1982; Vlayeyen, Haazen, Schuerman, & Kole-Snijders, 1995) as well as acute pain patients at risk for chronicity (e.g., Hasenbring, Ulrich, Hartmann, & Soyka, 1999).

The literature on headache pain patients is somewhat mixed. Some studies indicate that cognitive therapy is more effective than behavior therapy with headache patients (e.g., Holroyd & Andrasik, 1982; Murphy, Lehrer, & Jurish, 1990; Sorbi, Tellegen, & du-Long, 1989; Tobin et al., 1988), whereas other studies found that cognitive therapy or the addition of cognitive therapy components to relaxation or biofeedback training was not as effective as these behavioral interventions alone (see review by Emmelkamp & van Oppen, 1993).

In a meta-analysis study of behavioral treatments (i.e., cognitive behavioral therapy, behavior therapy, and biofeedback), no one type of therapy stood out as being the most effective for patients with chronic low back pain (van Tulder et al., 2000). More research is needed to explore whether cognitive therapy or behavior therapy is superior with chronic pain patients in general and for what types of problems or outcomes. No such meta-analytic study has explored this research question.

Overall, it appears that the cognitive-behavioral approach has a positive additive effect to active treatments (e.g., medications, physical therapy, and medical treatments) for chronic pain patients in general. In one meta-analysis study of randomized controlled trials of cognitive-behavioral and behavioral therapies with chronic pain patients (excluding headache patients), cognitive-behavioral therapy was more effective than active treatments in treating pain, cognitive appraisals, and pain behavior problems (Morley et al., 1999). However, in another meta-analysis of randomized controlled trials of cognitive-behavioral therapy, behavioral therapy, and biofeedback with chronic low back pain patients only, the addition of behavior therapy (i.e., cognitive-behavioral therapy, behavior therapy, and biofeedback) to other active treatments did not significantly improve outcomes (van Tulder et al., 2000). Further research in this area is recommended to verify the benefits of adding the cognitive-behavioral approach to active treatments for chronic pain patients, especially for those with low back pain problems.

Some of the criticisms of the research on cognitive-behavior therapy or behavior therapy with chronic pain patients include the intraparticipant variability in chronic pain conditions, small sample sizes, attrition, and the short-term nature of the therapy (on average, 5 to 6 sessions, with a range of 1 to 15 sessions; see Keefe & Van Horn, 1993; Parker et al., 1993). In addition, cognitive-behavioral therapy methods vary considerably from study to study. Miller (1993) argues that various treatment approaches should be viewed as complementary rather than competing, because the evidence suggests that a great therapeutic effect may result from more treatments being combined. Thus, the more important question is not which treatment is most effective, but which treatments are most effective for which patients with which conditions.

Patients' compliance with treatment is an important consideration when conducting these types of studies because it can influence behavioral and cognitive-behavioral therapy outcomes. For example, chronic pain patients who were more compliant with therapy recommendations experienced more significant improvements than patients who were less compliant (patients with multiple pain diagnoses, see Basler & Rehfisch, 1990; headache patients, see Gutkin, Holborn, Walker, & Anderson, 1992; miscellaneous pain, see Parker et al., 1988).

In summary, cognitive-behavioral therapy has strong empirical support as an effective treatment for chronic pain patients. It is just as effective as, and, in some cases, more effective than behavior therapy for this population.

RECOMMENDATIONS FOR FURTHER RESEARCH AND CLINICAL APPLICATION OF COGNITIVE THERAPY WITH CHRONIC PAIN PATIENTS

More research is needed to explore the effectiveness of specific cognitive therapy approaches with the chronic pain population. Despite the fact that research on cognitive-behavioral therapy interventions with specific pain patient populations uses some combination of focus on thought monitoring and modification processes as well as behavior change (e.g., relaxation), what is meant by *cognitive-behavioral therapy* may be unique to each study and therefore may not represent a coherent theoretical model of treatment. Therefore, more research is needed to support the efficacy of different theoretical approaches to cognitive behavioral therapy with chronic pain patients. In addition, a better of understanding of which interventions are most effective for which types of patients with chronic pain may provide researchers and clinicians with more answers about what really works in cognitive therapy with this population. It is hoped that this book serves not only as a treatment manual for practice but also as a source for researchers to study the efficacy of Beck's cognitive therapy with specific chronic pain patients.

2

The Cognitive Conceptualization of Pain

Phil, a 37 year old Caucasian man, experiences burning and numbing sensations in his lower back and legs. He feels frustrated and sad and thinks, "This pain is horrible; it's unbearable. I can't go on like this." Next, Phil imagines the pain taking over his whole body. His pain worsens. He becomes even more absorbed in his pain, frustration, and sadness. He decides to go back to sleep to escape from this pain.

Why is Phil feeling horrible? It isn't simply because he is experiencing severe pain. It is because of what he is telling himself about the pain—in other words, the meaning he has given his pain. Phil has interpreted his pain as being uncontrollable and unmanageable. He thinks of himself as a victim, as powerless to stop his pain. His negative thoughts start taking on a life of their own.

Junko, a 49 year old Japanese woman, experiences burning and numbing sensations in her lower back and legs. She feels slighted irritated and thinks, "Here comes that pain again. Okay, I know it's going to hurt. So, what can I do? I need to catch my breath and focus on something else if I can. It's really hurting. [pause] I have to remember that the pain will eventually subside in the next hour if I take steps to manage it. I have to focus on relaxing my body and moving through the pain. It's not time yet for my next pain pill. So I will have to wait." Junko exhibits more realistic and helpful thoughts about her pain compared with Phil. Whereas Junko is experiencing significant levels of pain, just like Phil, she is choosing to think differently about her pain. She realizes that her pain is hurting. She knows how difficult it can be to "get through the pain." However, Junko focuses on her efforts to cope with it. She reminds herself of what she can do to manage her pain, for example, to relax and distract herself. She remembers that her pain has subsided in the past and that it won't last forever. The way Junko thinks about her pain will help her focus less on her physical suffering and more on her efforts to cope. Junko will be less prone to negative emotions than Phil because of the meaning she has given to her pain—that she has some ability to cope with it and that the duration of her pain is typically time-limited. She feels in charge of her pain and her life because she is thinking more realistically about her pain.

Our thoughts, images, and beliefs can have a direct bearing on how we cope with pain and other life experiences. This is known as the cognitive model of pain. There are several important components of the cognitive model that need to be communicated to patients:

- Pain includes not only physiological sensations but also our emotions, behaviors, and thoughts; all of these experiences are interrelated.
- Pain also includes the personal, social, and environmental influences or stresses in our lives, including our individual characteristics, personality styles, physical limitations, relationships with others, medical care, and life roles, as well as aspects of our physical environment (e.g., weather and climate).
- People can have negative, unrealistic thoughts and beliefs about their pain, themselves, their personal world (including their relationships with others and life roles), and their future given their current chronic pain condition.
- Our negative, unrealistic thoughts about pain and other life events can have a significant and negative impact on how we perceive pain sensations, how we feel emotionally, and what we do when we are in pain.
- There are identifiable types of errors in our thinking (or cognitive distortions) that negatively impact pain.
- The thoughts and images we have about our pain and life events in the moment are related to underlying beliefs. There are three levels of cognition about pain and life circumstances: automatic thoughts (e.g., self-talk and imagery), intermediate beliefs, and core beliefs. In cognitive therapy, we work on automatic thoughts first, then on the underlying beliefs related to these thoughts.

Each of these key components of the cognitive model of chronic pain will be discussed in further detail below.

COMPONENTS OF PAIN

Pain includes sensations, emotions, thoughts, behaviors, and social/environmental influences; they are interrelated experiences.

PAIN SENSATIONS

What do patients experience physiologically when they are in pain? What adjectives do they use to describe their pain (e.g., *throbbing, pounding, stabbing, tight, sore, tender, achy, shooting, burning, and cramping*)? How often does the pain occur? How long does the pain last? Each patient has his or her own unique experience of pain sensations, which needs to be understood by the therapist.

EMOTIONS

What emotions are patients in touch with when they are in pain? Chronic pain patients may experience a variety of emotions when they are in pain, for example, anxiety, frustration, despair, depression, and psychological numbness. Identifying emotions connected to pain is important because emotions may be difficult to distinguish from pain and changes in emotions are often indicators of significant shifts in thinking.

THOUGHTS AND BELIEFS

What thoughts and underlying beliefs are activated when patients are in pain? Chronic pain patients tend to have specific thoughts and beliefs about their pain as well as the impact of pain on their lives. For example, they might be distressed about their ability to engage in activities, their relationships with others, their work and family roles, and their sense of identity, given their chronic pain condition.

It is not uncommon for these thoughts and beliefs to have negative, unrealistic, and potentially catastrophic qualities. For example, a chronic pain patient might think, "The pain has taken away my life. I can't get beyond this pain. God must be punishing me for my sins." Catastrophizing thoughts are often associated with psychological distress and increased pain intensity among other variables (see reviews by Boothby, Thorn, Stroud, & Jensen, 1999; Sullivant et al., 2001). In fact, depressed chronic pain patients are more at risk for catastrophic thinking than are depressed patients without pain (Lefebvre, 1981).

BEHAVIOR

What are patients doing when they are in pain? Chronic pain patients may behave or act in specific ways when they are in pain. Some people may wince when they feel intense pain, or they may lie down to rest. Others might complain about their pain to someone else. Some people will take pain medication immediately to alleviate their pain. These have been identified in the research literature as "pain behaviors" (Fordyce, 1976). In many cases, these behaviors solicit attention and support from others, which may reinforce the pain behaviors (e.g., Fordyce, Fowler, & DeLateur, 1968) as well as pain disability and distress (e.g., Paulsen & Altmaier, 1995; Romano et al., 1995).

OTHER PHYSIOLOGICAL SENSATIONS

What other physiological sensations do patients experience when they are distressed because of their pain? If patients are depressed, they may feel more tired or fatigued than before. If they are anxious, they may experience muscle tension, hyperventilation, or dizziness, among other symptoms. If they are angry or frustrated, they may feel hot, tense, and physically agitated. Some of these physiological sensations/states can exacerbate pain further. Becoming aware of these physiological sensations and states will help patients identify their moods and thoughts as well as signal the need for relaxation and cognitive coping responses to reduce pain and distress.

PSYCHOSOCIAL INFLUENCES

Pain is composed of personal, social, and environmental influences, including gender, race, sexual orientation, and socioeconomic status, personality factors, physical abilities and limitations, relationships with family, friends, health care staff, attorneys, and therapists, and environmental triggers, as well as life role problems, including work stress, unemployment, financial difficulties, and legal matters. These psychosocial stressors will be discussed in more detail later in the manual.

BELIEFS ABOUT PAIN, SELF, WORLD, AND FUTURE

Chronic pain patients can have unrealistic and negative beliefs as well as realistic and healthy beliefs about their pain, themselves, their personal world (including relationships and life roles), and their future. Cognitive therapists focus their efforts on identifying, evaluating, and modifying negative and unrealistic thoughts, images, and expectancies (beliefs and assumptions) in these four areas.

PAIN BELIEFS

People who develop chronic pain conditions may begin to develop stable and global views of their pain and how their pain has affected their lives. Many patients entering therapy have negative expectancies about their pain. Examples of pain beliefs include "My pain is untreatable," "I cannot control my pain," "The pain is horrible and unbearable," "My life is full of pain," "I shouldn't have pain all the time," and "The pain has taken over my life."

BELIEFS ABOUT SELF

When people develop chronic pain conditions, their perceptions of their identity may change over time. For example, some patients who were highly productive in their careers may not be able to return to work because of their pain and their physical limitations. Some patients may come to believe that they are inadequate or incompetent because they are not able to do things they used to do. Examples of negative self-beliefs related to adequacy/competence include "My pain makes me a weak person," "I am vulnerable," "I shouldn't be such a needy person," "I am powerless," "This pain makes me useless," and "I cannot be helped." Other patients may question how liked or loved they are given their chronic pain. Examples of negative self-beliefs related to lovability include "No one cares about me or my pain," "I am socially defective," "I have let others down," "I'm not a good friend," and "I am unlovable." Patients may also develop certain beliefs about their body because of the pain. Examples include "My body is broken/not whole," "My body is dysfunctional," and "My body has turned old."

BELIEFS ABOUT THEIR WORLD

Some patients begin to question their relationships with others after their pain persists despite medical care or alternative treatments. They may become frustrated and impatient with their medical care. Some patients are very concerned about social support. They may fear that others will reject them because of their physical limitations. Examples of negative beliefs about their world include "My doctors don't care about my pain," "No one understands what I am going through," "People will criticize me," "The world moves too fast for me," and "People are disappointed in me [because of my pain]."

BELIEFS ABOUT THE FUTURE

Patients develop general views of what the future will look like given their chronic pain. They may anticipate negative, fatalistic, gloomy outcomes in the future. Examples of beliefs about the future include "I am doomed to be pain-ridden forever," "My future looks grim," and "All I can see ahead of me is pain, pain, pain."

COGNITIVE MODEL

Negative, unrealistic thoughts, images, and beliefs contribute to physical and emotional suffering as well as self-defeating behaviors. The essence of the cognitive model of chronic pain is that negative, unrealistic cognitions (i.e., thoughts, images, and beliefs) about pain and other life events have a significant, negative influence on emotions, behaviors, and physiological sensations of pain (i.e., pain perceptions).

Negative, unrealistic thoughts, images, and beliefs typically occur as the result of having chronic, unremitting pain. However, these negative cognitions can also exacerbate pain perceptions and negative mood states.

When we think negatively, we are more likely to feel emotionally distressed, which can result in (1) muscle tension, making the pain even worse, and (2) a hyperaroused state in the nervous system (e.g., sympathetic), activating more pain messages in our body (e.g., peripheral and central nervous system), leading to more pain. When we think negatively, we are also more likely to engage in self-defeating behaviors, such as inactivity, social isolation, or overreliance on pain medications, which can affect the pain.

ERRORS IN THINKING

When patients try to make sense of their pain and their lives, they may make mistakes or errors in their thinking. For example, patients may focus exclusively on the negative aspects of pain, how horrible it is, and how it prevents them from doing the things they want to do in their lives. They may blame themselves for their pain condition or feel punished for having pain. They may look for all of the evidence that supports how terrible their lives are with pain, or how bad they are, without looking at the bigger picture—considering their strengths, abilities, level of support, and how they are coping in more realistic ways. Unfortunately, these errors in thinking can negatively impact patients' pain and moods.

There are times when patients can have negative thoughts or images that are indeed accurate. In those cases, the goal is to help patients identify the problem and solve it. In therapy, patient will learn to catch these errors and identify more realistic and healthy thoughts.

LEVELS OF THOUGHT

Thoughts and images in the moment are related to underlying beliefs. In cognitive therapy, patients are introduced to the notion of levels of cognition. Automatic thoughts, or thoughts and images about pain and life events at a particular moment, are related to deeper, underlying beliefs known as intermediate and core beliefs.

AUTOMATIC THOUGHTS

Automatic thoughts are thoughts that run through our minds, whether we are consciously aware of them or not. Automatic thoughts may come in the form of a running commentary (i.e., self-talk) or images or pictures on pain and our lives in general. Automatic thoughts are like the words in the bubble captions next to characters in a cartoon. Sometimes, the cartoon characters are actually saying what they are thinking; other times, the words in the bubble captions represent the thoughts of the character. Patients are encouraged to think about their own "bubble captions" when they are in pain or when they notice a change in their pain intensity or their moods.

Therapist: Recall an image of the stock market indicator displays that continue to chart the rise and fall of commodity prices. The displays are typically ongoing and continuous in their reporting of stock market indicators. In a similar vein, our minds are constantly at work; whether we are aware of it or not, our thoughts and images are constantly being displayed in our minds. Sometimes we attend to them, and sometimes we don't.

Here is another analogy therapists can use to explain automatic thoughts:

Therapist: Imagine that we are commentators on our experiences, just like sports commentators on television as they announce to us the various happenings during a sporting event. We are always trying to make sense of our experiences moment to moment. But if we were always aware of every thought we had, we might go into overload mode. Therefore, we have probably been wired to attend to our thoughts only at certain times, as part of our survival and coping. Similar to autonomic functions of the body, we don't have to constantly focus on our thoughts to survive. However, when we are feeling intense pain or feeling an intense emotion, it will be helpful to do a quick check on our thoughts in the moment to find out how we perceive events.

To help explain images as a type of automatic thought, patients are encouraged to think of a time when they caught themselves in a daydream.

Therapist: When we daydream, we create images in our minds. The images that we conjure up can almost seem real to us at times. Some of these images are memories of real-life events. For example, if a person has been in a car accident before, it is possible that simply getting into a car or driving it around town may bring back vivid memories of the accident. Other images are fictitious. For example, you may never have been in a car accident; however, you may have imagined that you were going to hit a car or that a car was going to hit you.

When you are in pain, you may have certain images of the pain or an image of yourself in pain. You also may have images of your relationships with others and what the future will hold. Pain can also activate negative images in people's mind. Has this ever happened to you before?

It is important for patients to learn that about the nature of automatic thoughts.

Therapist: Automatic thoughts—self-talk and imagery—can be positive or negative in nature. Some examples of positive thoughts are "I can get through the pain" and "I know this pain won't last forever." Examples of neutral thoughts are "I am going to watch this pain to see what happens," "Okay, I am feeling the pain again," and "What am I going to do about it?" Examples of negative thoughts are "This pain is too much to bear," "I can't do anything with this pain," and "I am doomed to misery."

Automatic thoughts can also be realistic and unrealistic in nature, as we discussed earlier. The goal of cognitive therapy is to help you evaluate the accuracy and the helpfulness of your thinking and not to judge the morality of those thoughts. There is no such thing as a good thought or a bad thought in cognitive therapy.

INTERMEDIATE BELIEFS

Patterns in patients' negative thoughts often reflect underlying beliefs. There are two basic levels of beliefs: intermediate and core (Beck, 1995).

Intermediate beliefs fall between automatic thoughts and core beliefs and refer to those beliefs that are typically conditional in nature. Intermediate beliefs include rules, attitudes, and assumptions (Beck, 1995).

People develop certain rules for themselves and others. These conditions are developed over time as people try to make sense of themselves, their pain, their world, and their future. Examples of rules include "I shouldn't have to live with this pain," "My pain shouldn't last this long," "There should be a cure for my pain," "I should be perfect at everything I do despite my pain," "Life should be fair" (having pain is unfair), "Pain is for older people" (I shouldn't have pain until my later years), "People must like me," and "The future must be secure."

Attitudes are another type of intermediate belief. Typically, attitudes are value-laden judgments about life events. Examples of attitudes include "The pain is awful," "It's horrible that the doctors can't find a cure for my pain," and "It's terrible when I can't do things the way I used to." Typically, patients with negative attitudes are more prone to emotional distress and increased pain awareness.

Assumptions are inferences people make about causality ("If . . . then"). Examples of assumptions include "If I work hard enough despite my pain, then I will be justly rewarded," "If I have pain, then I will be doomed to a life of despair," and "If I go to the doctors and follow their recommendations, then I will be pain-free."

CORE BELIEFS/SCHEMAS

Core beliefs are the basic beliefs people have about their pain, themselves, their personal world, and their future. They are the deepest level of thought. Core beliefs are often characterized as global, rigid, and overgeneralized. Patients hold onto these general, all-encompassing beliefs very strongly despite evidence to the contrary and use them in a variety of contexts. Most patients are unaware of these pervasive beliefs until further exploration in therapy reveals them.

Schemas are basically hypothetical structures in the brain that organize incoming information. Core beliefs compose the content of schemas and are stored within them. The metaphor often used to explain schemas is of a filing cabinet. In order to store information, people organize experiences in meaningful ways by developing systems to make sense of their world. Schemas provide a framework for understanding our pain, who we are, what the world is like (e.g., how people relate to others, how you get a job, or how you find a partner), and what the future holds (e.g., expectations for happiness, prosperity, success, security, and comfort). For example, if a person develops a medical condition that results in tremendous chronic pain despite the person's efforts to lead a happy, productive, and full life, she may begin to develop a schema of unfairness or mistreatment. Within this schema could be core beliefs such as "My pain is a punishment for my sins" (negative core pain belief), "I am used merchandise" (negative core self-belief), "People don't care about me and my pain" (negative core world belief), and "I can't trust medical professionals, family, and friends to take care of me in the future" (negative core future belief).

When most health care professionals become acquainted with cognitive therapy, they often assume that this approach to therapy focuses solely on specific thoughts that are running through patients' minds at a given time or moment, (i.e., their stream of consciousness). Although automatic thoughts are the most basic level of cognition, their roots lie in the underlying belief systems (i.e., intermediate and core beliefs), or core imagery, that are by nature at preconscious or subconscious levels of awareness. Through therapeutic intervention, these underlying beliefs and imagery can be explored and worked through. The skills that patients learn to cope with negative automatic thoughts will serve as building blocks for these deeper cognitions.

COGNITIVE CASE CONCEPTUALIZATION OF CHRONIC PAIN PATIENTS

Case conceptualization is an important skill that all therapists must acquire in order to assist their patients. Cognitive case conceptualization is an integrated picture of the patient's presenting problems given his or her historical and cultural context from a cognitive therapy orientation (adapted from Morrison, 1995). It is the therapist's view of the larger picture of the patient's presenting problems and how they developed and are maintained. In particular, the therapist identifies the patient's key automatic thoughts, intermediate beliefs, and core beliefs related to the presenting problems. Significant environmental, cultural, and social forces that may influence the development or maintenance of the patient's problems are also identified as part of the conceptualization of those problems. Case conceptualization starts with the intake interview and continues throughout the course of psychotherapy and beyond.

Case conceptualization from a cognitive therapy approach includes relevant patient information, including (1) the patient's demographics, such as gender, age, racial/ethnic identity, sexual orientation, and educational and work status, as well as the referral source for entering therapy; (2) the patient's presenting problems and history of how these problems developed, including compensatory strategies (the patient's ineffective coping strategies); (3) the automatic thoughts (self-talk and images), intermediate beliefs, and core beliefs associated with presenting problems and the corresponding emotions, behaviors, and physiology (including pain and other physiological sensations) related to these thoughts and beliefs; (4) the patient's diagnoses according to the *Diagnostic and Statistical Manual of Mental Disorders* (*DSM-IV-TR*; American Psychiatric Association, 2000); (5) family history, including information about the patient's family of origin (parents or legal guardians, siblings, birth order, and family role) and extended family; (6) social history, including information about the patient's friendships, dating relationships, marriages/divorces, and relationships with authority figures; (7) educational and work history; (8) medical history, including significant past or current medical conditions or surgeries, medical diagnoses, the nature of acute and chronic pain conditions, over-the-counter and prescribed medications taken and their effectiveness (including side effects), and family history of medical conditions; (9) psychiatric/psychological history, including previous and current psychotherapy experiences, if any, the patient's perceptions of these experiences, psychiatric hospitalizations for emotional problems/mental illness and substance abuse, and previous *DSM* diagnoses; (10) significant events and traumas; and (11) the goals for therapy or the treatment plan. Figure 2.1 is an example of a case summary worksheet that is used to help cognitive therapists conceptualize patient's problems.

COGNITIVE CONCEPTUALIZATION DIAGRAMS

Diagrams can be very helpful in putting patients' experiences into full view. Cognitive model diagrams are graphic presentations of the relationship among patients' automatic thoughts, feelings, behaviors, and physiological sensations (including pain levels) in each situation encountered. These situational experiences are then tied to the patients' intermediate and core beliefs. (The process of completing this diagram will be discussed in more detail in chapter 10.) Therapists develop these diagrams during the psychotherapy session as patients explain their distressing circumstances related to pain and other concerns. This diagram helps patients learn more about the influence of negative thoughts and images (at the lowest level), intermediate beliefs (at the middle level), and core beliefs (at the deepest level) on his or her pain, moods, actions, and physiology. These types of diagrams can also help the therapist develop a cognitive case conceptualization of a patient. By connecting situational automatic thoughts, emotions, behaviors, and physiological sensations to common themes in patients' thought processes, specifically, intermediate and core beliefs, therapists can better understand how the intermediate and core beliefs "drive" or influence patients' negative automatic thoughts. The diagram allows therapists to outline relationships among automatic

---

FIGURE 2.1 Case Summary Worksheet

Patient's Name: Keisha

Objective Scores: BDI = 34
                        BAI = 23
                        BHS = 9

Diagnoses: Axis I: Major Depressive Disorder, Recurrent, Severe
                Axis II: No diagnosis
                Axis III: Carpal tunnel syndrome (bilateral)
                Axis IV: Psychosocial stressors: chronic pain in wrists and
                        hands, social isolation, difficulty completing work
                        tasks
                Axis V: General Assessment of Functioning: Current: 52

Identifying Information:
Keisha is a 43-year-old African American woman who is married and has
three children, ages 10, 7, and 2. Keisha works as an architect for a local
architectural firm.

Presenting Problems

Presenting Problems and Current Functioning:
Keisha presents with complaints of severe pain in her hands and wrists.
She has been diagnosed with carpal tunnel syndrome. Other concerns
include her loss of interest or pleasure in activities because of her pain.

Chronic Pain Condition (medical diagnoses, location of pain; duration;
intensity; intermittent or recurrent; adjectives used to describe pain; include
history of pain condition and previous treatments)
    Keisha was diagnosed with bilateral carpal tunnel approximately 1 year
ago. She experiences pain in her hands and wrists. She described the pain
as being intermittent in nature, most prominent when she is writing or
working with her hands. Her pain can last as long as several hours at a
time. On a pain severity scale from 0 to 10 (0 = *no pain*, 10 = *worst pain
possible*), she rated her average pain to be a 6, but it can range from 3 to
10. She described her pain as throbbing, numbing, sore, and achy. She
has had surgery on both of her wrists, with little or no success in alleviating her pain.

Developmental Profile

History (family, social, educational, work, medical, psychiatric)
Keisha was born and raised in Mississippi. She was the oldest of four children born to her parents. She married her husband, Zeke, 12 years ago. They have three children ages 10, 7, and 2. She has been a very socially active person in the community. However, since her pain worsened this past year, she has isolated herself. She graduated from college with a bachelor's degree in architecture. Keisha has worked at the same architectural firm for the past 15 years. She is concerned about her ability to do her work for much longer given her carpal tunnel condition. She reports no other significant medical problems. She has never been in therapy nor been hospitalized for emotional problems.

Relationships (parents, siblings, significant others, authority figures)
Keisha reported that she has good relationships with her husband and children. She was the oldest of four children in her family. She recalls feeling a lot of pressure from her parents to be successful. She took on a caretaking role with her brother and sisters growing up. She tends to get along with authority figures. However, she takes a great deal of responsibility in relationships. If things don't work out, she tends to blame herself. She has isolated herself from her friends and from her church lately. Keisha doesn't want people to know about her pain and her suffering.

Significant Events and Traumas
Keisha reported that having this chronic pain is her most significant trauma. She does not report a history of emotional, physical, or sexual abuse.

Cognitive Profile

Typical Problems at Present (identify situations)
1. Doesn't want to see friends or go to church
2. Having difficulty finishing projects at work
3. Dealing with her chronic pain

Typical Automatic Thoughts, Experience of Pain, Mood, and Behaviors in Those Situations
1. "I don't want people to pity me." → sore, achy pain in hands and wrists → sad → social withdrawal
2. "I can't keep up with my work projects."→ sore, numbing pain in hands and wrists → anxious → tries to work harder, takes work home at night
3. "I am overwhelmed by my pain. It's ruining my life." → throbbing, sore, and numbing pain in hands and wrists → depressed → social withdrawal, cries

---

FIGURE 2.1 *(continued)*

Intermediate Beliefs

Rules (shoulds/musts applied to self/others):

    I shouldn't share my pain with others.

    I shouldn't slow down. I must keep up.

    I should be responsible.

    Life should be fair. The surgery should have worked.

    This pain shouldn't be here in my life.

Attitudes (awful/horrible nature of events):

    It would be horrible if people pitied me.

    It would be horrible if I let my boss down.

    This pain is awful and unbearable.

    It will be awful if I can't keep up with my responsibilities.

Conditional assumptions (positive and negative):

    If I don't share my pain with others, then people will regard me highly
        as they always have.

    If people find out about my pain, they will pity me (think less of me).

    If I can keep up with my work, I can keep my job.

    If I try to keep up the pace, I may hurt worse later.

    If I slow down, then I might lose my job.

    If I can't stop the pain, then I am doomed to a miserable life.

    If I can get this pain out of my life, then I will feel happier.

Core Beliefs

    I am a failure. (can't keep up with work)

    I am pain-ridden.

    I am trapped.

    People will reject/abandon me. (I am unlovable)

    I am out of control.

Integration and Conceptualization of Cognitive and Developmental Profiles

Formulation of Self-Concept and Concepts of Others

Prior to her carpal tunnel condition, Keisha had a very positive view of
herself and of others. Since developing this chronic pain, Keisha tends to
think negatively about herself (e.g., rejected, failure, trapped, pain-ridden) and others (e.g., people will reject me; I will get fired if I cannot
keep up at work).

Interaction of Life Events and Cognitive Vulnerabilities

Keisha's drive for success has usually resulted in positive outcomes in the
past. There is some evidence that she has not handled "failures" well in

the past (e.g., not winning the spelling bee, not winning a track race). It was during those times in her life when she began to be very critical of herself, resulting in depression. She has a history of being encouraged by her parents to "be the best she can be." Keisha interprets this to mean that she cannot let people down. Her boss has noticed Keisha's difficulty in meeting deadlines. A couple of friends have become frustrated with her for not getting together with them.

Compensatory Strategies and Coping Strategies
Keisha has always been a high achiever. She holds high expectations of herself and works very hard. She has withdrawn from others and does not talk about her pain with others.

Development and Maintenance of Current Problems
Keisha has not received much positive social feedback because she has avoided social events (e.g., getting together with friends, attending church). She keeps her feelings to herself and does not open up to her husband, children, other family members, or friends. By not sharing her experiences, she tends to feel isolated and trapped. She doesn't see a way out.

Implications for Therapy

Suitable for Cognitive Interventions

Psychological mindedness: 1. . . .2. . . . 3. . . .4. . . .5. . . ⑥. . .7
low   high

Objectivity: 1. . . ②. . . 3. . . .4. . . .5. . . .6. . . .7
low   high

Awareness: 1. . . .2. . . . 3. . . .4. . . ⑤. . .6. . . .7
low   high

Belief in cognitive model: 1. . . .2. . . . 3. . . .4. . . .5. . . .6. . . ⑦
low   high

Accessibility and plasticity of
automatic thoughts and beliefs: 1. . . .2. . . . 3. . . .4. . . ⑤. . .6. . . .7
low   high

Adaptiveness: 1. . . .2. . . . 3. . . .4. . . ⑤. . .6. . . .7
low   high

Humor: 1. . . ②. . . 3. . . .4. . . .5. . . .6. . . .7
low   high

Personality Organization (sociotropic vs. autonomous)
Keisha prides herself on being very autonomous. In her efforts to "handle things on her own," her drive for success and autonomy has resulted

---

FIGURE 2.1 *(continued)*

---

in increased distress. Her chronic pain has affected her work behavior. Her need to appear competent has prevented her from getting support from others. She also had a high need for affiliation and social support. She is afraid of being rejected if people find out about her pain and her depressed mood (high in both autonomy and sociotrophy).

Patient's Motivation, Goals, and Expectations for Therapy

Motivation: high
Expectations: She wants to be "pain-free." She wants to deal with her problems as quickly as possible.
Goals:
1. learn pain management skills
2. learn how to cope with her depression
3. learn how to keep up with her work responsibilities

Therapist's Goals
1. Teach pain management skills (e.g., deep breathing, muscle relaxation, guided imagery; identify, evaluate, and modify thoughts and beliefs about pain).
2. Teach Keisha how to cope with her pain and depression via activity scheduling and pacing as well as cognitive restructuring techniques (i.e., identify, evaluate, and modify thoughts, images, and beliefs about her pain, her work role, her sense of responsibility, etc.).
3. Learn to pace work activities and set realistic work goals. Explore to what extent carpal tunnel will interfere with work.
4. Seek reasonable accommodations in the work setting if possible.
5. Teach communication skills, with an emphasis on communicating with others about her pain and her moods without "losing face."
6. Learn to set realistic goals for self (challenging her unrelenting standards).

Predicted Difficulties and Modifications of Standard Cognitive Therapy
Because Keisha has high standards for success, it is anticipated that she might become frustrated with the therapy experience and/or her therapist. Focus on pain management and activity pacing first to help Keisha experience some immediate relief in her pain, if that is possible. Then begin to work on thought processes related to her pain and depressed mood.

---

thoughts, intermediate beliefs, and core beliefs about patients' pain and how this pain affects their lives. Figure 2.2 is an example of the cognitive conceptualization diagram that summarizes the main points of the patient's cognitive conceptualization worksheet in Figure 2.1.

FIGURE 2.2 Cognitive Conceptualization Diagram

RELEVANT CHILDHOOD/HISTORICAL INFORMATION
Keisha was raised by her parents, who encouraged her to "be all you can be." She is the oldest of four children. She described herself as a very successful person during her childhood. When she did not win events (e.g., spelling bee, track race), she viewed herself as a "failure." She has been a successful architect at the same firm for 15 years.

CORE BELIEF(S)

People will reject/abandon me.   I am trapped.
I am a failure.   I am out of control.
I am pain-ridden.

INTERMEDIATE BELIEF(S)
POSITIVE ASSUMPTIONS: If I keep my experiences to myself, people will have high regard for me. If I keep up with work, I will keep my job.
NEGATIVE ASSUMPTIONS: If people find out about my pain, they will pity me. If I slow down, I might lose my job.
RULES: I shouldn't share my pain with others. I should be responsible and hardworking. This pain shouldn't interfere with my life.
ATTITUDES: It would be horrible if people pitied me. It will be awful if I cannot keep up with my responsibilities. This pain is awful and unbearable.

COMPENSATORY STRATEGIES

Social withdrawal   Holds high expectations of self
Being a high achiever   Works very hard
Not sharing pain or moods with
   others

FIGURE 2.2 *(continued)*

SITUATION #1	SITUATION #2	SITUATION #3
A friend calls asking if she would like to go out to a movie.	I am trying to finish a deadline at work.	I am very aware of the pain in my hands and wrists.

AUTOMATIC THOUGHT	AUTOMATIC THOUGHT	AUTOMATIC THOUGHT
I don't want to see her. I don't want her to pity me because of my pain.	I cannot keep up with my work projects because of my pain.	This pain is over-whelming me and ruining my life.

MEANING OF A.T.	MEANING OF A.T.	MEANING OF A.T.
I wouldn't measure up. She would reject me.	I'm a failure. I might lose my job.	I am pain-ridden. I am out of control.

EMOTION	EMOTION	EMOTION
Sad	Anxious	Depressed

PAIN AND BEHAVIORS	PAIN AND BEHAVIORS	PAIN AND BEHAVIORS
Pain: sore, achy in hands/wrists Behaviors: tells her friend, "No."	Pain: sore, numb in hands/wrists Behavior: tries to work harder	Pain: sore, achy, numbing; intense Behavior: cries, withdraws

From Judith S. Beck's *Cognitive Therapy: Basics and Beyond.* Copyright 1995 by Judith S. Beck, PhD. Adapted with permission by Guilford Press.

3

The Usual Course and Structure of Cognitive Therapy With Chronic Pain Patients

Most chronic pain patients initially seek therapy for pain management. In addition, they may have other concerns or issues to address in therapy, for example, depression, anxiety, low self-esteem, low frustration tolerance, stresses related to their medical care, work, and financial difficulties, and relationship issues. Chronic pain patients are unique compared with patients on therapists' general caseloads for several reasons: (1) A significant number of these patients have never been in therapy before; (2) they usually come to therapy because their physicians recommended it; (3) they tend to have busy schedules regarding healthcare appointments and interventions, which can be taxing at times; and (4) pain management is often one of their main presenting problems for therapy.

Based on our clinical experience, at least half of chronic pain patients referred for treatment have never been in therapy before. These patients thus have a lot of anxiety about what therapy is going to be like. Socializing them to the therapy experience will help ease their concerns about the process.

Since many chronic pain patients come to therapy based on their physicians' recommendations, they may not have considered what their own goals for therapy are. Therefore, helping patients to find their own personal motivations and goals for therapy is essential.

Chronic pain patients tend to see a number of health care professionals for their medical care. These patients are usually sitting in office waiting rooms for significant periods of time (which is difficult when a patient has chronic pain), seeing health care professionals for structured, brief periods of time, and following specific recommendations between appointments (e.g., taking medication, attending other appointments,

43

and practicing specific exercises). Some of these patients are very satisfied with this arrangement. Other patients tend to feel overwhelmed (by
the number and frequency of office visits and recommendations related
to medical care) or minimized (e.g., felt unheard or misunderstood,
usually because of time constraints). Unlike other health care services,
therapy provides a longer time frame (50 minutes) in which to set an
agenda, discuss patients' concerns, and work on solutions to their problems. Thus, therapy serves as an opportunity to learn and to grow, as
well as an opportunity to feel supported. Therapists who are flexible and
can adapt the course and structure of the therapy to each individual
patient will experience more success than those therapists who are more
concerned about being technical experts.

Chronic pain patients typically want some quick solutions in the early
phase of therapy so that they can experience some pain relief as soon as
possible. They want to learn specific techniques to reduce their pain and
to cope better with it. They are thus more motivated than the typical
patient because they are often dealing with the physical suffering of having pain. Although the goal of being "pain free" is usually not realistic,
managing pain is.

In this chapter, we present a general overview of cognitive therapy treatment for chronic pain patients. Although this chapter highlights the usual
course of treatment, therapists should adapt the format of cognitive therapy to meet the needs of each individual patient.

OUTLINE OF TREATMENT

Cognitive therapy with chronic pain patients includes (1) an intake interview, (2) the therapy sessions, (3) the last session (termination), and (4)
booster sessions. Most patients with chronic pain can complete therapy
within 9 to 12 sessions. However, the duration of therapy depends on the
number and nature (i.e., chronicity or severity) of the presenting problems. While some patients may be dealing with Axis I issues (e.g., major
depressive disorder, pain disorder, generalized anxiety disorder), other
patients have personality disorders that will require more extensive cognitive therapy (e.g., one to two years). Some patients may want only certain components of the therapy program (e.g., cognitive restructuring,
assertiveness training, problem solving, and relaxation), which will reduce
the number of sessions (as few as three or four). In general, it is recommended that patients receive all components of the cognitive therapy program in order to maximize their gains in therapy and prevent relapses.

INTAKE INTERVIEW

The therapist should conduct a thorough intake interview prior to the start of cognitive therapy. During this session, the therapist obtains a clear picture of the patient's presenting problems and history, including a thorough assessment of his or her pain. (Pain evaluation will be discussed in chapter 4.) At the end of the intake interview, the goals of cognitive therapy should be identified, the cognitive model of chronic pain can be introduced, and an overview of cognitive therapy should be given (socializing the patient to cognitive therapy). Appropriate referrals to other services may be recommended at the end of the intake interview, for example, neuropsychological testing or dietary planning.

COGNITIVE THERAPY SESSIONS

Therapy sessions focus on helping the patient learn (1) cognitive restructuring skills (i.e., identifying, evaluating, and modifying negative automatic thoughts and beliefs) related to the pain and his or her emotional distress, (2) relaxation techniques to cope with pain and stress, and (3) problem-solving skills to cope with pain and other psychosocial stressors.

The course of cognitive therapy typically starts with a focus on pain management, then moves to other concerns or issues. (This is assuming that pain management is the primary goal in therapy.) Because many patients want some immediate relief from their pain, the patient can be taught a series of relaxation techniques in the first two sessions, along with pain and activity monitoring/scheduling exercises. Automatic thought and core belief work comprise the majority of the therapy sessions. Assertiveness training and problem-solving skills are covered later in therapy (or interspersed throughout the therapy experience). These specific techniques will be covered in the chapters that follow.

Here is an overview of the typical course of cognitive therapy (12 session format) with chronic pain patients.

Session 1.

The patient learns specific relaxation techniques, including deep breathing, progressive muscle relaxation, and patient-guided imagery. The therapist asks the patients how he or she felt, both physically and emotionally, at the end of these exercises, as well as any thoughts or images that the patient had while doing the relaxation technique. This introduces the patient to the connection between pain and other physiological sensations, emotions, thoughts, and behaviors. (The therapist writes these experiences down in the automatic thought records, which will be shared later with the patient.)

The patient also learns how to monitor the pain as well as his or her activity levels over the next week. The purpose of pain monitoring is to see how the patient's pain varies over time (over the course of the day as well as day by day) and by activity. The purpose of activity monitoring is to assess how active the individual patient is. Does the patient have enough variety in his or her daily schedule? Does the patient's participation in these activities affect his or her perception of pain? (Too much activity may aggravate it; too little may result in deconditioning.) Pain and activity monitoring are combined as one homework assignment, usually at the end of session 1. The patient also practices relaxation techniques as a homework assignment (at least 3 or 4 times a week).

Session 2.

The therapist and patient review the relaxation techniques learned last session and discuss how effective the relaxation exercises were in managing the pain levels over the past week. The patient learns some other relaxation techniques, including guided muscle relaxation and therapist-guided imagery. The pain and activity monitoring forms are then reviewed and discussed. Activity scheduling may be recommended at this point if the patient is too active or underactive. The therapist should work with the patient's physicians, physical therapists, and recreational therapists to determine appropriate activity levels. The patient is encouraged to continue pain and activity monitoring over the course of the next week. As he or she engages in an activity that is scheduled, the patient is asked to be aware of how he or she feels physically and emotionally and to record what he or she might be thinking about during those activities. Typical homework assignments include scheduling new activities and activity pacing and practicing new relaxation exercises.

Session 3.

The therapist and patient review the homework assignments from session 2 to ensure that the patient is practicing the relaxation exercises (and experiencing some pain relief during the relaxation), monitoring pain and activities, and finding a good balance of activity levels given the pain. The primary focus of this session is to learn how to use the automatic thought record to help the patient see the connections between pain sensations, emotional states, and thoughts. Only the first four columns of this journaling are used (Situation, Automatic Thoughts, Emotions, and Pain). At the end of the session, the patient is given a blank automatic thought record to practice using the first four columns over the next week, especially when he or she notices a change in pain levels or moods.

Session 4.

The automatic thought records are reviewed. The patient is encouraged to view his or her thoughts as hypotheses or hunches instead of facts. To help evaluate negative thoughts, the patient is introduced to cognitive errors in thinking. He or she is asked to come up with some personal examples of each type of error. Next, the patient is asked to identify his or her hottest (most salient) negative thought about pain from journal entries and begin evaluating it. Alternative explanations are developed. The patient is encouraged to use all six columns of the automatic thought record as the next homework assignment.

Session 5.

The automatic thought records are reviewed. The patient continues to practice skills in evaluating negative thoughts: exploring evidence for and against thoughts; imagining the worst, best, and most realistic scenarios assuming the negative thoughts were true; assessing the helpfulness of these thoughts (advantages and disadvantages analysis); and identifying what he or she would tell a friend who had the same thought. Alternative explanations are generated. The patient is introduced to behavioral experiments (Chapter 8, p. 154). As a homework assignment, the patient is asked to conduct a behavioral experiment to test the validity and helpfulness of one of his or her negative thoughts about pain. This experiment is developed collaboratively in session before it is implemented.

Session 6.

The results of the behavioral experiment are presented. Based on the findings, alternative explanations are developed (or problem solving is implemented if the negative thoughts are true). The primary focus of this session is to focus on any images the patient may have about pain. The therapist introduces techniques to stop negative images, especially if they are distressing and traumatic. Next, the patient puts images to his or her pain sensations and is asked to change the image in some way as though he or she were the director of the image. Other imagery techniques are reviewed in session. The patient is asked to practice some of these imagery techniques over the next week. In addition, the patient will continue to use the automatic thought records, with an emphasis on identifying any negative images when he or she is in pain or emotionally distressed.

Session 7.

The automatic thought records are reviewed. Any significant images are discussed and modified in session. The therapist summarizes the techniques used to identify, evaluate, and modify negative automatic thoughts (i.e., self-talk and imagery). Next, the therapist introduces the patient to the other two levels of cognition: intermediate beliefs and core beliefs. The therapist and patient use the case conceptualization diagram to write three typical examples of situations when the patient had negative thoughts about pain, including its impact on his or her life. Next, the underlying meanings of these thoughts are explored in session using a series of open-ended questions (known as the downward arrow technique). This process identifies the core beliefs related to automatic thoughts. The patient is asked for historical information about how these core beliefs developed as well as their function and purpose. He or she also identifies overused coping strategies (i.e., compensatory strategies) in dealing with his or her beliefs and the pain. As a homework assignment, the patient is asked to think about one of the core beliefs that were discussed in session and to write down the evidence for and against that core belief.

Session 8.

The therapist continues to help the patient identify, evaluate, and modify automatic thoughts. The core belief worksheet is introduced. The patient's evidence for and against the core belief (from the homework assignment) is written down on this new worksheet. The therapist and patient review this evidence, identify possible errors or distortions, and consider other information that they had not considered before. Reframes (alternative explanations) are developed in response to the evidence that the core belief is true. If time allows, a rational-emotive role play might be incorporated to help the patient explore this core belief further as well as identify alternative core belief responses. As a homework assignment, the patient can practice using the core belief worksheet, or continue to do automatic thought records depending on what the therapist and the patient believe is appropriate.

Session 9.

Homework is reviewed. The same core belief may be further modified using imagery (e.g., go back to memories of the past that support the core belief). Other core beliefs may be identified to explore and work through. The problem-solving model is introduced during this session. Problem-solving strategies are typically used when a patient's negative automatic thoughts or core beliefs are indeed true, or when the patient is ready to take some behavioral action in resolving a problem. The patient learns how to identify key problems, brainstorm possible solutions, select a solution, implement it, and evaluate its effectiveness in resolving the problem. The patient agrees to try out a solution to a problem over the next week.

Session 10.

The solution strategy (behavioral experiment) is reviewed for its effectiveness in resolving the problem. If it was not effctive, another solution will be selected from the list generated during the last session or from new ideas that develop in this session. The patient will agree to carry out this new solution over the next week. The primary purpose of this session is to teach the patient specific assertiveness skills. Learning how to communicate openly and directly without offending others is a very important skill for this patient population, given the number of health care professionals involved in their care. In addition, some of these patients struggle with social support issues. People may not understand how such patients experience pain and how it affects them. Therefore, communicating these experiences to others helps chronic pain patients feel more supported and understood than before. In this session, the patient learns how to be a good listener, to own his or her feelings and thoughts, and to speak from the "I" perspective instead of blaming others for his or her pain and problems. The patient also practices being more specific and concrete in his or her communications. Role playing is used in session to demonstrate and practice assertive styles of communication. The patient practices these skills over the next week.

Session 11.

Assertive communications over the past week are reviewed. Further practice may be necessary if the patient still needs help in being assertive with others. The focus of this session is to explore and work through possible psychosocial stressors that may affect the patient, including social support, medical care, work and financial issues, and legal issues. Specific strategies to handle these stressors are discussed (e.g., implementing assertiveness skills, relaxation, and cognitive restructuring techniques). Assuming that therapy goals have been accomplished and that there are no new goals to be set, the therapist prepares the patient for the ending of therapy. The patient is encouraged to review all of the therapy notes and homework to consolidate his or her learning and to discuss prevention strategies next week.

Session 12.

During the last session, the therapist and patient review what has been learned over the course of therapy and what the patient needs to continue to work on after therapy is over. Self-help plans are created in session to prepare the patient for how to cope with pain and other stressors (relapse prevention). Potential barriers or pitfalls to the self-help plan are identified, and possible solutions are generated. Typically, at the end of therapy, the therapist and patient schedule a follow-up booster session in 1 to 3 months to see how the patient is coping with pain and current life events. Most patients appreciate knowing that posttherapy sessions can be scheduled as a check-in to ensure relapse prevention and to assist in generalizing the insights gained in therapy.

BOOSTER SESSIONS

Booster sessions are given posttherapy. The term *booster* is indicative of the purpose of these follow-up sessions, which is to "inoculate" the patient to current and future stressors. This is often accomplished by reviewing with the patient what he or she learned in therapy and how he or she is applying these skills to recent events. Booster sessions allow the patient the opportunity to check in with the therapist to ensure that he or she is able to continue generalizing what was learned in therapy to new obstacles in his or her life.

Note that this is a general guide to the typical course of cognitive therapy with chronic pain patients. A therapist should adapt the therapy experience to the needs of each individual patient. Therefore, it is more important that the content of the program be covered than to follow the session-by-session format exactly. Being adaptive and supportive is more important than being technical.

STRUCTURE OF COGNITIVE THERAPY SESSIONS

Now that readers have a general overview of the cognitive therapy program for chronic pain patients, we can review the structure of therapy sessions. Each cognitive therapy session should comprise the following (adapted from J. Beck, 1995).

1. Check on mood.
2. Check on pain levels.

3. Check on activity level and changes in functional abilities.
4. Bridge from previous session.
5. Set an agenda.
6. Review homework.
7. Discuss agenda items, establish new homework assignment, and provide periodic (capsule) summaries.
8. Give final summary and feedback.

MOOD CHECK

At the start of each session, a quick check on clinical states is recommended, in particular, on how the patient has been feeling over the past week. The therapist often asks the patient to fill out the Beck Depression Inventory, the Beck Anxiety Inventory, and/or the Beck Hopelessness Scale prior to the start of the session. These questionnaires provide the therapist with a brief evaluation of the patient's levels of depression, anxiety, and hopelessness, respectively. However, depending on the key emotions or moods of the patient, the therapist may also want to check the patient's levels of anger, guilt, and helplessness, among other emotions. The therapist can also check the patient's moods by simply asking, "How have you been feeling over the past week, including today?"

PAIN LEVEL CHECK

It is important to do a quick check on the patient's pain levels every session. The therapist can ask:

- How would you describe your pain over the past week? (or How has your pain been this past week?)
- How would you rate your pain over the past week on a scale from 0 to 10, with 0 being no pain at all and 10 being the worst possible pain?

If there have been any significant changes in the patient's pain levels, this could be a topic for discussion during the session.

The patient also can fill out a brief pain questionnaire every few weeks in the waiting room prior to the start of the session. The short form of the McGill Questionnaire (Melzack, 1987) is highly recommended.

ACTIVITY LEVEL AND CHANGES IN FUNCTIONAL ABILITIES

The therapist needs to know if there have been any significant changes in the patient's activity levels and functional abilities (i.e., ability to engage in certain physical activities). The therapist can ask:

- How active have you been this past week on a scale from 0 to 10, with 0 being not active at all and 10 being very active?
- Have you noticed a change in your ability to do certain physical activities over the past week?

If there are significant changes in activity levels or functional abilities, this may be a topic for discussion during the session.

BRIDGE FROM PREVIOUS SESSION

The therapist summarizes the main issues discussed in the previous session and mentions any self-help homework that was assigned over the past week as a way to bridge one session to another. Bridging is an important ingredient in cognitive therapy because it helps build connections between the topics that are covered from one week to the next, to emphasize what is learned in therapy, and to facilitate progress toward established goals in therapy.

The therapist usually provides the structure to bridge from session to session in the early phases of therapy. Here is an example of how a therapist can bridge between sessions 1 and 2:

Therapist: Last week, we discussed ways that you can monitor your pain and your activity levels, so that we can identify potential triggers to your pain. We also practiced some specific ways to relax, including deep breathing exercises, progressive muscle relaxation, and guided imagery. Did you have thoughts or feelings about our last session?

However, later in therapy, the patient is usually an active participant in the bridging process and summarizes what was covered in the last session at the beginning of the next session.

Therapist: What do you remember us covering in last week's session?
Patient: Well, I learned how my pain is related to how I think and how I feel. You also taught me how to use the automatic thought record, so that I can catch my negative thoughts when I am in pain. Overall, I thought it was a really productive session because I have been more aware of my negative thinking and how it affects my pain.

SET AN AGENDA

Following a review of the previous session, the therapist and patient set an agenda for the therapy session. In other words, they decide on the main issues that need to be discussed. Usually, patients have one or two issues they want to discuss in session. In addition, therapists may need to cover some information in the session (e.g., introduction to intermediate and core beliefs related to pain) or to discuss some issues (e.g., observations from the previous session and issues related to the therapeutic relationship). To set the agenda, the therapist can ask:

- What would you like to work on today in therapy?
- What would you like to put on the agenda to discuss today?

During the first session, the therapist introduces the concept of agenda setting:

Therapist: At the beginning of every session, I will be checking in with you to find out what you want to discuss and work on that day. There may be some topics I want to cover in session too. This helps us decide what we are going to focus on during our sessions. We call this "setting the agenda." [pause] So, what would you like to work on today? [Pause for patient's response] I'll make a quick list of these topics before we start. Okay, in addition to [patient's agenda items], I will teach you some relaxation techniques today to help you cope with your pain. I also want to talk with you about keeping track of your pain and your activities. So, let's add these items to the agenda.

After the agenda has been established, the therapist asks the patient where he or she would like to start first. If several topics for discussion are listed, the therapist must use his or her judgment in collaboration with the patient to determine which issues are the most important to discuss during the session, in case they cannot get through all of them.

Therapist: [summarizes agenda list] You mentioned two important concerns for us to work on today: coping better with your pain and a recent argument with your partner. In case we cannot get to both of these concerns in today's session, which one would be the most important for us to discuss first? [pause for patient's response] Let's be sure we also have time to cover relaxation techniques and ways to track your pain.

REVIEW HOMEWORK

Review of homework is typically the first issue to cover after the agenda is set. This socializes the patient to the importance of homework and rewards him or her for his or her efforts between sessions. In rare cases, particularly crisis intervention sessions, it may be necessary to postpone the review of homework until later in the session.

DISCUSS AGENDA ITEMS, ESTABLISH NEW HOMEWORK ASSIGNMENT, AND PROVIDE PERIODIC (CAPSULE) SUMMARIES

After the patient and therapist go over the therapy homework, they can begin to discuss the concerns listed on the therapy agenda. Throughout the session, the therapist provides occasional summaries of the issues discussed to highlight the important points covered and to demonstrate empathy and support. At the end of each therapy session, the therapist and patient work collaboratively to develop self-help homework assignments for the following week.

FINAL SUMMARY AND FEEDBACK

The therapist summarizes the main issues discussed before obtaining feedback from the patient on how he or she felt about the session. The patient will eventually learn to provide the final summary for the session as well as share his or her thoughts and feelings about the session without prompting. At the end of the session, the therapist asks the patient how he or she felt about the session, what he or she found helpful, as well as any concerns the patient had about the therapy session.

- How did you feel about our session today?
- What did you get out of today's session? What was helpful for you?
- Is there anything I said or did that upset you or offended you?

ONGOING ASSESSMENT/EVALUATION OF CHRONIC PAIN PATIENTS

The therapist is actively involved in evaluating the effectiveness of the therapy. There are a variety of ways to assess or evaluate its effectiveness, including the patient's self-reports of progress in therapy, mood and pain questionnaire scores, weekly evaluations of therapy sessions, and mutual termination following the completion of therapy goals.

PATIENT'S SELF-REPORT OF PROGRESS IN THERAPY AND FEEDBACK

The therapist regularly discusses the patient's views on his or her progress to date in therapy, particular as it relates to the therapy goals. For example, the therapist might do a quick check with the patient approximately every three sessions to explore how the patient thinks and feels about the focus of therapy and the progress made to date.

- How have you felt about our last three sessions?
- What stands out from those sessions?
- What progress do you believe you are making in therapy so far?
- What do you think we need to focus on over the next few sessions? (Relate this back to original goals or set new goals.)

In general, the therapist should consistently request the patient's feedback on therapy at the end of each session. If the patient is dissatisfied with the session, the source of this dissatisfaction should be explored. Based on this feedback, the therapist should make adjustments (to his or her style and/or the therapy plan) to meet the patient's needs. For example, some patients may have a difficult time journaling and may feel overwhelmed by the homework assigned. One possible solution is to break the homework assignment into smaller steps and work toward one of those smaller goals. Or the therapist and patient could come to a compromise about other ways of learning the same information. For some patients, self-help homework may need to be completed in the therapy session with the therapist's support, rather than between sessions, until the patient feels a sense of confidence in doing the homework on his or her own. Some patients do not like to write, so other possibilities could be explored, including the use of audiotaping between sessions to record journal entries or dictating ideas for someone else (e.g., a close friend or family member) to write in the journal forms. Thus, regular patient feedback is helpful to ensure that cognitive therapy interventions are individually tailored to the needs and the motivations of the patient to optimize positive outcomes.

At the end of therapy, the patient is asked to reflect on his or her pain, moods, beliefs, and coping strategies when he or she started therapy compared with where he or she is now. Many patients report less pain than before (i.e., frequency, duration, and intensity). Even for those patients whose pain does not improve over the course of therapy, they report managing their pain and their moods better than before.

PAIN AND MOOD QUESTIONNAIRES

Qualitative data (i.e., self-reports) are very important in assessing the effectiveness of therapy. For example, patients are asked about their pain levels, moods, and physical functioning on a weekly basis to assess their progress. In addition, quantitative data can be collected at different points in time during the therapy process to determine the patient's progress as well as the effectiveness of therapy. Self-report measures of moods, pain levels, physical limitations, and psychosocial functioning are administered at certain points throughout therapy. In particular, the Behavioral Assessment of Pain, the Beck Depression Inventory, the Beck Anxiety Inventory, and the Beck Hopelessness Scale are the measures typically used in our practice. These measures will be discussed in chapter 4.

PATIENT'S WEEKLY EVALUATIONS OF THERAPY SESSIONS

The therapist can assess the patient's perceptions of the therapy session on a weekly basis using the Patient's Report of Therapy Session form (see Appendix A). This form includes questions about the degree of progress made in today's session, perceptions of progress in future sessions, views about the therapist's level of helpfulness and support (and other descriptors), and skills gained in the session that day. The patient is told that this form is an opportunity to share any experiences of therapy in writing. The patient completes this form in the waiting area after the session is over. Most patients can finish this form in 5 minutes. After it is completed, the patient places the form in a folder at the reception desk to be reviewed later by the therapist. Content shared in these forms can be used as a guide to begin the following therapy session. This form ensures that the patient has the time to provide formal feedback to the therapist about the therapy process, what he or she appreciated and did not, and areas for improvement.

MUTUAL TERMINATION OF THERAPY FOLLOWING COMPLETION OF GOALS

When both the therapist and the patient agree that significant progress has been made toward the goals set, therapy is brought to a close. Therefore, in most cases of mutual termination, the ending of therapy is a sign of progress.

4

Pain Assessment

Just as patients' physical condition is evaluated prior to recommending specific medical interventions, therapists evaluate patients' pain experience and their emotional or psychological functioning prior to beginning a course of therapy. The assessment process typically involves conducting an intake interview, administering self-report questionnaires, and collecting information (e.g., medical diagnoses and prognoses) from other health care professionals involved in their patients' care.

The primary purposes of the intake interview are to (1) establish a good working relationship with the patient; (2) clarify what brings the patient in for therapy; (3) understand the events surrounding the development of the chronic pain condition as well as its consequences; (4) collect information on the presenting problems (e.g., chronic pain, depression, and relationship issues), including a history of these problems and other information regarding family, social, educational, work, medical, legal, and substance use histories, as well as significant events, and traumas (e.g., history of physical, sexual, and emotional abuse); (5) assess for suicidal and homicidal risk, psychosis, and mental status; (6) clarify the patient's goals for therapy; and (7) prepare the patient for the course of therapy, including an explanation of the cognitive model of pain.

Whether or not pain management is a presenting problem, the therapist should collect information on the patient's experience of pain, including pain sensations, emotional states, thought processes, and actions (i.e., pain behaviors, and efforts to cope), any physical limitations, and significant psychosocial stressors (personal, social, and environmental factors) related to the pain. Self-report questionnaires can be administered as part of the intake process to provide a baseline assessment of the patient's pain levels, emotional distress, thought processes, behaviors, personality, and psychosocial functioning.

Other critical information will further assist the therapist in treatment planning and case conceptualization, including medical evaluations of pain, as well as an understanding of the patient's participation and level of success with other pain treatments. The therapist can learn about the patient's chronic pain condition from a variety of sources, including his or her physicians, nurses, physical, occupational, and recreational therapists, vocational rehabilitation counselors, family members, and friends. The therapist also should review the patient's medical records or medical reports (depending on what is accessible, with the patient's written consent) to learn more about the medical aspects of the pain.

This chapter will focus on recommendations for interviewing patients about their experience of pain and conducting a thorough pain and mood assessment.

PRESENTING PROBLEMS

Many patients are referred to psychotherapy by other health care professionals (e.g., physicians, chiropractors, nurses, and physical therapists) as part of a comprehensive treatment facility to address their chronic pain problems. Therapists who are new to working with this patient population will learn that chronic pain is often one of the initial presenting problems; however, it is often the case that other problems emerge—some that are related to the pain (e.g., lack of support from family or friends, loss of identity, parenting issues, difficulties in fulfilling life roles, and grief and loss issues). and others that are not.

It is helpful to clarify what brings the patient into therapy, in other words, identifying the presenting problems. The therapist can use questions such as the following:

- What brings you here to therapy?
- What concerns or problems brought you here today?

Chronic pain patients may not have a clear understanding of why they are in therapy initially, and are typically not familiar with the therapy process in general. Sometimes, patients will answer, "Because my doctor told me to come—I don't know why." Others might say, "My doctor told me I should see you for pain management." Follow-up questions are helpful here:

- What were your doctor's reasons for recommending therapy for you?
- What do you hope to get out of therapy?

A significant number of these patients may have never been exposed to psychotherapy before and are depending on their health care professionals' recommendations to pursue this course of treatment. Therefore, socializing the patient to the therapy process and establishing rapport are critical events during the intake interview.

PAIN EVALUATION

The patient's experience of chronic pain need to be assessed, regardless of whether or not managing chronic pain is the primary focus of therapy. Understanding the subjective nature of the patients pain will promote empathy and facilitate treatment planning. The most common method of pain assessment is to use interview questions to guide the patient in describing his or her experience of pain. Self-report questionnaires and clinical observations (e.g., of pain behaviors) can also be used to assess pain. This will be discussed later in this chapter.

The therapist can ask a variety of questions regarding the patient's pain, including its location, duration, intensity, frequency, fluctuations, the patient's descriptions of it, "triggers" (antecedents), emotions, thoughts, behaviors, physical limitations, and psychosocial factors (e.g., personality, level of support, and environment). Historical information regarding the development of chronic pain, including the patient's medical treatment of pain, is also crucial. Here are some possible questions to ask:

- Tell me about your pain and how it developed. (Let the patient speak first without interruption, then follow up with specific questions as needed.)
- How long have you been in pain? (time frame)
- What specific events led to the development of your chronic pain condition?
- Where is the pain located in your body? (locations)
- How often do you have pain [in each pain location]? (frequency)
- How long does the pain usually last [in each pain location]? (duration)
- How intense is the pain [in each pain location] on a scale from 0 to 10, with 0 being no pain and 10 being severe, excruciating pain— the worse pain possible?
- What words would you use to describe your pain [in each location]?
- Are there any triggers to your pain? What makes the pain worse? What makes the pain better?
- What emotions tend to surface when you are in pain?
- What thoughts or images typically run through your mind when you are in pain?
- How do you tend to act or behave when you are in pain [compared to when you are not]?

- How would people know that you are in pain? What do they see? (identifying pain behaviors)
- What have you tried to do to cope with your pain?
- What solutions have worked? Which ones have not?
- What has your health care professional (e.g., physician or chiropractor) told you about your pain? What are his/her explanations?
- What medical conditions do you have?
- What is/are your medical diagnosis(es)?
- What types of treatments have you received for your pain (e.g., medical exams, physical therapy, medication, etc.)?
- What other treatments have been recommended?
- How has this pain affected your life? Tell me how it has affected your different life roles (e.g., worker, partner, parent, student, leisure role, citizen).
- How does the pain affect your ability to perform daily life functions?
- How do people in your life respond to your pain?
- Are there any other problems or concerns associated with your pain?

DEVELOPMENT OF CHRONIC PAIN

Chronic pain can develop as a result of motor vehicle accidents, other personal injuries (e.g., sports injuries or home accidents), work-related injuries (e.g., slip-and-fall accidents, lifting accidents, and repetitive movement injuries), surgeries and other medical procedures (i.e., medical interventions may inadvertently cause chronic pain), and chronic medical conditions (e.g., lupus, fibromyalgia, and complex regional syndrome). Sometimes, there is no one clear-cut event, but rather a series of events that led to the development of a patient's chronic pain. For some patients, chronic pain develops mysteriously, without any precipitating events. It is important to find out how long they have had chronic pain and to understand what the patient views as the cause(s) of the pain. Later, the therapist can uncover physicians' explanations and diagnoses.

LOCATION OF PAIN

For some patients, pain is located in one or two areas; for other patients, pain is located in a variety of places throughout the body. How the pain is experienced (e.g., duration and descriptions) may differ across these locations. For example, a patient may report feeling a constant numbing or tingling sensation in his lower back, but feel a shooting pain running down his legs on an intermittent basis.

FREQUENCY OF PAIN

Frequency refers to how often the pain occurs (e.g., continuously, intermittently, daily, once a week, etc.). There are some patients who have regular, constant pain, whereas other patients are in pain only once in a while. For example, intermittent pain (i.e., pain that comes and goes) is common for patients with migraine and tension headaches.

DURATION OF PAIN

Duration refers to the time span of the patient's pain experience—when it starts and how long it lasts. Acute levels of pain usually last for hours, days, or weeks, whereas chronic levels of pain usually last for months or years.

INTENSITY AND FLUCTUATION OF PAIN

Intensity refers to how much the pain hurts. Some patients identify it as the "volume" of the pain—how "loud" or "soft" it is. A patient can rate pain using a scale from 0 to 10, with 0 representing *no pain* and 10 representing *severe, excruciating pain—the worst pain ever.* Fluctuations in pain levels can occur, as it is rare for pain to stay at the same "volume" consistently over time. Therefore, it is important for the patient to share examples of when the pain gets worse (higher intensity) and when it gets better (lower intensity).

DESCRIPTORS OF PAIN

The therapist needs to understand the patient's perception of the physiological sensations of pain in the different parts of his/her body. As part of the pain evaluation, the patient is asked to listen to a list of adjectives that people use to describe pain and identify which adjectives best represent his or her pain in each body region (e.g., head, neck, shoulders, arms, chest, upper back, lower back, groin/pelvis, buttocks, legs, feet, and toes). The patient also may have adjectives of his/her own that are not on this list. Here is a list we use in our clinics:

- Throbbing
- Pounding
- Tight

- Heavy
- Shooting
- Sore
- Tender
- Aching
- Burning
- Stabbing
- Numbing
- Other

PAIN TRIGGERS

Certain foods, activities, weather conditions, and situations can trigger pain, for example, drinking caffeine or alcohol, strenuous exercise and other physical activities (e.g., bending, grasping, walking, sitting, or lifting), hot or cold weather, rainy days, humidity, lack of social support, and stress. There are a variety of circumstances unique to each patient that can trigger pain and heighten pain levels. It is important to explore situations or factors that may reduce pain levels (e.g., specific pain medications, medical procedures, distraction efforts, and talking with a close friend).

FUNCTIONAL LIMITATIONS

Chronic pain can affect or limit patients' abilities to complete certain tasks or activities, which is referred to as their functional limitations. Patients can usually identify their current physical and task limitations without much prompting. Many limitations are related to functions of daily living and tasks related to work and school. The therapist also needs to know, from the patient's perspective, what tasks and activities do not cause much pain. Awareness of the patient's physical abilities and limitations can help both the patient and the therapist have a more balanced view of what the patient can and cannot do. Examples of physical limitations include basic motor activities such as sitting, standing, bending, lifting, walking, running, climbing, pulling, pushing, grasping, and writing. Examples of specific daily living activities that may be affected by pain include bathing or showering, making meals, washing clothes, making beds, washing dishes, vacuuming, sweeping floors, and taking care of children (if applicable). Work-related activities are specific to each profession or trade but may include standing, sitting, or walking for periods of time, lifting or carrying objects, and using hands to perform repetitive activities (e.g., sorting papers/mail, assembly line work, and typing). School-related activities include sitting for long periods of time, taking notes, typing on the computer, walking to campus/school, getting in and out of vehicles, and participating in physical education and extracurricular activities.

Much of this information can be obtained via the use of questionnaires or checklists. However, it is often very validating for patients to discuss how their pain has affected their abilities and to realize that their therapist is there to listen to them without judgment. Allowing a patient to share his or her personal experiences within the context of the interview can be very powerful and healing.

EVALUATING PSYCHOLOGICAL ASPECTS OF PAIN AND ITS CONSEQUENCES

The psychological aspects of pain that need to be evaluated include the patient's (1) feelings about the pain; (2) thoughts, images, and beliefs about the pain; (3) behaviors related to pain (e.g., when in pain or as the result of pain), also known as pain behaviors, as well as his or her coping strategies; (4) the physiological experience of pain; and (5) how pain affects various life roles, including relationships with others.

FEELINGS ABOUT PAIN

The therapist can start this part of the interview by asking the patient about his or her emotions when he or she is in pain, for example, "What emotions tend to surface when you are in pain?" or "What emotions are you aware of when you are in pain?" Patients usually can identify a range of emotions associated with pain, including sadness, depression, fear, anxiety, anger, frustration, jealousy, resentment, despair, hopelessness, discouragement, grief, loss, and hatred. Sometimes patients can get stuck in these feelings for a while (mood states).

Referring to a recent pain episode will help a patient identify his or her emotions. For example, "Tell me about a recent situation in which your pain was really bothering you. What emotions were you in touch with then?" The therapist may also reflect the patient's feelings in specific situations: "Sounds like you felt scared when you fell on the ground." It will not be possible to explore the patient's emotions in much depth during the intake interview because there is a lot of information to collect in a short period of time. However, listening, reflecting, and validating the patient's feelings will help him or her feel supported and understood.

COGNITIONS ABOUT PAIN

Once specific feelings have been identified, the therapist can then move to an exploration of the patient's thoughts. It is important to identify key automatic thoughts about pain (usually negative and unrealistic in nature), which include self-talk and images regarding pain as well as possible attributions about the pain. A typical question is "What thoughts or images run through your mind when you are in pain?" The therapist also can go back to the recent episode of pain identified and ask the patient about his or her thoughts and images in that specific situation. Examples of negative thoughts about pain include the following:

- No one understands my medical condition or my pain. No one cares about me.
- My doctors cannot figure out what is the cause of my pain. They think that my pain is all in my head. That is why I am here today, I think.
- This pain is unbearable. I can't stand it.
- I am being punished. Why did this have to happen to me?
- I am useless now that I cannot work anymore. What am I going to do?
- I am no good to my family.

In general, it is recommended that the therapist avoid evaluating or modifying negative automatic thoughts and beliefs about pain during the intake interview. Intervening too early may damage the therapeutic alliance and distance or alienate the patient from the therapy process to come.

PAIN BEHAVIORS

The therapist needs to understand how the patient behaves or acts when he or she is in pain. Does the patient behave differently when he or she is in pain? Is the patient more reclusive, isolated, reserved, demanding, aggressive, dependent, or critical than before the pain syndrome developed? The therapist can observe the patient's pain behaviors during the interview and throughout therapy by noticing verbal and nonverbal (e.g., body posture, gait, facial expressions, and body language) communications of pain. (Keep in mind that observations may or may not reflect the patient's self-report of pain; Labus, Keefe, & Jensen, 2003.) Sometimes, significant others and friends can provide more information in this area, with the patient's permission. Here are some examples of questions the therapist could ask in this domain:

- How do these feelings and thoughts influence your pain, the way you take care of yourself, and the way you relate to others? (How does feeling sad and thinking you are no good and useless influence the way you take care of yourself or relate to others?)
- How do you tend to act or behave when you are in pain? (When you are in pain and say to yourself, "I am no good to anyone anymore. I am useless," how do you tend to act or behave?)
- Do other people notice a difference in you (e.g., your actions, your words, your level of participation in activities) when you are in pain?

PAIN COPING STRATEGIES

Another aspect of the behavioral dimensions of pain is how patients cope with their pain. Chronic pain patients can be very resourceful. For example, they may implement coping strategies recommended by health care professionals, such as taking their pain medication as recommended, following physical therapy regimens, making modifications in diet and nutrition to eat healthier than before, and setting realistic exercise plans. They may also use some of their own coping strategies, for example, distracting themselves from the pain, joining a chronic pain support group, doing yoga or meditation, and seeking psychotherapy services. Yet some coping strategies may exacerbate their pain condition, for example, overexertion (i.e., pushing their bodies to do more than is appropriate), hiding their pain from others, social isolation, and not following treatment recommendations (e.g., over- and underutilizing prescribed medication for pain and inflammation). To assess a patient's pain coping strategies, the therapist can ask the following questions:

- How have you tried to cope with the pain?
- What coping strategies have worked?
- What coping strategies have not worked?
- What new skills would you like to learn to cope better with your pain and your life right now?

PSYCHOSOCIAL STRESSORS

Another important aspect of pain assessment is evaluating how patients' pain affects their life roles and relationships with others. Potential psychosocial stressors can be identified by exploring the patient's (1) relationships with family/friends, (2) work/employment situation, (3) financial affairs, (4) level of involvement in leisure and community activities, (5) current medical treatment and concerns, and (6) legal issues related to the chronic pain condition. Patients are more likely to be at risk for severe mood problems and poor coping responses related to their pain and/or medical treatment if they have a number of stressors in their lives, such as poor social support, unemployment, financial problems, and legal difficulties. For some patients, these stressors and their interpretations of them may cause more psychological difficulties than the actual pain. Examples of questions related to psychosocial stressors include the following:

Medical/Health Care History
- What has your physician/health care professional told you about your pain? What are his/her explanations?
- What medical conditions do you have? What is/are your medical diagnosis(es)?
- What types of treatment have you received for your pain (medical exams, physical therapy, medication, etc.)?
- What other treatments have been recommended?
- What types of medication are you taking? What are the dosages for each? What are the medications for (e.g., pain, sleep, moods, or other medical conditions)? What are the potential side effects of these medications? Are you experiencing any of these side effects?
- Have you had any surgeries or hospitalizations [in the past]?
- How are you feeling about your medical care and other pain treatments?
- Do you have any concerns about your medical care/pain treatments?
- Have you communicated those concerns to your physician/health care professional?

Relationships
- How has the pain affected your relationships with others?
- How do people respond to your pain?
- What do you need from others, in terms of support?

Physical Limitations/Productivity
- How does the pain affect your ability to perform daily life functions?
- Are you currently employed? If yes, how has the pain affected your ability to work?
- Are you currently in school? If yes, how has the pain affected your ability to succeed in school or complete school?
- What work and/or school tasks/responsibilities are you still able to do with relative ease?

Leisure/Citizen Roles
- How has the pain affected your involvement in leisure and community activities?

Financial/Legal
- How has the pain affected your financial situation?
- Are you involved with the legal system in any way as a result of your chronic pain condition(s)?

Readers are referred to Figure 4.1 for a semistructured interview format that can be used during the intake session. It includes a series of questions to evaluate different aspects of pain as well as a series of questions to obtain historical information (e.g., family, social, work, educational, medical, counseling/psychotherapy, and substance use history; assessment for abuse and trauma; suicidal/homicidal ideation and possible psychosis). Therapists may choose to use only some of the questions listed for their intake interviews with patients. However, many of the pain assessment questions are very helpful.

FIGURE 4.1 Semi-structured Interview

Presenting Problems
- What brings you here to therapy? What concerns or problems brought you here today?

If referred by a physician:
- What were your physician's reasons for recommending therapy for you?

- This is what your physician told you. What do you hope to get out of therapy?

Pain Evaluation

Pain Experience
- Tell me about your pain and how it developed. (Follow-up with questions below.)

- How long have you been in pain?

- What specific events led to the development of your chronic pain condition?

FIGURE 4.1 *(continued)*

□ Motor vehicle accident:_____
□ Personal injury:_____
□ Work-related injury:_____
□ Medical condition:_____
□ Other:_____

- Where is the pain located in your body?
  ____head ____neck ____shoulder(s) ____upper arm(s)
  ____elbow(s) ____lower arm(s) ____wrist(s) ____hand(s)
  ____knuckle(s) ____finger(s) ____upper back
  ____midback ____lower back ____chest ____stomach
  ____hip(s) ____groin ____upper leg(s) ____knee(s)
  ____lower leg(s) ____ankle(s) ____foot (feet) ____toes
  other:_____

- How often do you have pain in your _____ (assess each
  pain location)?
  C = constant, I = intermittent
  ____head ____neck ____shoulder(s) ____upper arm(s)
  ____elbow(s) ____lower arm(s) ____wrist(s) ____hand(s)
  ____knuckle(s) ____finger(s) ____upper back
  ____midback ____lower back ____chest ____stomach
  ____hip(s) ____groin ____upper leg(s) ____knee(s)
  ____lower leg(s) ____ankle(s) ____foot (feet) ____toes
  other:_____

- How long does the pain usually last (in each location)?
  S = seconds, M = minutes, H = hours, D = all day
  ____head ____neck ____shoulder(s) ____upper arm(s)
  ____elbow(s) ____lower arm(s) ____wrist(s) ____hand(s)
  ____knuckle(s) ____finger(s) ____upper back
  ____midback ____lower back ____chest ____stomach
  ____hip(s) ____groin ____upper leg(s) ____knee(s)
  ____lower leg(s) ____ankle(s) ____foot (feet) ____toes
  other:_____

- How intense is the pain in each part of your body on a scale from 0 to 10, with 0 being *no pain* and 10 being *severe, excruciating pain*—the *worst pain possible.*

0. . . . 1. . . . 2. . . . 3. . . . 4. . . .5. . . .6. . . .7. . . .8. . . .9. . . .10
no pain   severe pain, worst

____head   ____neck   ____shoulder(s)   ____upper arm(s)
____elbow(s)   ____lower arm(s)   ____wrist(s)   ____hand(s)
____knuckle(s)   ____finger(s)   ____upper back
____midback   ____lower back   ____chest   ____stomach
____hip(s)   ____groin   ____upper leg(s)   ____knee(s)
____lower leg(s)   ____ankle(s)   ____foot (feet)   ____toes
other:_____

- What words would you use to describe your pain (in each location)?
Head:_____
Neck:_____
Shoulder(s):_____
Upper arm(s):_____
Elbow(s):_____
Lower arm(s):_____
Wrist(s):_____
Knuckle(s):_____
Hand(s):_____
Finger(s):_____
Upperback:_____
Midback:_____
Lower back:_____
Chest:_____
Stomach:_____
Hip(s):_____
Groin:_____
Buttocks:_____
Upper leg(s):_____
Knee(s):_____
Lower leg(s):_____
Anke(s):_____
Foot(feet):_____
Toes:_____
Other:_____

FIGURE 4.1 *(continued)*

Choose adjectives from this list:
- ☐ Throbbing
- ☐ Pounding
- ☐ Tight
- ☐ Heavy
- ☐ Shooting
- ☐ Sore
- ☐ Tender
- ☐ Achy
- ☐ Burning
- ☐ Stabbing
- ☐ Numbing
- ☐ Other:_____

Pain Triggers
- Are there any triggers to your pain?
- What makes the pain worse?
- What makes the pain better?

Psychological Aspects of Pain

Emotions
- What emotions tend to surface when you are in pain?

- Tell me about a recent situation when your pain was really bothering you. (Patient describes situation.) What emotions were you in touch with then?

Thoughts
- What thoughts or images were running through your mind then?

- What thoughts or images typically run through your mind when you are in pain?

Behaviors/Pain Behaviors
- How do these feelings and thoughts influence your pain? The way you take care of yourself, and the way you relate to others?

- How do you tend to act or behave when you are in pain (as opposed to when you are not in pain)?

- Do people notice a difference in you (e.g., your actions, words, level of participation in activities) when you are in pain? How would people know that you are in pain? What do they see? (Identifying pain behaviors)

- What have you tried to do to cope with your chronic pain?

- What solutions have worked?

- Which ones have not?

- What new skills would you like to learn to cope better with your pain and your life right now?

Medical History
- What has your physician/health care professional told you about your pain? What are his/her explanations? [Get name(s) of patient's physicians]

- What medical conditions do you have? What is/are your medical diagnosis(es)?

- What types of treatment have you received for your pain (medical exams, physical therapy, medication, etc.)?

- What other treatments have been recommended?

- What types of medication are you taking? What are the dosages for each? What are the medications for (e.g., pain, sleep, moods, or other medical conditions)? What are the potential side effects of these medications? Are you experiencing any of these side effects?

Medication	Dosage	Purpose/Condition	Side Effects

FIGURE 4.1 *(continued)*

- Have you had any surgeries or hospitalizations (in the past)?

- How are you feeling about your medical care and other pain treatments?

- Do you have any concerns about your medical care/pain treatments?

- Have you communicated those concerns to your physician/health care professional?

Psychosocial Stressors
- How has this pain affected your life? Tell me how the pain has affected your different life roles (e.g., worker, partner, parent, student, leisure roles, citizen].

  Relationships
- How has the pain affected your relationships with others (partner/spouse, children, family members, friends, employer and coworkers, physician and other health care professionals)?

- How do people respond to your pain?

- What do you need from others, in terms of support?

  Functional Limitations/Productivity
- How does the pain affect your ability to perform daily life functions?

- Are you currently employed? If yes, how has the pain affected your ability to work?

- Are you currently in school? If yes, how has your pain affected your ability to succeed in school or complete school?

- What work and/or school tasks/responsibilities are you still able to do with relative ease?

  Leisure/Citizen Roles
- How has your pain affected your involvement in leisure and community activities?

Financial/Legal
- How has your pain affected your financial situation?

- Are you involved with the legal system in any way as a result of your chronic pain condition(s)? If yes, tell me about more about that. [Get the name of patient's attorney.]

Other Problems Associated With Pain
- Are there any other problems or concerns associated with your pain?

History of Other Presenting Problems (Besides Pain)
- Have you had these problems in the past?

- How did they develop?

Family History
- Where were you born and raised?

- Who were the members of your family during childhood and adolescence?

- Where were you in the birth order?

- How would you describe your relationships with your family growing up?

- Who are the members of your immediate family?

- How would you describe your relationships with them?

- Is there a history of chronic pain or chronic illnesses in your family?

Social History
- Tell me about the nature of your relationships with friends and peers growing up.

- How would your friends describe you during childhood and adolescence?

- How many significant dating relationships did you have?

FIGURE 4.1 *(continued)*

- Are you currently married or partnered?

- Have you been married or in a partnered relationship previously? (If so, how many times?)

- Describe your current partnership/marriage (if applicable).

- Describe your current relationships with friends.

Educational History
- How far did you go in school? (What is the highest level of education completed?)

- Did you receive any diplomas or degrees? If so, what were they? Where did you receive them?

- Describe your experiences as a student.

Work History
- Are you currently employed?

- Where do you work?

- What is your position title?

- Tell me about your work responsibilities.

- Are you or have you ever been on disability leave? If so, how long?

- What do you enjoy about your work?

- What are some of your work values?

- What are your future career goals/aspirations?

- What are some of the most significant work experiences you have had in the past?

Substance Abuse History
- Do you drink alcohol? What is your beverage of choice?

- Do you use drugs? What do you use? What is your drug of choice?

- How often do you drink/use?

- How much do you consume/use on average?

- Where do you tend to drink/use?

- What are your reasons for drinking/using?

- How has drinking alcohol or using drugs affected your life?

- Have you ever tried to stop drinking/using?

- What previous treatment have you received for your drinking/drug use, if any?

- Have any health care professionals been concerned about your use of prescription or over-the-counter medications for pain or other medical problems?

Significant Events and Traumas

- What do you view as some significant events in your life?

- How were they significant to you?

- Have you experienced any trauma in your life? Describe those experiences for me.

- Have you ever experienced emotional or verbal abuse (feeling put down and/or manipulated by others to the point that it affected your self-esteem)? Approximately when?

- Have you ever experienced physical abuse (someone using physical means to control you, for example, throwing objects to threaten you, and/or hitting or kicking you to the point of being bruised or injured)? Approximately when?

- Have you ever experienced sexual abuse (being exposed to genitals or sexual activity without your consent, as well as other unwanted sexual experiences, for example, being touched, fondled, or having intercourse without your consent)?

- Approximately when?
  (If a child, elderly person, or incapacitated adults is currently being abused, this must be reported to the appropriate authorities according to State law.)

Counseling/Psychotherapy/Psychiatric History
- Have you had any significant emotional problems in the past?

- Have you ever received psychotherapy or counseling services? What were your experiences like?

- Have you ever been hospitalized for emotional problems? If so, for what?

- Have you ever had thoughts of harming yourself or other people?

- Have you ever developed a specific plan to harm yourself or others?

- Have you ever seen, heard, or sensed things that other people haven't experienced?

- Conduct a mini-mental status exam to assess the cognitive functioning of the patient.

Goals for Therapy
- What are your goals for therapy?

Note: Developed by Carrie Winterowd, PhD. Printed with permission of Carrie Winterowd, PhD.

ADMINISTRATION OF QUESTIONNAIRES

Questionnaires can be administered to assess patients' pain experiences, personality styles, mood states, and cognitions, as well as behaviors that may affect their chronic pain or other presenting problems. Readers are referred to *Handbook of Pain Assessment* (Turk & Melzack 2001) for a detailed account of pain assessment measures and procedures available. The ones specifically discussed in this book are those frequently used by therapists in our clinics.

A comprehensive pain assessment (e.g., Behavioral Assessment of Pain) and mood questionnaires (e.g., Beck Depression Inventory, Beck Anxiety Inventory, Beck Hopelessness Scale, and State-Trait Anger Expression Inventory) are usually administered at the beginning and end of therapy to help assess patients' progress and therapy effectiveness. Patients typically complete the Beck measures at the beginning of every therapy session. Personality measures are usually administered at the beginning of therapy (e.g., Minnesota Multiphasic Personality Inventory-2, or Personality Assessment Inventory) if significant psychopathology is suspected or if personality issues may be complicating patients' pain. Readers are referred to Tollison and Hinnatt (1996) for a critique of psychological tests used with chronic pain patients.

PAIN MEASURES

The Behavioral Assessment of Pain (Tearnan & Lewandowski, 1992) is highly recommended as a comprehensive assessment of pain that can be completed by patients at the end of the intake interview (or between the intake interview and the first therapy session) and at the end of therapy. It is a self-administered questionnaire that assesses different aspects of pain including demographic information (pain location, intensity, and description), pain behavior, activity interference, avoidance, spouse/partner influence, physician influence, physician qualities, pain beliefs, perceived consequences, coping, and mood. It is a 390-item questionnaire that takes approximately 1 hour to complete. A summary report of the information can be printed out for clinical purposes. Although the length of the questionnaire may be viewed as a drawback by some clinicians, patients are able and willing to complete this measure so that it can help therapists gain a comprehensive picture of their pain and its impact on their lives.

As mentioned in chapter 3, pain is assessed at the beginning of every session when the therapist asks the patient to verbally rate his or her pain on a 10-point scale and to describe the pain since the last session ("How has your pain been this past week?" "How would you rate your pain over the past week on a scale from 0 to 10, with 0 being *no pain at all* and 10 being *the worst possible pain?*").

Many pain clinics use the McGill Pain Questionnaire to assess patients' pain. We recommend the short form of this questionnaire if therapists want a brief self-report measure of patients' pain.

There are several other ways to assess pain including clinical interviews (such as the one mentioned in this chapter), visual analogue scales, numerical rating scales, adjective checklists, pain drawings, and pain diaries (Tollison & Hinnant, 1996). In chapter 5, readers will be introduced to the pain and activity monitoring forms.

MOOD INVENTORIES

The Beck Depression Inventory (BDI-II), Beck Anxiety Inventory (BAI), and Beck Hopelessness Scale (BHS) are self-report measures of depression, anxiety, and hopelessness states respectively. These instruments are typically completed by patients in the waiting room prior to the beginning of therapy sessions (every week or every other week). They can be completed on a weekly, biweekly, or monthly basis depending on the therapist's perceptions of the level of monitoring needed to assess progress or improvement in the patient's moods.

The BDI-II (Beck, Steer, & Brown, 1996) is a 21-item depression questionnaire. Patients are asked to circle the statement that best represents how they have been feeling over the past 2 weeks, including the day they filled it out. Each item includes several statements related to the intensity of a specific symptom, for example, sadness, pessimism, worthlessness, loss of energy, and suicidal thoughts, among others. The BDI and the BDI-II have been used extensively with chronic pain patients for clinical and research purposes. Higher scores on the BDI-II indicate higher levels of depression. Therapists who use the BDI-II will want to give particular attention to items 2 and 9. Item 2 indicates the patient's level of despair and hopelessness; item 9 indicates the patient's level of suicidal ideation and intention.

The BAI (Beck, Epstein, Brown, & Steer, 1988) is a 21-item anxiety questionnaire. Patients are given a list of 21 symptoms and are asked to rate the degree to which they have been bothered by those symptoms over the past week, including the day they filled it out, on a 4-point scale from not at all to severely. Examples of symptoms measured include "unable to relax," "fear of the worst happening," "numbness or tingling," and "faint." Item scores are computed (*not bothersome* = 0, *mildly bothersome* = 1, *moderately bothersome* = 2, and *severely bothersome* = 3) and summed up for a total score. Higher scores indicate higher levels of anxiety.

Therapists who use the BAI with chronic pain patients should remind them that it measures their level of anxiety and not their symptoms of pain. Therefore, when patients read a symptom item, they should ask themselves if they have been bothered by that symptom (e.g., numbness) when they felt anxious or nervous. Without this reminder, several items could potentially be misinterpreted by patients as symptoms of pain, such as "numbing" (symptom of nerve involvement/damage), "hands trembling" (patients could perceive this as a sign of muscle spasms in their hands), "indigestion or discomfort in abdomen," "wobbliness in legs" (patients could perceive this as a sign of muscle weakness), "feeling hot" (could be interpreted as burning pain sensations), and "shaky" (could be interpreted as feebleness or muscle contractions).

(For readers who are interested in assessing fear or anxiety about pain, the Pain Anxiety Symptom Scale, by McCracken, Zayfert, & Gross, 1992, is recommended.)

The BHS (Beck and Steer, 1988) is a 20-item hopelessness measure. Hopelessness, otherwise known as pessimism, can be an indicator of potential suicide risk. Patients read each of the 20 statements and rate them as true or false based on how they have been thinking over the past week, including the day they filled it out. Items that are endorsed in the hopeless direction (scoring key is provided with questionnaires) receive 1 point each. A BHS total score of 4 or more indicates significant levels of hopelessness (severity ranges are included in the manual).

These three instruments can be completed in approximately 10 minutes. Patients can complete them in the waiting room prior to the session. The instruments can be scored by the therapist just prior to the intake session as a quick check on a patient's mood. Significant mood scores can then be discussed sometime during the intake session. These Beck instruments should be completed by the patient prior to each (or at least every other) therapy session as a way to assess his or her current mood and to evaluate progress in therapy.

The State Trait Anger Expression Inventory-2 (STAXI-2; Spielberger, 1999) measures the experience and expression of anger in patients. Subscales include state anger, trait anger, anger expression in (suppression), anger expression out (aggression), anger control in (i.e., internal efforts to control anger, e.g., calming down or cooling off), anger control out (e.g., efforts to prevent the outward expression of anger), and anger expression index. The STAXI-2 (as well as earlier versions, e.g., the Anger Expression Inventory) has been used in research studies with chronic pain patients (e.g., Burns, Johnson, Mahoney, Devine, & Pawl, 1996). It can be administered at the beginning and end of therapy (including follow-up sessions) to assess a patient's progress in managing anger over time.

PERSONALITY QUESTIONNAIRES

The Minnesota Multiphasic Personality Inventory-II (MMPI-II; Butcher, Dahlstrom, Graham, Tellegen, & Kaemmer, 1989) is one of the most recognized personality inventories used with chronic pain patients. It is not uncommon for chronic pain patients to show elevations on scales 1

(*Hypochondriasis*) and 3 (*Hysteria*) of this instrument because many items are related to somatic complaints (Etscheidt, Steger, & Braverman, 1995). Scores may also be elevated on scale 2 (*Depression*) if patients are concerned about their pain symptoms. However, elevated scores on scale 2 may also reflect significant clinical depression. A lower scale 2 score with elevations of 1 and 3 may represent a patient who has significant pain but is not preoccupied or concerned about it (e.g., not significantly depressed; see Tollison & Hinnant, 1996). Scale 2 scores should be examined in relation to scales 1 and 3 when making interpretations. Chronic pain patients may be more at risk of having elevated scores on scale 6 (*Paranoia*) and scale 8 (*Schizophrenia*) given that these scales measure "sensory disturbances, confusion due to medications, or bizarre interpretations of their symptoms" (Tollison & Hinnant, 1996, p. 124). See Deardorff (2000) for more information on the use and interpretation of the MMPI-II with chronic pain patients.

Other personality questionnaires are available, including the Personality Assessment Inventory, the Millon Behavioral Health Inventory, the NEO-PI-R, the Millon Clinical Multiaxial Inventory-2 (for personality disorder assessment), the California Personality Inventory, and the 16PF. For more information on personality characteristics among chronic pain patients, see Gatchel and Weisberg (2000).

COGNITIVE MEASURES

The Behavioral Assessment of Pain (BaP; Tearnan & Lewandowski, 1992) has a *Pain Beliefs* scale, which is composed of 52 items. It measures negative beliefs about pain and its consequences. There are eight subscales of the Pain Belief scale including catastrophizing (e.g., "My pain problem is more than I can handle"), fear of reinjury (e.g., "When I do things that increase my pain, I am concerned that I might reinjure myself"), expectation for a cure (e.g., reverse score—"I have accepted that nothing further can be done to eliminate my pain"), blaming self (e.g., "I should be able to control the pain much better than I do"), entitlement (e.g., "I deserve better than to have chronic pain"), future despair (e.g., "I will never enjoy life again as long as I have pain"), social disbelief (e.g., "It bothers me that others might not believe my pain is real"), and lack of medical comprehensiveness (e.g., reverse score—"My doctors have left no stone unturned in their attempts to treat my pain"). The BaP also has a *Perceived Consequences* scale (24 items) that measures what patients anticipate will happen as a result of chronic pain. There are five subscales, including social interference (e.g., "When your pain increases sharply, how concerned are you that . . . your pain will negatively affect others?"), physical harm (e.g., ". . . you will cause a setback in your healing"), psychological harm (e.g., ". . . you will 'lose your mind'"), pain exacerbation (e.g., ". . . your pain will not settle down"), and productivity interference (e.g., ". . . the rest of the day will be shot"). These are the two scales of negative thoughts and beliefs that we commonly use with our patients.

Another highly recommended measure of pain beliefs is the Survey of Pain Attitudes (Jensen, Karoly, & Huger, 1987), which has 57 items and 7 subscales, including control (e.g., "There are times when I can influence the amount of pain I feel"), disability (e.g., "If my pain continues at its present level, I will be unable to work"), harm (e.g., "The pain I feel is a sign that damage is being done"), emotion (e.g., "Anxiety increases the pain I feel"), medication (e.g., "I will probably always have to take pain medication"), solicitude (seeking attention; e.g., "When I hurt, I want my family to treat me better"), and medical cure (e.g., "A doctor's job is to find pain treatments that work"). It has been used extensively in research with chronic pain patients and can be used for clinical purposes.

Both of these questionnaires can assess a patient's beliefs about pain and its consequences.

PAIN BEHAVIORS AND COPING

As mentioned earlier, a patient's pain behaviors can be assessed directly by the therapist in session. In addition, the patient and his or her significant friends and family members can identify the key pain behaviors that the patient uses.

The Behavioral Assessment of Pain measures certain aspects of behaviors, coping, and psychosocial stress, including pain behaviors, influences from partners/spouses and physicians, physician qualities, activity interference, activity avoidance, and coping (in addition to pain, beliefs, and mood, as mentioned earlier).

There are other measures of pain behaviors that clinicians may want to consider, including the Illness Behavior Inventory (Turkat & Pettegrew, 1983), as well as observations and rating measurements (see Keefe, Williams, & Smith, 2001).

Clinicians interested in assessing coping strategies may want to use the Coping Strategies Questionnaire (CSQ; Rosenstiel & Keefe, 1983). The CSQ measures different behavioral and cognitive coping strategies among chronic pain patients, including diverting attention, reinterpreting pain sensations, coping self-statements, ignoring pain sensations, praying or hoping, catastrophizing, increasing activity level, and increasing pain behavior. Principle components analyses of these coping subscales revealed a three-component structure: cognitive coping and suppression (i.e., reinterpreting, coping self-statements, and ignoring), helplessness (catastrophizing, increasing activity level, control over pain, and ability to decrease pain), and diverting attention and praying (i.e., diverting attention and praying or hoping; Rosenstiel, & Keefe, 1983). However, most professionals use the original subscales for scoring and interpretation of patients' coping strategies.

CONSULTATION WITH PROFESSIONALS AND REFERRALS

Chronic pain patients are often working with a variety of healthcare professionals, including primary care physicians, neurologists, orthopedists, chiropractors, nurses, physical therapists, occupational therapists, recreational therapists, vocational rehabilitation counselors, psychiatrists, and psychotherapists. It is important to obtain a comprehensive picture of a patient's health care from a variety of sources. The therapist needs to know how the patient is doing from a physical/medical standpoint, including a summary of findings regarding medical exams, laboratory diagnostic exams, imaging (e.g., MRI, CAT scan), other testing (e.g., neuropsychological assessments), medical diagnoses, recommended treatments (including medications prescribed), and response to treatments, as well as clinical impressions from health care professionals. Some patients have clear-cut medical diagnoses associated with their pain, whereas others do not. Therefore, the etiology of pain is not always clear. The patient can sign a release of information forms at the end of the intake interview to give the therapist permission to communicate with other health care professionals regarding his or her medical and psychotherapy care.

Sometimes, it may be necessary to refer a patient to other professionals for services (e.g., neuropsychological testing medical evaluations). For example, if the patient has not seen a physician yet for the chronic pain, at the very least they should be referred to a primary care physician for a checkup and an evaluation of the pain. The physician can then refer the patient to a pain specialist.

When health care providers refer a chronic pain patient for psychotherapy services, they often appreciate knowing that the patient did follow through with the referral and want to know the therapist's perception of the psychosocial stressors that are affecting the patient as well as the *DSM-IV* diagnoses of the patient's presenting problems. To facilitate a holistic approach to chronic pain treatment, the therapist should communicate the patient's status to the physician who referred his or her patient for therapy, along with the patient's diagnoses and prognosis for therapy (assuming the patient has provided written permission to do so). Many physicians simply want a brief summary of how their patients are doing in therapy. This can be done verbally or in report form.

SOCIALIZING PATIENT INTO COGNITIVE THERAPY

Near the end of the intake interview, the therapist explain the course of cognitive therapy treatment and clarify the patient's expectations of what will happen in therapy. Although the nature and severity of the presenting problems may vary, most chronic pain patients can learn new ways of coping better with their problems in four or five sessions, but most benefit from a minimum of 12 therapy sessions (preferably on a weekly basis). Some chronic pain patients will try to make the argument that they have so many healthcare appointments and would prefer to meet only on a biweekly or monthly basis. Although this is up to the discretion of the therapist, it is recommend that patients attend therapy weekly or every other week. Otherwise, this may negatively affect therapy outcomes. (This recommendation is working from the assumption that chronic pain patients are seen on a weekly or biweekly basis in private practice, community mental health centers, and pain clinics. Therapists in some pain clinics may see patients several times a week over a 4- to 6-week period as part of a short-term pain management program.)

Some patients with chronic pain assume that cognitive therapy will help them become "pain-free." Although this is an ideal, most patients will learn how to cope with their pain and other stressful experiences in their lives and may experience some pain reduction. Some patients may be specifically interested in the behavioral management of pain, for example, biofeedback or relaxation training, because that is what their health care professionals recommended. Therapists can educate patients that pain management is not only about learning how to relax their bodies but also how to cope with their thoughts and emotions about their pain and its impact on their lives.

PART II

BEHAVIORAL
INTERVENTIONS

5

Monitoring Pain and Activity Levels and Activity Scheduling

During the early stages of therapy, patients learn specific behavioral strategies to cope with their pain as a lead-in to other cognitive therapy interventions (e.g., cognitive restructuring and problem solving). Behavioral approaches to pain management refer to skills such as pain monitoring (e.g., identifying and tracking pain and its intensity over time and across situations), activity scheduling and monitoring (e.g., tracking activity levels, adding more enjoyable activities to daily life, and modifying activities based on pain levels), relaxation training (e.g., deep breathing, guided imagery, and progressive muscle relaxation), and distraction techniques (e.g., focusing on other stimuli to "tune out" experiences of pain). Pain monitoring and activity scheduling and monitoring will be discussed in this chapter. Relaxation training and distraction techniques will be covered in chapter 6.

MONITORING PAIN

During the first therapy session, the patient learns how to track pain, so that he or she becomes more aware of how often the pain occurs, what his or her experience of pain is like (e.g., intensity), and factors that may affect it both positively and negatively. Pain monitoring promotes awareness of the multidimensional aspects of pain, including pain sensations and intensity, triggers, emotions, thoughts, and behaviors. It also helps the patient observe changes or improvements in pain levels over time. The Pain Monitoring Form is introduced during the first therapy session and is one of the first self-help homework assignments in cognitive therapy.

PAIN MONITORING FORM

The Pain Monitoring Form (see Figure 5.1) helps the patient to

- Identify when the pain occurred and its location
- Rate pain intensity, on a scale from 0 to 10, with 0 being *no pain* and 10 being *the worst pain possible (severe, excruciating)*
- Identify any triggers to the pain (situations, activities, foods/beverages, etc.), as well as factors that may exacerbate the pain (after it starts)
- Identify coping strategies used, particularly pain medications and dosage levels, as well as the level of exertion used to complete a task or activity
- Identify any emotions and thoughts related to pain (this process will be explored in further detail in chapter 7)

The patient should be encouraged to monitor the pain at least three times a day (i.e., morning, afternoon, and evening) over the next week to get a "baseline" of his or her pain experiences. In the first five columns, the patient enters the date, the time of day, the location(s) of the pain sensations, descriptions of the pain, and pain intensity.

In the sixth column, the patient identifies triggers to the pain—in other words, possible factors that may activate the pain. The patient also can write down any events or factors that make the pain worse (pain exacerbators). Pain may emerge seemingly out of nowhere. However, certain events or factors can activate or exacerbate pain including biological factors (e.g., muscle tension, nerve impingement, and soft tissue damage), physical factors (diet and activity level), psychological aspects (e.g., thoughts, feelings, and actions), and social situations (e.g., other people's reactions to the pain and level of support).

In the seventh column, the patient writes down his or her efforts to cope with pain, including the effectiveness of these strategies. Some patients already have some healthy means of coping, for example, taking medications as prescribed by their physician or participating in activities such as self-help groups, yoga, meditation, or some form of physical exercise adapted to suit their physical condition. However, some patients' coping efforts can have a negative impact and may serve as triggers for further pain, for example, inactivity (resulting in muscle deconditioning), overexertion when exercising or completing tasks, and isolation from others.

The last column of the Pain Monitoring Form provides an opportunity for the patient to identify any significant emotions and thoughts he or she had while in pain. This is one of the first steps in helping a patient connect physical sensations of pain with emotions, thoughts, and behaviors

FIGURE 5.1 Pain Monitoring Form

Date	Time of Day	Location of Pain	Describe the Pain	How intense was the pain? (0–100)	Triggers to Pain	Coping Efforts	Thoughts/ Emotions
	M = morning A = afternoon E = evening	Where did you experience the pain in your body?	What words would you use to describe the pain (throbbing, burning, aching, tender, etc.)?	0 = *no pain* 100 = *excruciating pain*	What brought on the pain? (situations, activities, foods, environment, stress, etc.) What made it worse? What made it better?	What did you do to cope with your pain? How effective was it? 0 = *not at all* 10 = *very effective*	What were your emotions at that time? What were you thinking about when the pain kicked in?

Note: Developed by Carrie Winterowd, PhD. Printed with permission of Carrie Winterowd, PhD.

(coping efforts). As a general rule, the therapist should not attempt to evaluate or modify the patient's thoughts at this point in the therapy process. This is simply an opportunity to help the patient establish the relationships among these pain phenomena.

During the second session, the patient can continue to track pain with this form, or the patient can combine pain and activity monitoring using the Weekly Activity Chart.

WEEKLY ACTIVITY CHART

Patients can monitor their pain levels and activity levels at the same time using the Weekly Activity Chart (see Figure 5.2). Pain can be monitored (intensity ratings only) on an hourly basis or three times a day (morning, afternoon, and evening). If this is too tedious, pain ratings can be "sprinkled" throughout the chart to represent examples of severe, moderate, and low levels of pain while participating in activities during the week.

Pain intensity ratings are designated by the letter *P* and are followed by a number on a scale from 0 to 10, with 0 representing *no pain*, and 10 representing *severe, excruciating pain*. So, for a particular patient, mopping the floors might be a P9 activity, whereas watching television might be a P6 activity, on a given day.

In the next section, we describe how to combine pain and activity monitoring using this chart.

ACTIVITY MONITORING AND SCHEDULING

ACTIVITY MONITORING

Patients' participation and involvement in daily activities can have a direct bearing on their pain and their moods. Oftentimes, patients are not as active as they were before their pain condition started. In addition, they may not enjoy these activities as much. The goal of activity monitoring is to assess a patient's daily activities on an hourly basis over the course of a week to see how active the patient is and to assess his or her level of mastery and pleasure when participating in activities. As mentioned earlier, pain ratings can be incorporated in this monitoring process.

Activity monitoring teaches patients to be aware of what they are doing, in terms of activity levels and their choice of activities. It also prepares them for scheduling more meaningful and realistic activities in their lives to increase their sense of mastery and pleasure and to reduce their pain levels. For therapists, knowing what patients do during a typical week can help them identify potential activity problems related to pain interference and psychological distress. For example, patients often want to maintain the same activity level they had before they developed chronic pain, which may not be realistic for some patients given their condition. If these patients push their bodies to do too much, they may put themselves at risk for further injury and pain. Being overly active can reinforce psychological problems such as denial (of their chronic pain condition), perfectionism, and an exaggerated need for independence (asking for help means being dependent). Alternatively, some patients become significantly less active because of their pain. Inactivity may worsen patients' physical condition (e.g., muscle deconditioning), leading to more pain. Inactivity can also reinforce psychosocial problems such as social isolation, apathy, and depression.

Activity monitoring is usually introduced during the second session. The patient is asked to try to write down the main activities he or she participated in each hour of the day for an entire week using the Weekly Activity Chart (see Figure 5.2). Most individuals find the evening best for reviewing the events of the day.

Next, the patient rates these activities in terms of pleasure and mastery. *Pleasure* refers to the extent to which the patient experienced a sense of enjoyment while participating in an activity. *Mastery* refers to the extent to which the patient experienced a sense of accomplishment while participating in an activity. The primary purposes of these ratings are to find out which activities, if any, are enjoyable and pleasurable, and which ones lead to feelings of mastery to assess the patient's ability to enjoy activities and to feel a sense of accomplishment, and to prepare for scheduling more enjoyable and mastery-oriented activities into the patient's daily life. Low ratings of pleasure and mastery may be indicators of moderate to severe psychological distress or pain interference.

The patient's perceptions of pleasure and mastery are rated on a 10-point scale, with 0 being *no enjoyment or sense of accomplishment* and 10 being *complete enjoyment or a total sense of accomplishment.* For abbreviation purposes, *E* represents enjoyment or pleasure, along with the rating number (0–10); M represents mastery or accomplishment, along with the rating number (0–10). It is possible for an activity to receive different mastery and pleasure ratings. For example, it may have taken a patient a couple of hours, off and on, to make the beds in the house given his pain levels (P8), and thus the task was not pleasurable (E1). However, the patient may have felt a sense of accomplishment in completing the task of making each bed (M8). In this case, the ratings of E1, M8, and P8 could be written next to the task, "making beds" on the Weekly Activity Chart.

FIGURE 5.2 Weekly Activity Chart

Time	Sunday	Monday	Tuesday	Wednesday	Thursday	Friday	Saturday
5 a.m.							
6 a.m.							
7 a.m.							
8 a.m.							
9 a.m.							
10 a.m.							
11 a.m.							
noon							
1 p.m.							
2 p.m.							
3 p.m.							
4 p.m.							
5 p.m.							

6 p.m.									
7 p.m.									
8 p.m.									
9 p.m.									
10 p.m.									
11 p.m.									
midnight									
1 a.m.									
2 a.m.									
3 a.m.									
4 a.m.									

Ratings: M = mastery, E = enjoyment/pleasure, P = pain, on a scale from 0 to 10. Provide morning, afternoon, and evening pain ratings.

Activity monitoring and ratings are combined as one homework assignment. (In traditional cognitive therapy, patients monitor activities for 1 week, then add their mastery and pleasure ratings to the chart during the following week.) The therapist can decide whether the patient should add pain ratings to this chart or have the patient continue to use the Pain Monitoring Chart mentioned earlier as a separate homework assignment.

> Maria, a 60-year-old Hispanic woman, has daily migraine and tension headaches and intermittent low back pain. She has been very anxious and depressed about her pain and its impact on her life. During the first therapy session, Maria acknowledged that she was spending most of her days lying in bed or sitting in front of the television to cope with her pain. To get a clearer picture of her daily activities in relation to her pain, Maria was asked to complete a Weekly Activity Chart for the next week (see Figure 5.3).
>
> As can be seen from her chart, Maria spent some of her mornings sleeping or lying in bed and most of her afternoons in front of the television. She did make time to clean her house, but she would do it all at once (2 hours straight). This activity triggered headaches and exacerbated her low back pain. Maria spent most of her time at home; and very little time was spent interacting with other people. Completing this chart and reviewing it in session helped Maria realize how isolated she had become. Her primary activities were sedentary in nature or involved cleaning or running errands, with no time allocated for pleasurable or fun activities. In addition, Maria did not participate in an exercise program despite her physical therapist's recommendation. Maria and her cognitive therapist discussed ways in which she could (1) diversify her activity experiences, adding new, meaningful as well as fun activities; (2) pace her household work; (3) incorporate a daily exercise plan; and (4) combat her pain, depression, and anxiety by getting out of bed (and staying out of bed) earlier in the day.

When pain and activity monitoring are combined, patients can observe the reciprocal relationship between their activities (e.g., activity levels, pace, and type) and their pain. Some activities may trigger or exacerbate pain levels, whereas other activities may alleviate pain or temporarily distract patients. Pain can prevent patients from participating in certain activities. In fact, some patients choose certain activities so they do not aggravate their pain. Some activities may not be affected by pain at all.

The therapist and patient can review how pain levels and activity involvement varied over the course of a week and make note of interesting relationships. The therapist could start this discussion by asking the patient

FIGURE 5.3 Weekly Activity Chart

Time	Sunday	Monday	Tuesday	Wednesday	Thursday	Friday	Saturday
5 a.m.	Sleep	Sleep	Sleep	Sleep	Sleep	Sleep	Sleep
6 a.m.	Sleep	Sleep	Sleep	Sleep	Sleep	Sleep	Sleep
7 a.m.	Sleep	Sleep	Sleep	Sleep	Sleep	Sleep	Sleep
8 a.m.	Sleep	Sleep	Sleep	Sleep	Sleep	Sleep	Sleep
9 a.m.	Got up and ate breakfast, showered	Got up and ate breakfast	Got up and ate breakfast	Got up and ate breakfast	Got up and ate breakfast	Got up and ate breakfast	Got up and ate breakfast
10 a.m.	Went back to bed, in pain. E0 M0 P8	Lay on sofa P7–8 Watched TV E3 M0	Went out to check the garden M5 P6	Went back to bed, in pain E0 M0 P9	Paid bills M6 P7	Took pet to vet M8	In pain, went back to bed E0 M0 P9
11 a.m.	Lying in bed	TV	Early lunch	Lying in bed	Went to post office and ran errands M5	Lay down in bed, in pain E0 M0 P8	Lay in bed
noon	Made lunch	TV	Ran a few errands (grocery store) M6	Made lunch	Made lunch	Sleep	Made lunch
1 p.m.	Watched TV all afternoon	Cleaning the house (mop) M10	Watched TV all afternoon	Cleaned the bathrooms M7	Watched TV	Ate a late lunch	Cleaned the house all at once M10

FIGURE 5.3 (*continued*)

2 p.m.	TV E5 M3 P5	Washing clothes, dishes, dusting M9	TV E4 P5–6	Lay down to rest, in pain E0 P10	TV	Watched soap operas	Cleaning M10 P10
3 p.m.	TV	Vacuuming M9 carpets P9	TV	Watched TV	TV E4	TV	Tired, took a nap
4 p.m.	TV	Lay down to rest, had a headache E0	TV	Watched TV E4	TV, fell asleep	TV E3 P5	TV E5
5 p.m.	Prepare dinner for friend's visit M5	Sleep	Made dinner M4	Didn't fee like cooking	Slept	Made dinner	TV
6 p.m.	Same	Made dinner	Ate dinner	Ordered dinner to go and ate M0	Made dinner	Went to a movie with husband E10 P5	Went to dinner party with husband
7 p.m.	A friend came over for dinner E10	Read a book	We went to a bridge game E0	Read a book	Played cards with husband E7 P5	Movie	Dancing— too much pain E3 P8
8 p.m.	Same P6	Read a book E5 P5	Bridge game, was bored E0 P7	Read a book E3	Read a book	Movie	Sat there listening to boring talk E0

9 p.m.	Friend left, watched TV E5	Had an argument with husband P9	Bridge game, was bored E0	Went to bed early, in pain P8	Watched TV	Wrote in journal E5 M9	Went home, wrote in journal M6
10 p.m.	Went to bed	Headache; tried to go to sleep	Went to bed	Sleep	Called a friend E10 P4	Went to bed	Went to bed
11 p.m.	Sleep	Sleep	Sleep	Sleep	Sleep	Sleep	Sleep
midnight	Sleep	Sleep	Sleep	Sleep	Sleep	Sleep	Sleep
1 a.m.	Sleep	Sleep	Sleep	Sleep	Sleep	Sleep	Sleep
2 a.m.	Sleep	Sleep	Sleep	Sleep	Sleep	Sleep	Sleep
3 a.m.	Sleep	Sleep	Sleep	Sleep	Sleep	Sleep	Sleep
4 a.m.	Sleep	Sleep	Sleep	Sleep	Sleep	Sleep	Sleep

Ratings: M = mastery, E = enjoyment/pleasure, P = pain, on a scale from 0 to 10.

From Judith S. Beck's *Cognitive Therapy: Basics and Beyond.* Copyright 1995 by Judith S. Beck, PhD. Adapted with permission from the Guilford Press.

such questions as "What did you notice as you kept track of your activities and your pain levels this past week?" "Did you see any patterns in your pain levels over the course of the day or the week? and "Did you see any patterns in your pain levels when you participated in certain activities?" In Maria's case, her pain was more severe in the mornings after waking up and late at night, when she was doing a lot of household chores, when she was bored, and when she was arguing with her husband. Her chart summary revealed that she tends to cope with her pain by resting or going to sleep, especially when she has headaches. Maria's pain lessened when she got together with friends, read a book, or watched TV. These activities appeared to distract Maria from her pain.

Activity levels and pacing can also affect patients' pain levels. Although patients chart their activities, it is sometimes unclear how they paced themselves when they were involved in specific activities. The therapist can follow up with questions to explore activity pacing such as "Were you working on that task continuously or were you taking breaks in between?" and "How long did it take to complete that task?"

On Maria's chart, it was clear that she would do her household chores all at once, rather than breaking them down into smaller tasks. She also admitted that she did not take breaks between chores. Although she felt a great deal of mastery in completing these chores, it also resulted in a lot of pain.

As another example of pacing problems, Maria went dancing with her husband one night last week (Saturday). She stayed on the dance floor with her husband for 30 minutes straight, which was 15 minutes too long for Maria, given her low back pain (according to the patient). But she didn't want people to think she was disabled and she didn't want pity, so she pushed herself to continue dancing despite the pain. In the short run, she saved face. In the long run, she was in pain for the rest of the night.

ACTIVITY PACING AND SCHEDULING

Once activity levels and pain levels have been monitored and reviewed (typically during the second therapy session), activities can be scheduled to help the patient cope better with his or her pain and moods. For some patients, this means scheduling more activities. For others, it means scheduling fewer activities and pacing their activities.

Using metaphors and analogies can help patients better understand the importance of activity pacing. For example:

Therapist: I would like for you to think about pacing your life activities
    just as long-distance runners pace themselves in a race. If you run

at sprint speed from the beginning of the race, you won't be able to make it across the finish line because you can't keep up that fast pace for long. A long-distance runner plans out a specific strategy for each part of the race and sets a more realistic pace to complete the race. The same is true in your situation, as well as for others who have chronic pain. You want to successfully cross the finish line in a number of activities. However, your eagerness to do so at your previous pace may result in more frustration, more pain, and more suffering in the long run, which may not allow you to experience the same success. We will need to explore different ways to complete tasks as well as different ways of enjoying your life.

In the past, patients probably did not have to give much thought to their choice of activities or how long they would participate in them. However, given their chronic, unrelieved pain, some patients may need to break certain activities into smaller steps. They should also be careful not to "overbook" their schedules with too many activities.

For those patients who continue to push themselves despite the pain and their doctors' recommendations, the potential advantages and disadvantages of continuing their previous pace versus adapting their pace could be explored. This will help therapists understand the underlying motivation for patients to maintain such a fast pace in their daily lives. Engaging their willingness to experiment with a different activity schedule and pace followed by an assessment of their productivity, enjoyment, and pain levels might be quite enlightening for some patients. In many cases, prioritizing activities and tasks, scheduling in slightly fewer activities, and finding ways to accomplish those tasks in healthy ways may help patients become even more productive than before. Given the fast-paced lives many people lead, getting permission to slow down a little or streamline a schedule (prioritizing activities and scheduling slightly fewer activities) seems inconsistent with mainstream culture in many industrialized societies. However, adjustments to schedules can lead to a number of positive outcomes.

In Maria's case, her tendencies to complete her housework "in one fell swoop" and dance for long periods were targeted activities for pacing. Maria's therapist recommended that she break her household chores into smaller steps. The first step was to create a hierarchy of household chores, from the least painful to the most painful. From this hierarchy, Maria could identify those chores that could be completed with little or no pain. Then, to handle the more difficult chores, Maria was asked to break these chores into smaller steps. For example, "doing laundry" was a chore that was ranked as a "high pain" activity, given her chronic low back pain. Maria was asked to describe step-by-step how she performed this activity. Maria stated that she tended to pick clothes off the floor (bending at the waist instead of bending her knees) and throw them into a large hamper. She dumped out the hamper into the laundry basket, then carried the basket to the washer. When she transferred the clothes from the washer to the dryer, she typically picked up large armfuls of clothes at a time. When the clothes were dry, she bent over (at the waist, not bending her knees to lower herself) to take out the laundry. Next, Maria and her therapist discussed ways she could break this household chore into smaller steps. Here was the new plan for doing laundry:

1. Put dirty clothes into a laundry basket (placing basket on a chair).
2. Don't let the clothes fill the basket.
3. When the basket is half-full, pick it up (bending with knees and not bending at the waist) and carry it to the washer.
4. Set the basket on top of the dryer, and slowly put the clothes (a few pieces at a time) in the washer.
5. When the wash is done, run the spin cycle one more time to draw out any excess water on the clothes. Then remove one to two pieces of wet clothing at a time and put them in the dryer.
6. When the laundry is dry, remove a few pieces at a time, focusing on good posture.
7. Don't carry more than one load of laundry at a time.
8. At any step along the way, take a break if you are in pain.

Maria was encouraged to take breaks between steps when needed as well as between chores. Although Maria did prefer to finish the chores all at once, she acknowledged that having a chore left unfinished temporarily was less stressful than being in more pain for having pushed it too much.

In terms of her dancing, Maria and her husband participated in a weekly dance class. Maria was encouraged to talk with her dance teacher about her pain and how the dance moves might affect her pain. In addition, she was encouraged to practice dancing for shorter blocks (e.g., 10 minutes instead of 30 minutes) with breaks in between. This was identified as an experiment to see if scheduling her dancing in this way might ease her pain and how others may respond. If someone pointed out her breaks, Maria developed a response: "I just need to take a break" or "I have low back pain, so I need to pace myself."

Maria and her therapist also explored other ways to cope with her morning migraine pain besides going back to bed. For example, she would implement one of the relaxation techniques she was learning in therapy as her first course of action to manage her pain. If Maria still needed to lie down and rest to help the migraine pain subside, she agreed to limit her rest time (e.g., 30 minutes).

Maria also agreed to add more social activities to her schedule. Her physician and physical therapist had recommended low-impact exercises to strengthen her back and to reduce her stress levels. She decided to explore some possible fitness centers to join over the next week. In this case, Maria and her therapist were trying to schedule activities that would combat her isolation and stress and encourage physical fitness. Joining a fitness center would promote a sense of accomplishment, enjoyment, and possibly reduce pain in the long run.

As a general rule, therapists should consult with their patients' physicians, physical therapists, and recreational therapists to establish activity schedules that are realistic and conducive to pain management and health promotion. In fact, patients can bring their activity and pain monitoring forms to their other healthcare appointments to get their independent feedback on activity scheduling and pace.

When Maria returned for her third session, she reported that activity pacing and activity scheduling did make a difference in her pain and her moods. Breaking difficult tasks into smaller steps helped Maria manage her pain more effectively than before. She also "sprinkled" chores throughout the week instead of doing them all at once, which seemed to make a difference. When Maria consulted her dance teacher and set boundaries regarding her dancing (taking breaks when needed; asserting herself with others), she was able to enjoy the experience and felt less pain than before. She also felt a sense of accomplishment for facing her fears of rejection. No one made a big deal about her occasional breaks from dancing. Maria practiced her relaxation exercises in the morning, which helped her cope better with her headaches and low back pain. She did lie down on occasion when her migraines were really bothering her, but limited her resting to 30 minutes.

In summary, pain monitoring and activity monitoring help therapists and patients understand how patients' pain levels and activities vary over the course of a week. Monitoring activities can assist in establishing more realistic schedules to promote mastery and enjoyment while reducing or managing pain. Part of activity scheduling involves integrating new activities related to pain management, for example, relaxation and distraction exercises. These other behavioral interventions will be discussed in the next chapter.

6

Relaxation Training and Distraction Techniques

Relaxation training and distraction techniques are common behavioral interventions for pain management. Relaxation training helps patients cope with their pain by reducing muscle tension and stress. Distraction techniques help patients shift their focus of attention away from their pain and other bodily sensations, which is usually a temporary solution to pain management.

RELAXATION TRAINING

There are a number of relaxation techniques that patients can learn, including deep abdominal breathing, progressive muscle relaxation, autogenic relaxation, and guided imagery. Although biofeedback can also be used, this strategy will not be discussed in this book, as strategies that people can use everyday are emphasized. The following is a script that therapists can use to introduce relaxation techniques.

Therapist: During part of our session today, you will learn some relaxation exercises to help you manage your pain (and stress). The specific exercises include deep abdominal breathing, progressive muscle relaxation, and some guided imagery. You will learn how to breathe using your diaphragm and abdominal muscles. Breathing correctly is an important first step in relaxing your mind and body. Progressive muscle relaxation is an exercise that involves tensing and relaxing different muscle groups in your body. I will demonstrate how to do each exercise with you. We will tense muscle groups just to the point of tension, not pain, then release these muscles, focusing on the relaxation there. Guided imagery involves picturing relaxing images. Next week, we will focus on guided muscle relaxation and guided imagery. I want you to learn a variety of relaxation skills, so you can pick and choose which ones help you the best in managing your pain and your moods. These exercises will reduce muscle tension and stress in your body and may provide some pain relief for you. After we try out these exercises, I encourage you to practice them on a daily basis. Relaxation is a skill just like any other, which means that it takes time and practice to learn it. Most patients find that they are able to achieve a more relaxed state over time as they practice these exercises in the privacy of their homes. If you use relaxation regularly, you may notice positive changes in your stress, tension, and pain levels, as well as positive changes in how you think, feel, and act.

Not every patient benefits from one type of relaxation. Therefore, it is important to teach patients a variety of relaxation strategies so that they can find the ones that work and fit best with their personalities and coping styles. Deep abdominal breathing is the first relaxation technique taught to patients because it is a skill that can be used at any time; it is also a building block for the other relaxation exercises. Because each person is unique, some patients will respond better to guided muscle relaxation imagery, whereas others will respond better to progressive muscle relaxation. All three of these techniques will be described below.

Probably the most concrete technique is progressive muscle relaxation, which involves tensing and relaxing different muscle groups in the body. In contrast, guided muscle relaxation, an abstract method, incorporates autogenic relaxation and guided imagery. Autogenic relaxation refers to words or phrases patients can repeat to themselves to help them relax, for example, "I am beginning to feel very relaxed," "My muscles are feeling relaxed," "I am at peace with myself," and so on. Guided imagery refers to specific images that help patients achieve a state of relaxation. Therapist-guided images are images that therapists ask patients to picture. Patient-guided images are images that patients create themselves. For guided muscle relaxation, patients are asked to focus on one part of their bodies at a time and imagine relaxation moving into those muscle groups.

In general, it is recommended that patients bring in audiotapes to use for recording purposes during the relaxation training sessions. Therapists should provide a high-quality tape recording device for use in the sessions. The deep breathing, guided muscle relaxation, progressive muscle relaxation, and guided imagery exercises can all be recorded on audiotapes to be used by patients between sessions to practice these relaxation techniques. As a homework assignment, patients should practice their relaxation skill daily between sessions before learning a new relaxation skill. Relaxation techniques are usually covered in the first two therapy sessions. In the first relaxation training session, deep breathing, progressive muscle relaxation, and patient-guided imagery exercises (e.g., special place image) are covered. In the second session, guided muscle relaxation and therapist-guided imagery (e.g., nature scenes) exercises are covered. (Note: If patients like imagery, they may prefer to learn guided muscle relaxation first).

RELAXATION TECHNIQUES

DEEP BREATHING

Deep breathing refers to slow, deep breathing using the abdominal and diaphragm muscles. Most people, whether they are aware of it or not, tend to use their chest or shoulder muscles when breathing. To learn abdominal breathing, patients are asked to put one hand on their stomach while they are breathing. With each inhale, they should notice their stomach pushing out toward their hand (the diaphragm moves downward, pushing the abdominal muscles out). With each exhale, they should notice their stomach moving inward toward their body (the diaphragm moves upward, allowing the abdominal muscles to move back toward the body). Patients are asked to focus on their breathing for a minute or two, making sure that they do not use their chest or shoulders, but rather their diaphragm and stomach muscles to breath. Patients are asked to breathe in and out deeply, gradually slowing down their breathing. Therapists may tell patients to say, "Relax" with each inhale, and to imagine pain and tension leaving their bodies with each exhale.

The following is a suggested script:

Therapist: The first relaxation skill is deep breathing. Let's take a moment now to focus on your breathing. [pause] When you inhale, what part of your body expands? Your shoulders? Your chest? Your stomach? [Get the patient's response.] Most people tend to notice that they breathe using their chest muscles. However, the most relaxing type of breathing involves the use of your stomach or abdominal muscles. In fact, when people learn how to sing or play a musical instrument, they are asked to use their stomach muscles and diaphragm to breathe, not their chest muscles. Deep breathing is basically abdominal breathing. Do you have any questions so far?

To learn abdominal breathing, place one hand on your stomach muscles and begin taking a slow breath in and out [pause] and in and out. If you are breathing with your abdominal muscles, you should notice your stomach pushing toward your hand when you inhale. When you exhale, your stomach muscles are moving in toward your body. Take a few moments to focus on breathing using your stomach muscles. As you breathe in, notice your stomach pushing out; as you breathe out, notice your stomach moving back into your body. [Pause for 15–20 seconds.] Your stomach is pushing out toward your hand when you inhale because your diaphragm, a muscle underneath your rib cage, is pushing down on your abdominal muscles when you breathe in oxygen. When you exhale, your abdominal muscles move back into the abdominal cavity because your diaphragm muscle lifts up toward your rib cage as you breathe out carbon dioxide. Do you have any questions so far?

The next step in deep abdominal breathing is to develop a slow rhythm to your breathing. Find a pace that is comfortable for you. Most people try to slow down their breathing by breathing in three or four counts and breathing out three or four counts. Why don't we try this? So, breathe in 1, 2, 3, and breathe out 1, 2, 3. Breathe in three counts and out three counts. Just slow down your breathing.

To help you relax a bit more, you can add some words to your breathing to remind you to relax. As you inhale, say to yourself: r-e-l-a-x. As you exhale, imagine pain and tension leaving your body . . . just slipping away from your body.

Most patients are very responsive to the deep abdominal breathing and can learn it with ease. For those patients who have respiratory problems, it is recommended that they breathe in and out through their mouths and not through their noses. Teaching patients to place one hand on their abdominal muscles in the early stages of relaxation training helps them to stay in tune with how their abdominal muscles push outward with each inhale and pull inward with each exhale. It also helps them stay focused on breathing with their abdominal muscles and not with their chest or their shoulders. If needed, patients who still breathe primarily from their shoulders or chest could be instructed to watch themselves in the mirror as they practice their deep abdominal breathing to ensure that neither their shoulders are lifting nor their chest is expanding with each inhale.

PROGRESSIVE MUSCLE RELAXATION

Progressive muscle relaxation (Jacobson, 1938) involves tensing and relaxing different muscle groups. Patients learn progressive muscle relaxation while sitting, starting with the deep breathing exercise just described as the first step. Before moving to the script, several recommendations are offered. After asking patients to release each muscle group, say the following phrases: "Notice the difference between tensing and relaxing your _____," or "Focus on the relaxation in your _____." Occasionally repeat autogenic relaxation messages throughout the exercise, such as "You are feeling more and more relaxed with each moment," or "Enjoy the deep relaxation in your body," or "How good it feels to be this relaxed and calm." Patients typically will experience more success with this exercise if the therapist demonstrates the tensing and relaxing positions for each muscle group.

Progressive muscle relaxation should be adapted to the individual needs of each patient. For example, some patients may not be able to tense certain muscle groups because of severe pain in a particular location. The goal of progressive muscle relaxation is to tense muscles and then release them (focusing on the contrast of tightening and relaxing each muscle group), not to induce pain or to increase pain levels. Patients can decide which tension exercises they want to try. Most patients find that they can do the majority of them or all of them. They can experience a strong relaxation response by working around severe pain locations and focusing on tensing and relaxing the other muscle groups.

In general, it is recommended that patients keep their eyes open during this relaxation exercise so that they can learn the positions for tensing and relaxing each muscle group. Although closing one's eyes can deepen the relaxation response, it is not necessary in order to achieve a relaxation response.

Here is a script that therapists can use to teach progressive muscle relaxation.

Therapist: During the next part of our relaxation exercise, we will be tensing and relaxing different muscle groups in our bodies. This is an exercise called progressive muscle relaxation. When I ask you to tense each muscle group, be sure to tense it only to the point of feeling tension, not pain. We will be holding each muscle group by tensing it for 4 or 5 seconds and then releasing it, focusing on the relaxation. If there is a muscle group that you do not believe that you can tense because of severe pain, then tense the previous muscle group again. You know your body better than anyone else, and you know what your limits are.

  Let us begin our relaxation exercise by focusing on the toes. (If you have pain in this part of your body, you may want to skip this exercise. However, I will demonstrate it for you.)

  Toes/feet: Curl your toes underneath your feet and hold 2, 3, 4, 5 and release. Focus on the relaxation in your toes. [pause] Again, curl your toes under your feet and hold 2, 3, 4, 5 and release, noticing the difference between tensing and relaxing the muscles in your toes. [pause]

Now we are going to focus on the lower legs, starting with the shin muscles. [Point to them.] (If you have pain in this part of your body, you may want to skip this exercise. However, I will demonstrate it for you. While I am showing you this exercise, you can practice the feet exercises we just completed.)

Shins: Keeping your heels on the floor, lift your toes and feet up, pointing (flexing) your toes toward the ceiling and hold 2, 3, 4, 5 and release. Focus on the relaxation. [pause] Again, keeping your heels on the floor, lift your toes and feet up, pointing (flexing) your toes toward the ceiling, and hold 2, 3, 4, 5 and release, noticing the difference between tensing and relaxing the muscles in your shins. [pause]

Now we are going to focus on the calves. [Point to them.]

Calves: In a moment, I am going to ask you to lift your heels off the floor while keeping the balls of your feet on the ground. Ready, lift your heels off the floor, and hold 2, 3, 4, 5, and release. Focus on the relaxation in your calves. [pause] Again, lift your heels up while keeping the balls of your feet on the ground, and hold 2, 3, 4, 5, and release, noticing the difference between tensing and relaxing the muscles in your calves. [pause]

Now we are going to focus on the upper legs and buttocks.

Thighs and buttocks: Bring your legs and feet together, press your knees and upper legs together while squeezing your buttocks and hold 2, 3, 4, 5 and release. Focus on the relaxation in your upper legs and buttocks. [pause] Continue to breathe deeply in and out. Breathe in relaxation. Breathe out pain and tension. You feel more and more relaxed with each moment during this exercise. [pause] Again, bring your legs and feet together, press your knees and upper legs together, creating some tension there, squeezing your buttocks and hold 2, 3, 4, 5 and release, noticing the difference between tensing and relaxing your upper legs and buttocks. [pause]

Now we are going to focus on the muscles in your stomach.

Stomach: In a moment, you will take a deep breath and hold your stomach in, like you are trying to squeeze into a tight pair of pants. Ready? Take a deep breath, hold your breath and hold your stomach in 2, 3, 4, 5, and release. Focus on the relaxation in your stomach. [pause] Again, you are going to take a deep breath and hold it while holding in your stomach muscles, and hold 2, 3, 4, 5, and release. Notice the difference between tensing and relaxing the muscles in your stomach. [pause]

Now we are going to focus on the lower back.

Back: In a moment, I am going to ask you to lift your back and shoulders slightly off the back of your chair, arch your back slightly while pulling your shoulders back, and hold this position for 5 seconds. [Demonstrate this]. Okay, lift your back and shoulders slightly off the back of your chair, arch your back slightly while bringing your shoulders back, and hold 2, 3, 4, 5, and release. Focus on the relaxation in your back. [pause] Again, lift your back and shoulders away from the chair while arching your back slightly and pulling your shoulders back, and hold 2, 3, 4, 5, and release. Notice the difference between tensing and relaxing the muscles in your back. [pause]

Now we are going to focus on the chest muscles.

Chest: Bring the palms of your hands together in front of your chest (or clasp your hands together in front of your chest), pushing your hands together, keeping your arms at chest level, and hold 2, 3, 4, 5, and release. [repeat]

Now we are going to focus on the upper back and shoulders.

Upper back/shoulders: Press your shoulders back toward the chair behind you and hold 2, 3, 4, 5, and release. [repeat]

Shoulders: Next, lift your shoulders up toward the ceiling and hold 2, 3, 4, 5, and release. [repeat]

Now we are going to focus on the muscles in the hands.

Hands: I want you to make a fist with both hands and hold 2, 3, 4, 5, and release. Focus on the relaxation moving through your hands. [repeat]

Now we are going to focus on the muscles in your arms.

Right arm: To relax your right arm, make a fist with your right hand. Then bring that fist up to your right shoulder, while pressing your arm firmly against your chest. Ready and hold 2, 3, 4, 5, and release. [repeat]

Left arm: To relax your left arm, make a fist with your left hand. Then bring that fist up to your left shoulder, while pressing your arm firmly against your chest. Ready and hold 2, 3, 4, 5, and release. [repeat]

Now we are going to focus on the muscles in your neck.

Neck: Slowly bring your chin down toward your chest while at the same time trying to resist this movement and hold 2, 3, 4, 5, and release. [repeat]

Another way to tense and relax the muscles in your neck is to slowly turn your head to the right and to the left. Let's start by slowly turning your head to the right as though you were looking for traffic . . . just to the point of feeling a stretch or some tension there. Ready and hold 2, 3, 4, 5, and release. Focus on the relaxation in your neck. Now, slowly turn your head to the left (as though you were looking for traffic . . . just to the point of feeling a stretch or some tension there). Ready and hold 2, 3, 4, 5, and release. Notice the difference between stretching and relaxing the muscles in your neck.

Moving to the muscles in our face, we will begin by . . .

Face: Smiling really big and wide with your teeth showing and hold 2, 3, 4, 5, and release. Feel the relaxation in your cheeks and jaw. [repeat]

With your eyes closed, squint your eyes and wrinkle your nose and hold 2, 3, 4, 5, and release. Focus on the relaxation in your eyes, nose, and temples. [repeat]

To relax the forehead and the top of your head, raise your eyebrows high and hold 2, 3, 4, 5, and release. Feeling the relaxation in your forehead and the top of your head. [repeat]

Continue to enjoy this relaxation throughout your body now. [pause] If there is any part of your body that needs further relaxation, go to that part of your body now, tense or stretch that muscle group, and then relax it, focusing on the difference between tensing and releasing it. [pause] Now your entire body is relaxed. Enjoy this peaceful state.

[Add patient-guided imagery here, "Favorite or Safe Place," or end the exercise.] In a few moments, we will be ending this relaxation exercise. I will be slowly counting back from 3 to 1. When I say, "One," we will end this relaxation exercise. However, do not make any quick movements right away. Just sit there quietly and calmly and enjoy the relaxation. 3-2-1.

Adapted with permission from *Stress Management Training: A Group Header's Guide* (p. 20), by N. Norvell and D. Belles, 1990, Sarasota, FL: Professional Resource Exchange, Inc. Copyright 1990 by Professional Resource Exchange.

Patient-guided imagery ("Favorite or Safe Place") is usually added to the end of the progressive muscle relaxation exercise. However, some therapists may wish to stop the exercise here. At the end of the exercise, patients can be asked about their relaxation experience and their pain ratings.

GUIDED MUSCLE RELAXATION

Guided muscle relaxation differs from progressive muscle relaxation in its emphasis on imagery (e.g., visual or kinesthetic) and words to induce relaxation rather than the physical aspects of tensing and releasing muscle groups. This relaxation exercise includes autogenic relaxation, which are statements encouraging patients to relax. In guided muscle relaxation, patients are asked to focus on different muscle groups and imagine relaxation entering these muscles. They may actually feel the relaxation (e.g., warmth, coolness, or tingling) or put a visual image to their relaxation. They are also asked to imagine pain or tension slipping away from their body.

Some patients prefer this type of relaxation instead of the progressive muscle relaxation discussed earlier because this technique does not involve any physical manipulation of muscles. This type of relaxation is recommended for patients who are visually or kinesthetically inclined (i.e., they can visualize or sense what their pain and relaxation might look or feel like), who have a good imagination, or who want to learn more relaxation techniques. It is also recommended for patients who are unable to do progressive muscle relaxation because of their pain. This exercise works well with most patients, even those who tend to be concrete thinkers. Whether or not patients actually visualizes the relaxation is not as important as their ability to attend to their entire exercise in general and their ability to feel relaxed. Patients who are able to incorporate the relaxation comments in this exercise will achieve a significant relaxation response, even without any visualization of relaxation. In rare cases, patients may not achieve a state of relaxation with this exercise during the session. These patients tend to be anxious or skeptical about trying this exercise in session. However, when they practice this exercise regularly during the week between sessions, they can develop a relaxation response to it in their own environment, free from distractions and in the privacy of their own home.

As with progressive muscle relaxation, patients begin with deep abdominal breathing. Here is a guided muscle relaxation script.

Therapist: Now that you are breathing slowly and beginning to feel relaxed, we will further relax your muscles . . . allow relaxation to move into the different parts of your body . . . no room for pain or tension . . . only room for deep relaxation. During this exercise, I want you to focus on my voice . . . and my voice only. Any sounds that you may hear in and around this room . . . move farther into the background . . . my voice is moving more and more into the foreground of your awareness. You will always be aware of what I am saying to you and what we are doing during this relaxation exercise. Put aside any worries or concerns for the next 15 minutes to allow your mind and body to relax. Focus only on my voice . . . on your deep breathing . . . and on the deep relaxation in your body. We will begin our exercise by focusing on the different parts of your body, one at a time, to experience deep relaxation. Focus your attention first on the toes . . .

Toes: Allow the toes to go very limp and relaxed. Sometimes people feel warmth or heaviness in the toes; other people feel a lightness or a cool sensation in their toes. Whatever you feel is a sign of relaxation. [pause] The toes are feeling very, very relaxed.

Feet: Allow that relaxation to move up into the muscles in your feet. There is no room for pain and tension. There is only room for deep relaxation in your feet. They are feeling very relaxed and limp.

Your toes and feet are feeling very relaxed. You may decide to put an image to the relaxation in your toes and feet. Some people imagine that the relaxation is a ball of light, moving around the muscles in the toes and feet. Other people imagine relaxation as a waterfall, cascading over the toes and feet. Find an image of your relaxation now. Imagine it slowly taking over your feet and toes.

Lower legs: Move the relaxation into your lower legs. Feel the positive energy of deep relaxation taking over the muscles in your legs. There is no room for pain and tension. Pain is slipping away from the lower legs. Deep relaxation moves into the muscles in your lower legs.

Upper legs/buttocks: The feelings of relaxation slowly move into the thighs—the top of your legs, on around to the hamstrings—underneath your upper legs, and to your buttocks. Imagine the pain slipping away from the muscles in your upper legs and buttocks . . . relaxation circulating deeper into the muscles there.

Always remember your deep breathing . . . breathing in and out . . . enjoying the slow, easy rhythm of your breathing as you continue to focus on the relaxation in your body.

Stomach: Imagine the relaxation moving into the muscles of your stomach . . . breathe in relaxation . . . breathe out any pain or tension in your stomach. You are moving deeper into a state of relaxation.

Lower back: Allow the pain and tension to slip away from your lower back now. Move the relaxation into the muscles in your lower back. Imagine the relaxation shining down on your back, like the sun. Or you might imagine the relaxation as a cool sensation, like snow or ice on your back.

Upper back/shoulders: Feel the relaxation moving into your upper back and shoulder blades . . . on into the shoulder muscles. You are feeling more and more relaxed with each moment. Your upper back, shoulder blades, and shoulders are feeling heavy and relaxed . . . very, very relaxed.

Hands/fingers: Allow the relaxation to flow down into your upper arms, into your lower arms, down into your wrists . . . your hands . . . the tops of your hands and the bottom of your hands . . . on down into your fingers. Feel the relaxation radiating from your finger-tips. Enjoy the deep relaxation circulating throughout your arms, hands, and fingers now. Breathe in and out . . . feeling content and at peace with yourself.

Neck: Relax the muscles in your neck. Give special attention to your neck . . . allow pain and tension to slip away . . . slip away from your neck. Relaxation is flowing into the muscles here.

Face: Imagine the relaxation slowly flowing into the muscles in your face, starting with your chin and jaw. Open up your lips just a little to allow your jaw and chin to relax. There is no room for pain . . . it's slipping away from the muscles in your face. Move the relaxation into your cheeks . . . nose . . . eyes . . . eyebrows. Relax your forehead and temples. Imagine the relaxation flowing over the top of your head and down the back of your head . . . on into the muscles in your neck. Imagine the relaxation moving deeper and deeper into the muscles in your head and face.

Summary: Enjoy now the deep state of relaxation throughout your body. If there is any part of your body that feels pain or ten-sion, go to that part of your body now . . . allow relaxation to take over. Move that relaxation deeper into the muscles in your body. [pause] And now your whole body is limp and relaxed . . . as though you were a rag doll. [pause] [Add therapist-guided images next or end the exercise.] In a few moments, we will be ending this relax-ation exercise. I will be slowly counting back from 3 to 1. When I say, "One," we will end this exercise. However, do not move your body right away. Just sit there quietly and calmly and enjoy the relax-ation. 3-2-1. Slowly begin to open your eyes and orient yourself to the room. Become aware of my voice as well as other sounds around you, inside and outside of this room, yet continue to feel relaxed. Feel the chair beneath you and the floor beneath your feet. You have done a wonderful job of relaxing your mind and body. Enjoy the deep relaxation in your body. In a moment, we will discuss what the relaxation exercise was like for you.

As with any relaxation exercise, it is important to query patients about their experience of relaxation, including any difficulties they encountered during the exercise.

If the patient has migraine or tension headaches or neck and shoulder pain, the therapist may want to reverse the order of this guided muscle relaxation exercise, starting with the head first and then moving down the body (i.e., head, neck, shoulders, arms, hands, chest, back, stomach, buttocks, upper and lower legs, feet, and toes). The same is true for the progressive muscle relaxation exercise. In other words, the therapist can adjust the starting point of the exercise based on where the patient's pain is located. This gives particular areas in the body more time to relax throughout the exercise.

As a general rule, therapists should start the relaxation exercise from one end of the body—either the toes (and have the patient mentally move relaxation up the body) or the head (and have the patient mentally move relaxation down the body), rather than starting in the middle (e.g., abdomen or lower back). Many patients with low back pain also have pain radiating into their legs, so starting with the toes and feet will help them experience relaxation in an area highly related to their low back pain.

Starting the relaxation exercises in the areas of the body with the most pain may be too difficult for some patients to focus on because the pain is so unbearable. Other patients look forward to working on the area with the most severe pain first. So, therapists should ask patients where they want to start the relaxation—from the head down or from the toes up, keeping in mind where the worst pain is located.

This guided muscle relaxation exercise may be difficult for some patients because they have spent so much time trying to distract themselves from pain rather than focus on their bodies. Typically, those patients who have low frustration tolerance for this exercise respond more favorably to the progressive muscle relaxation exercise. Given the individual differences of patient preferences for relaxation exercises, it is recommended that therapists teach all of these exercises so patients can decide which ones best suit their needs.

If therapists notice that their patients still seem to be oriented to their bodies (e.g., eyes are still closed, still focused on the relaxation), have fallen asleep (try to watch for this when it happens to help patients wake up), or are not clearly aware of their surroundings after the relaxation exercise is over (seems somewhat disoriented—in a daze), they should give the patients some time to become reoriented to the room by reminding them of the sounds around them, making them aware of the feeling of the chair or sofa beneath them, and reminding them that the exercise is over. If a patient still does not respond, the therapist can let the patient know that he or she is going to gently touch his or her arm or shoulder to signal that the exercise is over. Some patients experience an altered state of consciousness during this exercise—they are so involved in the experience of relaxation that they may not wish it to end. Thus, therapists may need to help patients get reoriented to their external environments as a way of bringing them out of the internal focus on relaxation.

GUIDED IMAGERY RELAXATION

Guided imagery relaxation exercises can be used in conjunction with the progressive muscle relaxation or the guided muscle relaxation exercise mentioned above. At the end of either exercise, guided imagery relaxation can be used to help patients achieve stronger, deeper states of relaxation. However, these guided imagery relaxation techniques can also be combined with deep abdominal breathing and serve as separate relaxation techniques in and of themselves.

Chronic pain patients can experience a great deal of temporary relief from their pain by focusing on relaxing images in their minds. For example, they might imagine a place they have been before, such as a beach, a national park, a mountain range, or a favorite spot with friends. Patients can also use their imagination to create a "safe haven" from their pain and discomfort—a place that is free from pain. With guided imagery relaxation techniques, therapists can guide patients to create relaxing images they have chosen for themselves (patients' images) or provide specific, vivid images for patients to visualize (therapist-directed imagery).

As with the relaxation exercises mentioned earlier, guided imagery exercises should be audiotaped during the therapy sessions so that patients can take the tapes home to practice these exercises regularly. Although some therapists may choose to make these tapes in advance, it is recommended that these exercises be taped live during the session. In this way, each audiotaped relaxation exercise can be individually tailored to the needs of each patient (i.e., considering the pain locations, noticing what images are powerful). For example, therapists working with patients who have chronic shoulder pain may decide to incorporate the shoulders more often in imagery exercises to help patients relax that area of the body. In addition, therapists can specifically refer to patients by name during these exercises, making these tapes more personal and meaningful to them.

FAVORITE OR SAFE PLACE (PATIENT-DIRECTED IMAGES)

In this guided imagery exercise, patients are asked to think of a favorite or safe place to help them feel relaxed. This is a place that is free from pain and worries. The following is a script that therapists can use with patients following deep breathing and other muscle relaxation exercises. (This exercise usually follows the deep breathing and progressive muscle relaxation.)

Therapist: Now that you are enjoying this deep state of relaxation, take a moment to think of a favorite or safe place that you have been to before . . . a place that is free from pain . . . free from tension . . . free from any worries. Or use your imagination to create such a place . . . a place that is a safe haven for you . . . a sanctuary of relaxation. Take a moment now to see this place in your mind. [pause] You are now here in this special place. Become aware of what you see in this favorite place. [pause] As you take a look around you, you also notice the relaxing sounds that you hear in this place. [long pause] Fully sense the sights and sounds here. [pause] Notice the comforting smells here in this special place. [pause] Become aware of anything you may taste that is satisfying and relaxing. [pause] Notice anything you may feel or touch in this place that is soothing to you. As you enjoy being here in this place, you realize how comfortable you feel . . . there is no room for pain or discomfort here . . . no room for worries . . . only room for deep, calming moments of relaxation.

After this exercise, therapists should discuss patients' favorite or safe place in some detail (i.e., where was it, who was there with them, what patients were sensing that was relaxing, and so on). Again, guided imagery is a skill just like deep breathing and muscle relaxation. Patients should be encouraged to practice getting in touch with their favorite or safe place at least three times over the next week prior to the following therapy session.

THERAPIST-DIRECTED GUIDED IMAGERY

Another guided imagery task involves therapists directing patients to visualize specific images that are relaxing. Here are two examples of imagery scenarios that can be used with patients. (This exercise usually follows the deep abdominal breathing and guided muscle relaxation).

Beach Script

Therapist: Let's take a moment now to imagine that you are standing on a beautiful beach. As you look out at the ocean, you notice the rays of sunlight glistening on the ocean. The water is so crystal clear and blue. Watch the waves lap the shore, crashing softly against the beach. Feel the cool water run across your feet as you walk along the shore. Take in all of the beauty and wonder around you. The smells of salt from the ocean come into your awareness now. Seagulls are flying over the water . . . hear their calls . . . watch their wings move while in flight. Feel the warm sand beneath your feet as you walk farther down the beach. With each step, you feel more and more relaxed. You notice the sun shining down on your body . . . feel the warm sun on your face, neck, and shoulders [or any other part of the patient's body that is in pain]. The sun's warmth and energy move through your body, deep into the muscles and nerves. Feeling very relaxed and calm, you soak up the sun and the cool breeze that blows through your hair and around your body. You decide to lie down on the warm sand to take a rest. Feel the warm sun beating down on your body. Feel the warm sand underneath you. As you lie there, your body feels connected to the sand . . . as though you cannot separate your body from the sand beneath you. Listen to the rhythmic sounds of the waves as they meet the shore. Feel yourself drifting into a state of deep relaxation . . . how peaceful it is here.

Forest Script

Therapist: Imagine that you are walking on a nature trail in a forest near a mountain range. It is a refreshing day . . . the temperature is cool yet comfortable for a late morning in the fall. As you continue down the path, you fully sense and enjoy the lush, green scenery around you. You notice that some of the leaves are turning red, orange, and yellow. You can hear the sounds of leaves crunching under your feet as you walk down the nature trail. With each breath you take, the crisp, clean air fills your lungs with deep relaxation and pure satisfaction. You notice two deer nearby, both unaware of your presence. You stop to take a rest under a tree, sitting near a small stream. Listen to the sounds of the water rushing over the rocks and pebbles in this stream. A few fish in the stream swim past you, one leaping out of the water and diving back in. You enjoy the sights and sounds as you rest here . . . looking up through the overlapping branches of the tall trees around you . . . seeing the sun peeking through the tops of the trees. The clear, blue sky above is so inviting. You become aware of the smells of pine and morning dew in the air. After a bit, you begin to walk down the path some more. You feel more and more relaxed with each step you take down that path.

Soon, you come to an opening in the forest and discover a magnificent mountain range. Colorful trees grace the mountainside. You can feel the beauty before you. What a breathtaking view. You enjoy the peace and quiet of this moment . . . being at one with nature.

OTHER FORMS OF RELAXATION

Other techniques can be developed based on the unique needs of each patient. In addition to the deep breathing, muscle relaxation, and guided imagery, patients can use other methods to help them relax, including but not limited to music, art, literature, yoga, meditation, exercise, and travel. Many patients enjoy listening to music as a way to relax. There are also relaxation compact discs and tapes available that include the sounds of nature (e.g., ocean, birds, whales, etc.) and specific relaxation or meditation exercises.

Artistic endeavors can help patients relax and enjoy moments of solitude. Art allows patients to use their senses and promotes an awareness of their surroundings, which may distract them from their pain. Drawing, painting, sculpting, ceramics, and other media allow patients to express their thoughts and feelings in different ways than therapy can. Participation in the arts allows patients to focus on something other than themselves and to produce some meaningful and beautiful projects, thus fostering their sense of creativity and resourcefulness.

Patients can also experience relaxation by reading. Literature can provide patients with a quick escape from their own realities for a period of time. Patients can also read a variety of books on the topics of relaxation, meditation, nutrition, and cognitive therapy to further develop their pain management skills.

Meditation and yoga are forms of mental, physical, and spiritual exercises specifically designed to help patients increase their awareness, facilitate relaxation, and increase fitness. Meditation involves an internal focus on oneself while sitting in solitude or with a group of people—allowing thoughts, feelings, and physical sensations to move in and out of an individual's awareness. It is an exercise in being an observer of oneself without trying to solve or do anything about those inner experiences. Meditation may be difficult for some patients because they may focus on their pain. Yoga is a form of exercise devoted to physical strengthening and stretching, deep breathing, and inner awareness. Some people find that yoga helps them build physical, emotional, and spiritual strength through the deep breathing and stretching exercises that are part of this form of exercise.

Physical exercise in general can help patients increase their muscular strength, flexibility, conditioning, and range of motion, as well as facilitate relaxation. (The act of flexing and releasing muscle groups while exercising produces a relaxation response.) In fact, endorphins, natural opiates in the brain, can be activated and released when people engage in physical exercise. Patients can develop a realistic and appropriately paced exercise plan in consultation with their physicians, physical therapists, and recreational therapists.

DISTRACTION TECHNIQUES IN COPING WITH PAIN

Patients can learn to use a variety of approaches to distract themselves from their pain. Distraction is a short-term (or temporary) coping strategy to help patients cope with their pain. Engaging in pleasurable activities and relaxation training are examples of distraction mentioned earlier in this manual.

Patients can also learn to distract themselves from their pain by turning their attention and focus toward their environment. One of the first ways to learn this strategy is to have a patient learn how to describe all of the things he or she sees in the therapy room. (This is assuming that the person does not have a significant visual impairment, such as blindness.) This distraction technique can be introduced in session with very little explanation of its rationale at the beginning. The therapist should encourage the patient to rate his or her pain levels (on a scale from 0 to 10, with 0 being *no pain* and 10 being *severe, excruciating pain*) just prior to and following this exercise. After the exercise is over, the patient is asked if he or she noticed a change in pain levels and/or a change in their focus on the pain while describing the room. Many patients tend to notice being temporarily distracted from their pain and report lower pain ratings after the exercise. However, some patients may find that this distraction technique is not very helpful for them. Regardless, this distraction exercise prompts important discussions on distraction techniques for coping with chronic pain, including patients' current distraction methods as well as brainstorming new ones. Here is an example of a therapist–patient dialogue using this distraction technique. Dewayne is a 54 year old Caucasian man who has neuropathy in his right arm and hand from years of repetitive work as a postal delivery person. He has been so absorbed in his pain and is searching for some relief.

Therapist: Dewayne, you seem to be feeling more pain than usual this week [average pain rating is 9 on a scale from 0 to 10]. We identified several factors that may have influenced this increase in pain intensity, for example, your activity level and the recent change in your pain medication. Before we continue to discuss this issue in session, I am wondering if you are willing to do an exercise with me in session right now. [pause]

Patient: Okay. What is it?

Therapist: I would like to see if you can describe in detail what you see around you in the therapy room, as though you are describing it to someone who has not been here before.

Patient: [hesitates briefly] Okay, well, I notice that you have a new picture on your wall today . . . a picture of some beautiful flowers—it looks like a Georgia O'Keefe piece. And there are bookshelves on both sides of the room, filled with a number of books. It looks as though you are running out of space to put your books here. [laughs] I am sitting in a very comfortable chair, with good back support. And there are three other chairs here in this room. I am looking at the window behind you . . . you have a great view of some trees and buildings nearby. [long pause]

Therapist: What else do you see around you in this room?

Patient: I notice that you have some piles of papers on your desk and a desktop computer. There is a tile floor beneath my feet and a soft rug covering most of the floor.

Therapist: As you are describing what you see, feel free to comment on the colors, sizes, and shapes.

Patient: Oh . . . the flowers in the picture are pink, lavender, yellow, and blue. The room is very bright with the sun shining through the window. . . . [Patient talks for a few more minutes about the details.]

Therapist: Okay. Thanks, Dewayne, for doing this exercise with me. Now, let's talk about what it was like to describe what you saw around you.

Patient: Oh, no problem. I guess it made me aware of some things that I hadn't noticed about your office until now.

Therapist: Okay, that's great. Now, I'd like you to rate the level of pain right now in session.

Patient: Oh, I would say, it's about a 7 [on a scale from 0 to 10].

Therapist: So, before we started, the pain was at level 9. What do you think led to the slight drop in your pain level?

Patient: I don't know. Maybe getting caught up in the exercise . . . I just wasn't as aware of my pain at the time.

Therapist: So, when you were focused on describing the therapy room, you were temporarily distracted from your pain?

Patient: Yeah, I guess so. I was aware of the pain some, but not as much as when I was telling you how frustrated and worried I was about my pain this past week.

Therapist: Well, thanks Dewayne for doing the exercise with me. The reason I asked you to do this was to see if it would temporarily distract you from your pain, lowering your pain awareness, by focusing on your surroundings . . . your environment.

Can you think of times when you have been able to distract yourself from your pain because you were really focused on an activity or something else in your environment?

Patient: Hmm. I do notice that when I'm watching TV, especially if it's one of my favorite shows, I might experience some escape from the pain.

Therapist: That's great. Is there anything else that you do to distract yourself from your pain?

Patient: Well, I enjoy traveling to new places, when they're not too far away. It's also nice to get out of the city and go to the shore. I love the ocean! I also enjoy inviting friends over for a drink on occasion.

Therapist: Okay, so it sounds as though you already have some things that you enjoy doing that keep you distracted from your pain, including visiting with friends, traveling, and watching a favorite TV show. It might be helpful to journal about other ways you try to distract yourself from the pain. How does that sound?

Patient: Sounds fine. Sometimes I forget what really "works" for me when I'm in the middle of all of this pain.

Therapist: Do you think this distraction exercise is something that you could practice between now and next week?

Patient: Yes, definitely. I think I'll have lots of opportunities to practice distraction. I'm not sure how much it will help, but it's worth a try.

Therapist: Well, you did notice that your pain levels went from 9 to 7 in just a few minutes by doing the distraction exercise in session, which I think is significant. One way to find out how much distraction helps you is to rate your pain before you attempt any distraction efforts and then rate your pain afterwards to see if it reduces your pain awareness at all. If you distracted yourself by doing something pleasurable, then it probably was beneficial, even if your pain level doesn't change. Does that make sense?

Patient: Yes, because sitting around focusing on my pain and feeling sorry for myself isn't going to make me feel better. Distracting myself while doing things I enjoy should make a difference.

Therapist: Great. Remember, the goal is to try and describe your surroundings in as much detail as possible. Learning how to distract
yourself from your pain is a skill . . . just like the relaxation techniques you learned in session today. So, practice it regularly, at least
a few times over the next week. You can also distract yourself by
calling a friend, watching TV, or taking a drive to some travel des-
tination of interest.

Patient: Okay, sounds good to me. I'll give it a try.

During the next session, Dewayne reported that the relaxation and distraction techniques helped him cope better with his pain. Turning his
attention away from his pain and bodily sensations provided some temporary relief. However, the relaxation techniques were the most helpful
in managing his pain.

In the next section of the book, readers will learn how to identify, evaluate, and modify patients' negative thoughts about their pain.

PART III

COGNITIVE INTERVENTIONS

7

Identifying Automatic
Thoughts About Pain

Negative thoughts and beliefs about pain can have a significant and negative impact on patients' physical and psychosocial functioning. In cognitive therapy, patients learn how to identify, evaluate, and modify self-talk, imagery, and core beliefs related to pain and distress. As mentioned earlier, automatic thoughts include both self-talk and imagery. Self-talk interventions will be covered in this chapter and imagery work will be described in chapter 10.

It has been our experience that patients who have chronic pain are very sensitive to the terms, "dysfunctional thoughts" and "irrational thoughts." However, "negative automatic thoughts" or "automatic thoughts" are terms often accepted by these patients because they are not judgemental in nature. Therefore, throughout this manual, we will refer to negative thoughts as "negative automatic thoughts" or "automatic thoughts."

IDENTIFYING AUTOMATIC THOUGHTS RELATED
TO CHRONIC PAIN

Negative automatic thoughts often accompany fluctuations in pain intensity and moods. However, these thoughts are not always in our immediate awareness. A variety of events or experiences can "trigger" negative self-talk or imagery, for example, the onset of pain, elevations in pain levels, negative mood states, lack of a clear-cut diagnosis, lack of social support, and financial problems, to name a few. Once these situations are identified, therapists can explore how their patients were feeling at that time, both physiologically (e.g., pain intensity and locations) and emotionally (e.g., sad, mad, glad, scared, or guilty), followed by an exploration of their thoughts. Exploring patients' pain levels and their emotional states during specific situations primes them to access these automatic thoughts.

In the following therapist–patient dialogue, automatic thoughts related to pain will be identified. Bemice, a 67 year old African American woman, has been diagnosed with degenerative disc disease in her back. Despite medical intervention, she continues to be bothered by pain. Bernice feels depressed and anxious about her pain and how it limits her ability to do things. In particular, she doesn't believe she can do anything to control her pain, which leads her to feel hopeless.

Therapist: Automatic thoughts are often hard to catch at the beginning. Because they are so automatic, you may not be aware of them when they occur. Negative thinking can get activated in stressful situations or when you are in pain, especially when the pain kicks in or intensifies. Do you think this might fit you?

Patient: Yes, I think I probably do think negatively about my pain. I really wish I did not have to deal with this pain.

Therapist: To help us catch your negative thoughts, we need to identify situations when you were really bothered by your pain or other upsetting events. Can you remember a time this past week when your pain was really bothering you or when you were upset about an event?

Patient: Yes. The pain was really bothering me yesterday. It all started when I bent over to pick a sock off the floor [situation]. I felt a sharp, stabbing pain in my lower back [pain] that really took my breath away. It just wouldn't go away.

Therapist: On a scale from 0 to 10, with 0 being *no pain at all* and 10 being *the worst possible pain*, how intense was your pain?

Patient: Oh, definitely an 8.

Therapist: And what emotions were you in touch with when you felt the pain?

Patient: I was very upset, very frustrated. [emotions].

Therapist: How upset and frustrated were you, on a scale from 0 to 100, with 0 being *not at all*, and 100 being *the most upset and frustrated you have ever been?*

Patient: I was very upset and frustrated, probably 100.

Therapist: So, when you were in pain, feeling upset and frustrated, what thoughts or images were running through your mind?

Patient: [pause] I remember thinking to myself, "I cannot stop this pain. I cannot control it" [automatic thoughts]

Therapist: Any other thoughts?

Patient: I couldn't even pick up a sock without hurting!

Therapist: How strongly did you believe that you could not stop the pain? That you could not control it?

Patient: Oh, a lot.

Therapist: Using a scale from 0 to 100, with 0 being *you did not believe it at all* and 100 being *you believed it totally,* how strongly did you believe that you could not stop or control the pain at the time when you bent over to pick up the sock?

Patient: Probably about 90.

Therapist: And how strongly did you believe then that you couldn't even pick up a sock without hurting, using that same scale, 0 to 100?

Patient: Definitely 100.

Therapist: Okay. What did you do after the pain came on?

Patient: Well, I was in so much pain, it was unbearable. So, I laid down on the recliner to rest [behavior]. The pain subsided a few hours later.

Therapist: Did you try any of the relaxation techniques you have learned in therapy?

Patient: I did play the relaxation tapes, and it helped.

Therapist: Great! I'm sorry to hear that the pain lasted so long. But I am glad to hear that you took some steps to cope with your pain. [pause] So far today, we have explored a situation in which you felt tremendous pain, identified the emotions you felt at the time, the thoughts that were running through your mind, and what you did to cope with the pain. Your thoughts, "I am not in control of my pain" and "I can't do anything," are actually very common for people in pain.

Patient: Well, it's good to know I'm not alone. I just wish I could take control of my pain and do more in general.

Therapist: One way to take control of your pain is to continue practicing the relaxation techniques. Catching your negative thoughts will also help you take charge of your pain. The meaning you give to your pain can have a significant impact on your pain and your emotions. Negative thoughts can keep us focused on our pain and suffering. Does that make sense?

Patient: Yes, it does. I try to tune out my negative thoughts. But I find that really doesn't help much.

Therapist: Well, one of the goals of cognitive therapy is to help you begin to face those thoughts and experiences, so that you can learn how to cope better with them. The focus of today's session is to help you catch your negative automatic thoughts "in action"—when they happen. When you notice a change in your pain levels or your mood, those are times when you can ask yourself, "What thoughts or images were running through my mind." This question will help us catch those negative thoughts.

Patient: That sounds good to me! I really want to find ways that I can deal with my pain and the stress in my life. My negative thinking probably does affect my pain and stress.

AUTOMATIC THOUGHT RECORD

The Automatic Thought Record (ATR) is an essential tool that therapists use in session to teach patients how to identify, evaluate, and modify their negative thoughts. It provides patients with a structured format to chart their pain, emotions, and automatic thoughts related to significant events and situations (e.g., onset of pain and recent doctor's visit). There are six columns in the ATR (see Figure 7.1). Therapists should teach patients how to use the first four columns—Situations, Automatic Thought(s), Emotions, and Pain—in one or two sessions before using the last two columns—Alternative Responses and Outcome. Once patients learn to identify and describe their pain, emotions, and automatic thoughts in a variety of situations, they can learn how to evaluate and modify their thoughts.

When patients complete the ATR, they should write down the situation first, then the pain/physical sensation, then the emotions, and finally the automatic thoughts. This order is recommended because many patients can identify their pain experience and emotional states better than their automatic thoughts. In addition, having them recall the situation, their pain levels, and their emotional states primes them to identify their negative self-talk and imagery.

As patients complete the first four columns of the ATR for a given situation, they are encouraged to rate their pain in that situation on a scale from 0 (*no pain*) to 10 (*severe, excruciating pain*); to rate the intensity of their emotions in that situation on a scale from 0 (*no emotion*) to 100 (*the most intensity possible*); and, finally, to rate the strength of their beliefs in the thoughts or images in the Aautomatic Thought(s) column on a scale from 0 (*don't believe at all*) to 100 (*believe it totally*). These scales are designed to help patients see the continuous nature of their pain, emotions, and the strength of their beliefs, rather than view them as all-or-nothing phenomena. These indices of physical and emotional distress can also direct

FIGURE 7.1 Blank Automatic Thought Record

SITUATION	AUTOMATIC THOUGHT(S)	EMOTION(S)	PAIN	ALTERNATIVE RESPONSE	OUTCOME
1. Describe the actual event or the experience of pain that led to the unpleasant emotion.	1. What thought(s) and/or image(s) went through your mind? 2. How much did you believe each one at the time? (0–100)	1. What emotion (sad, anxious, angry, etc.) did you feel at the time? 2. How intense (0–100) was the emotion?	1. Where did you experience the pain in your body? 2. How intense (0–10) was the pain? 3. What words would you use to describe the pain (throbbing, burning, aching, tender, etc.)?	1. What cognitive distortion did you make? 2. Use questions at bottom to compose a response to the automatic thought(s). 3. How much do you believe each response? (0–100)	1. How much do you believe each original automatic thought? 2. What emotion(s) do you feel now? How intense (0–100) is the emotion? 3. Describe your pain now. How intense (0–10) is your pain now?

Questions to help you compose an alternative response: (1) What is the evidence that the automatic thought is true? Not true? (2) Is there an alternative explanation? (3) What's the worst that could happen if the automatic thought were true? Could I live with it? What's the best that could happen? What could be the most realistic outcome? (4) What's the effect of my believing the automatic thought? What could be the effect of changing my thinking? (5) What should I do about it? (6) If _____ (friend's name) was in this situation and had this thought, what would I tell him/her?

From Judith S. Beck's *Cognitive Therapy: Basics and Beyond.* Copyright 1995 by Judith S. Beck, PhD. Adapted with permission by the Guilford Press: New York.

patients and therapists to the most relevant (e.g., distressing) thoughts/beliefs, emotions, and situations to discuss and address in the therapy session. "Hotter" cognitions (higher strength values) are usually associated with "hotter" (more intense) emotions and pain.

Patients learn to ask themselves a series of questions to complete the first four columns of the ATR, which are provided on this worksheet.

Situation Question
• What was the actual event or the experience of pain that led to my unpleasant emotion?

Pain Questions
• What was my pain like then?
• Where did I experience it in my body?
• How intense was the pain, on a scale from 0 to 10, with 0 being *no pain at all* and 10 being *the most severe, excruciating pain ever experienced?*
• What words would I use to describe the pain?

Emotion Questions
• What emotions did I feel at the time (e.g., sad, mad, glad, scared, guilty, ashamed)?
• How intense was my emotion on a scale from 0 to 100, with 0 being *no emotion at all* 100 being the *highest level of intensity?*

Automatic Thought Questions
• When I was feeling _____ pain and experiencing _____ emotion in that situation, what thoughts or images went through my mind then?
• How much did I believe each thought or image on a scale from 0 to 100, 0 (*not believing it at all*) to 100 (*believing it totally*)?

In the next therapist–patient dialogue, the therapist shows the patient how to use open-ended questions and the Automatic Thought Record to identify key negative automatic thoughts related to her pain (see Figure 7.2).

Therapist: Let's begin by teaching you how to journal your thoughts when you are in pain or when you are experiencing a distressing situation. While we were talking, I wrote some of the main points from our discussion on a special worksheet called the Automatic Thought Record. Here is a blank copy for you to keep so that you can make copies of it to use between our sessions. This form will help you to chart situations that are bothersome or distressing to you [pointing to the first column Situation], your experience of pain at that time [pointing to the fourth column, Pain], how you were feeling, that is, your emotions [pointing to the third column,

Emotion(s)], and lastly what thoughts or images were running through your mind at the time [pointing to the second column, Automatic Thought(s)].

Let's take a look at what I wrote down on this form. You will notice in the Situation column, it says, "Describe the actual event or the experience of pain that led to the unpleasant emotion." In the space below, I wrote down the situation we discussed, "Bent over to pick up a sock on the floor." I also wrote "Felt a sharp, stabbing pain in my lower back" in that same column because sometimes pain is the event that activates the negative thoughts. In this case, it sounds like bending over *and* experiencing pain best describes the "trigger situation" that led to your frustration. Does that seem to fit?

Patient: Definitely.

Therapist: I wrote down in the Pain column your experience of pain at that time—"Sharp, stabbing pain in my lower back"—with your rating of 8 on a scale from 0 to 10, with 0 being *no pain* and 10 being *the most excruciating pain imaginable.* Next, I wrote down "Upset" and "Frustrated" in the Emotion column, along with your intensity rating of 100 for each emotion. In the Automatic Thought(s) column, I wrote down your thoughts, using your own words, "I can't stop my pain. I can't control it" and "I can't even pick up a sock without hurting." I also wrote down how strongly you believed each of those thoughts at the time, 90 for the first set of thoughts and 100 for the next thought. Do you see how we were able to chart your experiences on this worksheet?

Patient: Yes. That's pretty neat. I like how this lays out what I just shared with you. It helps me see what I was experiencing then.

Therapist: Great! It really helps people to write down their experiences on paper so that they can see the bigger picture of what happened. Many people find that the Automatic Thought Record helps them see how their pain is related to their emotions and thoughts in particular situations. Once you understand this connection, your negative automatic thoughts will become easier to identify. Now, as we look at the Emotion(s) column, you identified two emotions, being upset and feeling frustrated. Do you think those were two separate emotions or really one emotion?

Patient: I think they were two separate emotions.

Therapist: Okay. Now, as we look at the Automatic Thought(s) column, you identified some specific thoughts. Which thoughts do you think were connected to feeling upset and which to feeling frustrated?

FIGURE 7.2 Bernice's Automatic Thought Record

(1) SITUATION	(4) AUTOMATIC THOUGHT(S)	(3) EMOTION(S)	(2) PAIN	ALTERNATIVE RESPONSE	OUTCOME
1. Describe the actual event or the experience of pain that led to the unpleasant emotion.	1. What thought(s) and/or image(s) went through your mind? 2. How much did you believe each one at the time? (0–100)	1. What emotion (sad, anxious, angry, etc.) did you feel at the time? 2. How intense (0–100) was the emotion?	1. Where did you experience the pain in your body? 2. How intense (0–10) was the pain? 3. What words would you use to describe the pain (throbbing, burning, aching, tender, etc.)?	1. What cognitive distortion did you make? 2. Use questions at bottom to compose a response to the automatic thought(s). 3. How much do you believe each response? (0–100)	1. How much do you believe each original automatic thought? 2. What emotion(s) do you feel now? How intense (0–100) is the emotion? 3. Describe your pain now. How intense (0–100) is your pain now?
Bent over to pick up a sock on the floor and felt a sharp, stabbing pain in my lower back.	I can't stop my pain. 90 I can't control it. 90 I can't even pick up a sock without hurting. 100	Upset 100 Frustrated 100	Sharp, stabbing pain in my lower back 8		

Questions to help you compose an alternative response: (1) What is the evidence that the automatic thought is true? Not true? (2) Is there an alternative explanation? (3) What's the worst that could happen if the automatic thought were true? Could I live with it? What's the best that could happen? What's the most realistic outcome? (4) What's the effect of my believing the automatic thought? What could be the effect of changing my thinking? (5) What should I do about it? (6) If _____ (friend's name) was in this situation and had this thought, what would I tell him/her?

Numbers above the first four columns indicate the recommended order in filling out this chart.

From Judith S. Beck's *Cognitive Therapy: Basics and Beyond.* Copyright 1995 by Judith S. Beck, PhD. Adapted with permission by the Guilford Press: New York.

Patient: I was upset that I couldn't control my pain, and I was frustrated that I couldn't pick up the sock without the pain.

Therapist: Great! So you can see how specific thoughts are connected to specific emotions. If you identify more than one emotion to a situation, be sure to ask yourself the thoughts or images that ran through your mind when you were feeling each emotion. Does that make sense to you?

Patient: Yes.

Therapist: I would like for you to try and journal your experiences this week using the Automatic Thought Record I just showed you. I recommend that you journal for about 20 to 30 minutes several times this week. It will help you make more progress in coping with your pain and distress. Would you be committed to journal using this form over the next week?

Patient: Yes, I will. I think it will really help me.

Therapist: When you experience pain or distress, I want you to describe the situation or event you experienced and write it in the Situation column. Second, write down your experience of pain in the Pain column. Then, write down what emotions you felt in the Emotion(s) column. Last, I want you to ask yourself, "What thoughts or images were running through my mind then?" Write down your thoughts in the Automatic Thought(s) column. If you have an image, write it down too.

Be sure to use the questions under each column heading to guide you in writing your responses, and don't forget to rate the intensity of your pain and your emotions as well as the strength of your thoughts at that time using the scales provided. Does that make sense?

Patient: Sounds good to me.

Therapist: Becoming aware of the thoughts you have when you experience pain or a distressing situation is the first step toward understanding the impact they have on your pain and your life.

Patient: I have a feeling I will have a lot written down on this form to share with you next week.

Patients who have difficulty accessing their emotions or thoughts in session can be asked to imagine a recent time when they experienced pain or distress as though they were experiencing it again to access these experiences. This process is described in the next example.

Logan, a 28 year old Caucasian man, has chronic lower back pain. So far, his physician have not been able to diagnose his pain problem, which is discouraging to Logan. He has become agitated and frustrated with his pain and tends to berate himself—focusing on his inadequacies. In this part of the session, Logan describes how hard he is on himself.

Patient: I was pulling up into the parking lot for our appointment today, and I was in a hurry to get out of the car. I twisted my back a little, and, boy, did I feel that sharp, throbbing pain.

Therapist: How would you rate that pain on a scale from 0 to 10, with 0 being *no pain at all* and 10 being *the worst pain imaginable?*
Patient: Definitely a 10.

Therapist: And what emotions were you in touch with then?
Patient: [pause] I can't really remember.

   [Because the patient is having difficulty accessing his emotions in that situation, the patient will be asked to imagine himself back in that situation to help him access his emotions and thoughts more readily.]

Therapist: Take a moment now to get in touch with a picture in your mind . . . an image of you getting out of your car and feeling that sharp, throbbing pain. Imagine that you are back there in that moment. [pause] Do you have that picture in your mind?
Patient: Yes.

Therapist: What emotions are you in touch with as you were trying to get out of the car? Sad, mad, glad, scared, guilty, ashamed? [The therapist can provide some emotion options if the patient does not identify them readily.]
Patient: Oh, I was angry with myself.

Therapist: How intense was that anger on a scale from 0 to 100, with 0 being *not angry at all* and 100 being *the most angry?*
Patient: Probably 85.

Therapist: And what thoughts or images were running through your mind when you were feeling angry and having that sharp, throbbing pain?
Patient: [pause] I think I was telling myself how stupid I was for rushing like that.

Therapist: Okay, so let's write that thought down on the paper here. What do you think were your exact words in that moment?
Patient: How stupid I am!

Therapist: How strongly did you believe you were stupid for rushing, on a scale from 0 to 100, with 0 *not believing it at all* to 100 *believing it totally?*
Patient: Oh, about 95.

Therapist: Any other thoughts or images that ran through your mind then?
Patient: Yes, I was thinking, "I am such a klutz."

Therapist: How strongly did you believe that you were a klutz?
Patient: Definitely 100.

Therapist: Any other thoughts? [It is important for the therapist to access all of the thoughts.]
Patient: No. I think that covers it.

Therapist: When you thought you were a klutz, what emotions were you experiencing then? [The therapist is clarifying what emotion was connected to this new thought.]
Patient: I was embarrassed.

Therapist: And how intense was your embarrassment on a scale from 0 to 100.
Patient: Definitely 100.

Therapist: Okay, let's stop here for a moment. This is a great example of how your pain is related to your emotions, in this case, anger and embarrassment, and your negative automatic thoughts, like "I'm stupid" and "I'm a klutz."

Sometimes, in our efforts to motivate ourselves, to coach ourselves, we think negatively, hoping it will force us out of a rut. However, in many cases, these types of thoughts are not helpful to us. In fact, they may encourage us to stay in a rut—to not change at all!.
Patient: I think that is very true of me. I want to do my best, and when I don't, I feel like such a failure. So, I push myself, which probably means I put myself down, which doesn't help me feel better.

Therapist: That is a great insight for us to explore some more.

The therapist continues to demonstrate how to use the ATR over the next couple of sessions to be sure that patient know how to fill it out correctly. Logan brought his ATR homework to the next therapy session (see Figure 7.4).

FIGURE 7.3 Logan's Automatic Thought Record

SITUATION	AUTOMATIC THOUGHT(S)	EMOTION(S)	PAIN	ALTERNATIVE RESPONSE	OUTCOME
1. Describe the actual event or the experience of pain that led to the unpleasant emotion.	1. What thought(s) and/or image(s) went through your mind? 2. How much did you believe each one at the time? (0–100)	1. What emotion (sad, anxious, angry, etc.) did you feel at the time? 2. How intense (0–100) was the emotion?	1. Where did you experience the pain in your body? 2. How intense (0–10) was the pain? 3. What words would you use to describe the pain (throbbing, burning, aching, tender, etc.)?	1. What cognitive distortion did you make? 2. Use questions at bottom to compose a response to the automatic thought(s). 3. How much do you believe each response? (0–100)	1. How much do you believe each original automatic thought? 2. What emotion(s) do you feel now? How intense (0–100) is the emotion? 3. Describe your pain now. How intense (0–100) is your pain?
Pulled into parking lot for our appointment. I twisted my back as I was hurrying to get out of the car. I felt a sharp, throbbing pain in my back.	How stupid I am for rushing like that. 95 How stupid can I be? 95 I am such a klutz. 100	Angry 85 Embarrassed 100	Sharp, throbbing pain in my lower back. 10		

Questions to help you compose an alternative response: (1) What is the evidence that the automatic thought is true? Not true? (2) Is there an alternative explanation? (3) What's the worst that could happen if the automatic thought were true? Could I live with it? What's the best that could happen? What's the most realistic outcome? (4) What's the effect of my believing the automatic thought? What could be the effect of changing my thinking? (5) What should I do about it? (6) If _____ (friend's name) was in this situation and had this thought, what would I tell him/her?

From Judith S. Beck's *Cognitive Therapy: Basics and Beyond.* Copyright 1995 by Judith S. Beck, PhD. Adapted with permission by the Guilford Press: New York.

FIGURE 7.4 Logan's Automatic Thought Record for the next Session

SITUATION	AUTOMATIC THOUGHT(S)	EMOTION(S)	PAIN	ALTERNATIVE RESPONSE	OUTCOME
1. Describe the actual event or the experience of pain that led to the unpleasant emotion.	1. What thought(s) and/or image(s) went through your mind? 2. How much did you believe each one at the time? (0–100)	1. What emotion (sad, anxious, angry, etc.) did you feel at the time? 2. How intensE (0–100) was the emotion?	1. Where did you experience the pain in your body? 2. How intense (0–10) was the pain? 3. What words would you use to describe the pain (throbbing, burning, aching, tender, etc.)?	1. What cognitive distortion did you make? 2. Use questions at bottom to compose a response to the automatic thought(s). 3. How much do you believe each response? (0–100)	1. How much do you believe each original automatic thought? 2. What emotion(s) do you feel now? How intense (0–100) is the emotion? 3. Describe your pain now. How intense (0–100) is your pain?
Going for a walk in the park. Felt sharp pain in my lower back. Sat down on a bench. Got up and walked again. I tripped on a crack in the sidewalk. My back arched, but I regained my balance and didn't fall.	I feel so humiliated. 100	Embarrassed 100	Sharp, stabbing pain in my lower back when walking 5 When I tripped, sharp, stabbing pain in my lower back 95		

Questions to help you compose an alternative response: (1) What is the evidence that the automatic thought is true? Not true? (2) Is there an alternative explanation? (3) What's the worst that could happen if the automatic thought were true? Could I live with it? What's the best that could happen? What's the most realistic outcome? (4) What's the effect of my believing the automatic thought? What could be the effect of changing my thinking? (5) What should I do about it? (6) If _____ (friend's name) was in this situation and had this thought, what would I tell him/her?

Therapist: Okay, last week, we agreed that you would try to identify your automatic thoughts when you noticed changes in your pain levels or in your moods. How did that go last week?

Patient: Well, I found out how mean I was to myself. I didn't realize how much I really put myself down in a lot of situations. Like, last week, I was going for a walk in the park next to my house, and I felt a sharp pain in my lower back. So I sat down on a bench nearby. Then, later on, when I continued my walk, I tripped on a crack in the sidewalk, my back arched, and I regained my posture, but I was so embarrassed. I wrote it down on the Automatic Thought Record.

Therapist: Let's take a look at what you wrote. So, the situation was that you tripped on a crack in the sidewalk. You felt a sharp, stabbing pain in your lower back and you felt embarrassed. In the Automatic thought column, you wrote "I feel so humiliated."

[At this point, the therapist realizes that the patient may be confused about the difference between an emotion and a thought.]

Therapist: Okay, so you were *feeling humiliated.* That is an emotion, so let's move that to the Emotion column. When you felt humiliated, what thoughts or images were running through your mind?

Patient: [pause] I cannot even walk three blocks without this pain controlling me. I am clumsy and cannot do anything right. You see what I mean? I am so hard on myself.

Therapist: Okay, let's take this one step further. What emotions are you in touch with right now in session?

Patient: Um, I don't know.

Therapist: You just told me a moment ago that you were hard on yourself. How were you feeling then?

Patient: Really sad and discouraged. I just feel like I cannot do anything right these days.

Therapist: How sad and discouraged are you on the 0 to 100 scale?

Patient: 75.

Therapist: And how strongly you believe that you can't do anything right?

Patient: Oh, probably 95.

Therapist: Well, I noticed that you did a good job of identifying some important feelings and thoughts that we can work on today. It sounds like you've developed a new insight about yourself—that, at times, you're hard on yourself when you experience pain and feel humiliated or embarrassed.

Patient: Yes, I would really like to work on that today.

Therapist: Sounds good. Let's take a look again at the Automatic Thought Record you brought into session today. Earlier in session, I helped you clarify the difference between an emotion and a thought. "I feel humiliated" is a statement of your feelings, so it belongs under the Emotion(s) column. When I asked you about your thoughts when you feel humiliated, we identified some new ones like "I cannot even walk three blocks without the pain controlling me," "I am clumsy," and "I cannot do anything right." These are all examples of negative thoughts that were activated when you tripped and felt humiliated. Identifying your negative thoughts when you experience pain or an upsetting emotion is the first step in teaching you not to be so hard on yourself. The next step will be to help you learn to evaluate how realistic these thoughts are. This is something we will focus on later in this session.

As a second example, I wrote down what you experienced in session with me a moment ago. You were telling me how hard you are on yourself, and I asked you what you were feeling. You said sad and discouraged. Then I asked you what you were thinking about. You said, "I cannot do anything right." So, here is an example of how I graphed out the situation, your emotions at that time, and your thoughts then. Did you feel any pain in your body when we were talking about how hard you were on yourself?

Patient: Only some minor achy, tight pain in my back . . . about a 3.

Therapist: Okay, let's add that to the Pain column. Do you have any questions about how to fill out the form or about the difference between emotions and thoughts?

Patient: No. It makes sense to me.

Therapist: Okay. We were talking earlier about how hard you are on yourself. Let's look back at this form to see where you might have been hard on yourself in these two examples. [See Figure 7.5.]

IDENTIFYING THE "HOTTEST" COGNITIONS RELATED TO PAIN AND DISTRESS

Once patients have learned how to identify their automatic thoughts using the ATR, the next step is to help them identify which thoughts were the most distressing to them—the ones that bothered them the most. We call these thoughts "hot" cognitions (Padesky and Greenberger, 1995) because

FIGURE 7.5 Logan's revised Automatic Thought Record

SITUATION	AUTOMATIC THOUGHT(S)	EMOTION(S)	PAIN	ALTERNATIVE RESPONSE	OUTCOME
1. Describe the actual event or the experience of pain that led to the unpleasant emotion.	1. What thought(s) and/or image(s) went through your mind? 2. How much did you believe each one at the time? (0–100)	1. What emotion (sad, anxious, angry, etc.) did you feel at the time? 2. How intense (0–100) was the emotion?	1. Where did you experience the pain in your body? 2. How intense (0–10) was the pain? 3. What words would you use to describe the pain (throbbing, burning, aching, tender, etc.)?	1. What cognitive distortion did you make? 2. Use questions at bottom to compose a response to the automatic thought(s). 3. How much do you believe each response? (0–100)	1 How much do you believe each original automatic thought? 2. What emotion(s) do you feel now? How intense (0–100) is the emotion? 3. Describe your pain now. How intense (0-100) is your pain?
Going for a walk in the park. Felt sharp pain in my lower back. Sat down on a bench. Got up and walked again. I tripped on a crack in the sidewalk. My back arched, but I regained my balance and didn't fall.	I cannot even walk three blocks without this pain controlling me. I am clumsy. I cannot do anything right.	Embarrassed, humiliated 100	Sharp, stabbing pain in my lower back when walking 5 When I tripped, sharp, stabbing pain in my lower back 9		
Talking about the tripping accident in session. I am thinking about how hard I am on myself.	I cannot do anything right these days. 95	Sad, discouraged 75	Achy, tight pain in lower back 3		

Questions to help you compose an alternative response: (1) What is the evidence that the automatic thought is true? Not true? (2) Is there an alternative explanation? (3) What's the worst that could happen? What's the best that could happen? What's the most realistic outcome? (4) What's the effect of my believing the automatic thought? What could be the effect of changing my thinking? (5) What should I do about it? (6) If _____ (friend's name) was in this situation and had this thought, what would I tell him/her?

From Judith S. Beck's *Cognitive Therapy: Basics and Beyond.* Copyright 1995 by Judith S. Beck, PhD. Adapted with permission by the Guilford Press: New York.

they are the ones that are most upsetting and the most closely tied to patients' pain and emotional suffering. In reality, it may not always be possible to evaluate and modify every automatic thought that a patient has. Identifying the hottest cognitions will conserve time and help patients make progress more quickly than if every possible automatic thought was examined.

One way to figure out which negative automatic thoughts are the "hottest" is to look at the ATR, under the Emotion(s) column, to identify emotions with high-intensity ratings (e.g., 80 or higher). Alternatively, therapists may look under the Pain column to examine when the pain was most intense (e.g., ratings of 8 to 10 on a scale from 0 to 10). However, this assumes that the hottest cognitions are primarily associated with the most intense emotions or pain levels, which may or may not be the case. Therapists can also look at the strength of patients' thoughts, particularly those that patients believe in the most (e.g., 90 or higher), to gauge which ones are the "hottest." One of the best methods of identifying the hottest cognitions is to simply ask, "Which thought is the most distressing or bothersome to you?" However, some patients do not have the ability or the motivation to make this determination. For example, they may be so overwhelmed that they view all of the thoughts as equally troubling. In such cases, therapists should start with the thoughts that are the most malleable to therapeutic intervention. When moving to the evaluation stage of automatic thought work, therapists need to balance the "hot cognition" criteria with the "easiest to intervene" criteria to determine the best course of action. In the next chapter, we will discuss evaluating automatic thoughts about pain.

8

Evaluating Automatic
Thoughts About Pain

Once patients have learned to identify their automatic thoughts about their pain and other distressing events (especially the most salient, or the "hottest" ones), then these thoughts can be evaluated to determine how realistic, accurate, or helpful they are. There are a variety of steps in the evaluation process. Patients start this process by viewing their thoughts as hypotheses or assumptions rather than facts. Next, therapists and patients explore possible errors in patients' thinking to determine how realistic or accurate their thoughts may be. This is followed by a review of the evidence for and against a particular automatic thought. Some thoughts may be tested, using behavioral experiments, to see if indeed they hold true. Therapists and patients may also explore the worst, best, and most realistic scenarios assuming the negative thought is true. This allows patients to move their thinking in different directions—to anticipate the best, the worst, and what might be a realistic outcome. The underlying motivations for thinking negatively and the consequences for doing so can be clarified using the advantages/disadvantages analysis. Each of these steps will now be discussed.

VIEW AUTOMATIC THOUGHTS AS HYPOTHESES OR ASSUMPTIONS TO TEST OUT

Patients are taught to view their thoughts as hypotheses or assumptions to explore and test out, rather than as facts. Patients are encouraged to think of themselves as scientists or investigators. Cognitive therapy uses the scientific method to help patients evaluate their thought processes. Once hypotheses are established, patients can then learn to test them to see if they are accurate.

USE GUIDED DISCOVERY

Therapists can use one or more of the following interventions to help patients evaluate the accuracy and the usefulness of their negative thinking. The experienced cognitive therapist will use a variety of questions to evaluate negative automatic thoughts with patients. Therapists should not presume that they know what their patients' answers will be to those questions. Cognitive therapy is different from other cognitive-behavioral approaches in the use of questions, within the collaborative therapeutic relationship, to guide patients to make new discoveries about themselves, their experiences of pain, their emotions, and their thoughts. Patients are not told what or how to think. Questioning helps patients see not only the grain of truth but also the unrealistic nature of their thought processes (thus putting these cognitions in a more realistic context).

IDENTIFY ERRORS OR LOGICAL DISTORTIONS IN THOUGHTS

Patients can learn about the basic types of errors people make in their thinking after they have learned to identify and monitor their thoughts, emotions, and pain levels in distressed situations (first four columns of the Automatic Thought Record [ATR]). A list of these common cognitive distortions is reviewed in session. Each cognitive distortion category is explained, and examples are provided. Patients often find it helpful to identify their own examples for each type of cognitive distortion. Figure 8.1 provides a list of these cognitive distortions. (This list was adapted from Beck, Rush, Shaw, & Emery, 1979; Beck, 1995; and Burns, 1989.)

After introducing these distortions, therapists can help patients catch these cognitive errors when negative automatic thoughts arise. Some common questions used by therapists to help patients identify errors in thinking are

- Let's look at the list of errors in thinking and tell me which ones might fit with this thought.
- What cognitive distortion(s) did you make?

Patients should be encouraged to identify the cognitive distortion(s) from the list. If a patient is having difficulty identifying these errors, the therapist can review the list until both are clear on which distortion most accurately describes the type of error(s) made in the patient's thinking. More than one cognitive error usually can be found in negative automatic thoughts.

FIGURE 8.1 Cognitive Distortions (Errors in Thinking)

1. *All-or-nothing thinking.* You view your pain, yourself, people, or events as falling into extreme, opposing categories (e.g., good or bad, beautiful or ugly, perfect or defective, pain-free or pain-ridden) instead of seeing them as falling along a continuum.

> Examples: "I can't do *anything*. Having this chronic pain makes me feel like a *total* failure."
>
> "I am in pain *all* of the time. It *never* stops hurting. It *never* ends."
>
> "*Nothing* you say or do is going to help me cope with this pain."

2. *Overgeneralization.* You make sweeping negative conclusions based on little evidence. Or you view one negative event as a never-ending pattern of defeat.

> Examples: "If this doctor can't help me, no one can." (All physicians are the same.)
>
> "This first epidural injection didn't help my lower back pain. This just goes to show you that you cannot trust medicine to help you. What's the point of trying?" (If one medical intervention won't work, nothing will.)

3. *Negative mental filter (selective abstraction).* You tend to focus selectively on negative details taken out of context (tunnel vision) while ignoring the bigger picture of the situation, which may include positive experiences (disqualifying the positive). Mental filtering relates to your attention and focus on information in your environment (e.g., attending vs. not attending to your pain or your ability to cope with pain).

> *Tunnel vision:* You see only the negative aspects of a situation.
> Example: "All I can see is bad things happening to me."
> *Disqualifying the positive* (type of mental filter). You filter out positive experiences, so they do not enter your awareness. You don't give yourself credit for the good things you do or the positive aspects of life.
> Example: "Even if I did complete the project, it took me five times as long to finish it because of the pain."
> "If my doctor was being nice to me, it was because she had to. It was her job."

4. *Magnification (of the negative) and minimization (of the positive).* You magnify or exaggerate the significance of negative qualities in yourself (e.g., weaknesses), someone else, or an event; you minimize or shrink the significance of positive qualities in yourself (e.g., strengths), others, or an event.

Examples: "When I'm in pain, I tend to be absorbed in my sense of failure—in my insecurities." (magnifying)
"My efforts to achieve don't count for much now that I am disabled with this pain." (minimizing)

5. *Catastrophizing (jumping to conclusions).* You tend to assume the worst and fail to consider more realistic possibilities. You may jump to conclusions and assume the worst in your relationships (by "mind reading") or in general (by "negative forecasting" or "fortune-telling").

Mind reading: You assume people are reacting very negatively toward you without sufficient evidence. In assuming you can read other peoples' minds, you misread or misinterpret verbal and nonverbal cues in relationships as signs of rejection or failure. Example: "My partner doesn't care about me and my pain. I can tell even if he/she hasn't said it in so many words."

Negative forecasting (fortune-telling error): You anticipate negative outcomes in the future without sufficient evidence.
Examples: "I am doomed to be stuck with this pain forever."
"Having this chronic pain is a catastrophe. There is nothing to look forward to."

6. *Emotional reasoning.* When you reason with your emotions, you assume they reflect the way things really are. If you feel emotions, you assume that they must be true, without considering other possible explanations or discounting them. When some people experience pain, they use their pain and their emotions to explain why they cannot engage with the world around them or take control of their lives.

Examples: "Even though I'm taking steps to cope with my pain, I still feel like such a failure."
"I feel like this pain has robbed me of my identity."
"The pain reminds me of what I cannot do. Why even try?"
"I feel as though people don't want to be around me when I'm in pain."

7. *"Should" statements.* You have precise, fixed ideas of how events occur in life and how you or other people should behave. When your expectations of yourself, others, or events are not met, you view this as horrible or bad. In expressing "shoulds," you may be attempting to motivate yourself or someone else. However, your "should" often ends up punishing, rather than motivating, yourself or others. "Shoulds" directed toward oneself typically result in guilt. "Shoulds" directed toward others or situations in general typically result in anger.

FIGURE 8.1 *(continued)*

Examples: "I should not have to deal with this chronic pain. No one should. It's unfair."

"My doctor should help me find a solution to my pain. It shouldn't take this long."

"Life just isn't fair. People shouldn't have to suffer with this chronic type of pain."

"I should be able to work again."

8. *Labeling.* You tend to use simplistic, fixed, global terms to describe yourself, others, or a specific situation without acknowledging the bigger picture or the complexity of the situation.

Examples: "I'm *stupid* for thinking I can trust others."

"My friend is a *jerk* for telling someone else about my chronic pain problem."

"I am a *cripple.*"

9. *Personalization (self-blame).* You tend to assume responsibility for negative events or interactions, without considering other possible explanations or evidence to the contrary.

Examples: "My doctor was very short with me during my last office visit. I must have done something to make him/her mad."

"My friends haven't called me in weeks. It's my fault because all I ever talk about is my pain and suffering."

From J. Beck's *Cognitive Therapy: Basics and Beyond.* Copyright 1995 by Judith S. Beck, PhD. Adapted with permission by the Guilford Press: New York.

In Logan's case, he caught himself saying, "There I go again. How stupid can I be!" He and his therapist reviewed the list to identify the errors or distortions he might be making. Calling oneself "stupid" is an example of the "labeling" error. However, as the therapist and Logan explored how he came to the conclusion that he was "stupid," Logan said, "Well, that is how I was feeling then. I felt so embarrassed." The therapist could then point out how Logan used his feelings of embarrassment to reason that he was stupid. This is an example of the "emotional reasoning" error. In the Alternative Response column of the Automatic Thought Record, Logan wrote, "Cognitive errors— labeling and emotional reasoning."

The cognitive distortions can also be written down on a separate form, along with the answers to the other evaluation questions listed at the bottom of the ATR, to allow enough room to record information. See Figure 8.2.

FIGURE 8.2 Thought Evaluation Form

Automatic thought:

What is the evidence that the automatic thought is true?

What is the evidence that the automatic thought is not true?

Is there an alternative explanation?

What is the worst that could happen if the automatic thought were true? Could I live with it?

What's the best that could happen?

What is the most realistic outcome?

What's the effect of my believing the automatic thought? (advantages/disadvantages of believing it)

What could be the effect of changing my thinking? (advantages/disadvantages of letting go of it)

What should I do about it?

If _____(friend's name) was in this situation, what would I tell him/her?

From "Worksheet Packet," Bala Cynwyd, PA, Beck Institute for Cognitive Therapy and Research, Copyright 1996. Used with permission from Judith S. Beck, PhD.

In an earlier example, Bernice felt out of control with her pain. The thought "I cannot control it [the pain]" was identified as a hypothesis to be tested out. Bernice and her therapist reviewed all of the cognitive distortions on the list (i.e., reading each error and its description, one at a time, asking if this thought could fit in the categories). Bernice identified "negative mental filter" (focusing on the negative) and "magnification/minimization" (not giving oneself credit for her abilities to cope with pain) as possible errors in her thinking. In addition, her therapist pointed out that she may be engaging in "all-or-nothing thinking" by assuming that she had no control whatsoever. In the Alternative Response column of the ATR, Bernice wrote, "Cognitive distortions—negative mental filter, magnification/minimization, and all-or-nothing thinking."

It can take patients some time to learn to catch the errors in their automatic thoughts. Patients should be encouraged keep this list handy—in their purses or wallets, on their refrigerators, on mirrors, or at other key locations—so that they will eventually memorize these errors in thinking. Knowing and remembering these types of errors in thinking will be helpful.

EXPLORE THE EVIDENCE FOR AND AGAINST AUTOMATIC THOUGHTS ABOUT PAIN AND OTHER DISTRESSING EVENTS

After patients learn to identify their cognitive distortions, they are taught how to put their automatic thoughts to the test by exploring the evidence for and against those thoughts to find out how realistic and accurate they are. The typical questions that therapists use in this part of therapy include

- What is the evidence that your thought is true?
- What is the evidence that your thought is not true?

In Bernice's case, "I can't control my pain" was identified as the "hottest" cognition to explore. The therapist asks Bernice, "What is the evidence that you cannot control your pain?" All of the experiences that confirm or support the hypothesis are written down as evidence for the automatic thought in the Alternative Response column of the ATR. The therapist could facilitate this process by asking Bernice to complete sentences such as "I cannot control my pain because . . ." and "I believe this because. . . ." An example of an entry here is "No matter what I do, the pain will still be there."

Here are some examples of questions therapists can use to explore the thought "I am not in control of my pain":

- What leads you to believe that you have no control over your pain?
- What is the evidence that you cannot control your pain?
- Give me some examples of when you had no control over your pain.

Patients are then asked to list the evidence against their automatic thoughts—evidence that their thoughts may not be true. This task is usually more difficult for patients because they have devoted a great deal of time (and practice) thinking of evidence to support their viewpoint, while they have given little time or energy to considering the evidence to the contrary. Here are some questions that address evidence against the negative automatic thought mentioned earlier:

- What's the evidence that you have some control over your pain?
- So you are telling yourself that you are not in control of your pain. How much control do you think you have? (The therapist could illustrate this by drawing a circle, or "pie," that represents the patient's pain and asking the patient to "cut out" from the "pie" how much of the pain he or she can control.)
- Let's explore the times when you have had some success, however small, in coping with or controlling your pain.
- Give me some examples when you had some control in managing your pain.
- What have you tried to help you cope with your pain?
- What pain management strategies have been recommended by your physician/nurse/physical therapist?
- How do you know when you have control of the pain?
- How much control do you think most people have over their pain?
- What do you think others do to cope with their pain so that it is more tolerable?

In asking these questions, the therapist is trying to highlight the ways in which the patient has tried to control or manage his or her pain or ways of managing the pain that he or she had not considered before.

It is often helpful for therapists and patients to develop a chart listing the evidence for and against the automatic thought. This can be entered under the Alternative Response column of the ATR or on a separate form as shown in Figure 8.2 mentioned earlier (includes all questions related to the Alternative Response column). This evidence can also be written on an index card, or coping card.

Here was the evidence Bernice and her therapist collected:

Automatic thought: "I cannot control my pain."
(all-or-nothing thinking)

Evidence that this thought may be true	*Evidence that this thought may not be true*
No matter what I do, the pain is still there.	When I push myself too hard, my pain gets worse, so pacing myself helps some.
My doctor said that I will always have this pain.	I am taking steps to better understand my chronic pain condition.
My medication does not take pain away for very long.	My medication helps dull the pain for a while. The relaxation exercises help me cope.

After the therapist and patient have gathered evidence for and against a particular negative automatic thought, each piece of evidence in the "Evidence for" column can be reviewed to see which ones are salient and valid and which are not. Is it really true that no matter what the patient does, the pain is still there, and that it is always of the same intensity? Or is this an example of emotional reasoning? When the patient in this case acknowledged that pacing does help the pain, she provided evidence that what she does really matters in relation to her pain. Although the physician may have told Bemice that she would always have pain, does that mean she has no control over it? The therapist could follow up with questions about the physician's perceptions of the patient's ability to control her pain as well as the physician's intentions in telling her that she will always have pain. Although the medication does not diminish the pain for very long, it does help dull it for a period of time. Some patients believe medical interventions are the only solution to pain. However, patients learn that their ability to cope with pain resides in their personal efforts as well—for example, activity pacing, their attitudes or outlook on their pain, and their efforts in learning as much as they can about their condition.

Through this guided discovery process, patients will also uncover the grain of truth in many of their automatic thoughts. No one can totally control whether he or she is going to experience pain or not, nor when the pain is going to occur.

On the other hand, people can control how they interpret and respond to their pain. Although people cannot control or manage their pain 100%

of the time, they can learn to cope with their pain. To hold the thought that one can have some degree of control over pain is in itself empowering.

IDENTIFY THE BEST, WORST, AND MOST REALISTIC OUTCOMES IF THE AUTOMATIC THOUGHT IS TRUE

Chronic pain patients tend to imagine the worst-case scenarios related to their pain and distress, rather than focusing on best-case scenarios or realistic outcomes. Patients can examine their notions of both extremes—the worst and best possible outcomes, and what they believe will realistically happen if their thoughts are true (usually this is somewhere between the best and worst possible outcomes). This technique helps patients evaluate the possible outcomes of their negative thinking.

Here are examples of questions that therapists can ask patients to identify the worst, best, and realistic scenarios assuming patients' automatic thoughts are true.

- What is the worst that could happen? Could you live with it?
- What is the best that could happen?
- What is the most realistic outcome?

The following is a therapist–patient dialogue that illustrates a discussion of best, worst, and most realistic scenarios assuming the patient's automatic thought is true.

Therapist: We have been talking today about the fears you have related to the thought "You cannot control your pain." Let's assume for a moment that it's true that you are not in control of your pain at all. What is the worst thing that could happen?

Patient: That I have to endure this miserable pain forever and that I won't be able to work.

Therapist: So the worst-case scenario is that you will be miserable and unemployed. Does it get any worse than that?

Patient: No.

Therapist: What will "miserable" look and feel like?

Patient: Just full of pain and suffering. I can see my face all crinkled up because the pain is so overwhelming. No one will want to be around me . . . that's miserable.

[Under the Alternative Response column of the Automatic Thought Record, the therapist writes down "Worst: Miserable and unemployed, full of pain and suffering, isolated from others."]

Therapist: Anything else?
Patient: No, I think that about covers it.

Therapist: So, if it were true that you had no control over your pain, the worst would be feeling miserable, full of pain and suffering, being unemployed, and feeling isolated from others. Does that describe the worst scenario you were talking about?
Patient: Yes. Gosh, when I hear you saying that, it sounds so pitiful.

Therapist: What is the best thing that could happen if you have no control over your pain?
Patient: I don't know. I've never thought about that before. [long pause] Maybe the doctors and my family will start to realize what I have been worried about for so long and will finally find the right treatment or medication for me to stop this pain and suffering. Maybe they would stop blaming me.

Therapist: Sounds like you feel hurt and believe that others don't understand your pain and suffering.
Patient: Yes, and all I get are quick fixes that don't work. Just take a pill; just do a little bit more physical therapy. When they see that all of this doesn't work, then they will appreciate what I have been saying. I have been trying, you know.

[Therapist writes a note as a reminder that the patient has been trying to cope with the pain. This will be explored further after the worst, best, and most realistic scenarios have been identified.]

Therapist: Sounds like you want people to understand that you are trying to cope with your pain.
Patient: Yeah. I just need a break. This is not all in my head. This pain really hurts, and I feel so out of control with it . . . not only the pain but also how people treat me. I am tired of people telling me it's all in my head.

[There are two important automatic thoughts the patient just shared that can be explored later—"I am not in control of how people treat me" and "People think my pain is all in my head"—implying that people do not treat her well.]

Therapist: Well, we can explore this more in a few moments. This seems important to your sense of control—feeling that people respect you and understand your pain. So, if it is true that you cannot control your pain at all, then the best that could happen is that your physicians, family, and friends will finally realize that you have tried to cope and that they will provide you with better support and helpful medical treatments.

Patient: Yes, I think that sums it up.

Therapist: What do you think is the most realistic outcome if indeed you have no control over your pain?

Patient: I guess we will continue to explore other medications, treatments, and such. But they probably won't find the "miracle cure" right now. I guess I'll continue to be in pain.

Therapist: What do you think is the most realistic outcome about how people will treat you if indeed it is true that you cannot control your pain?

Patient: I don't know. [pause]

Therapist: If you did know . . .

Patient: Maybe someone will understand me.

Therapist: How would that happen?

Patient: I guess I would probably have to tell people more about my experiences.

Therapist: Do you think that might help you cope better with your pain?

Patient: Um . . . maybe.

Therapist: You know, Bernice, there has been some research out there to show that perceptions of support have more of an impact on people than their actual levels of support. In other words, if you really believe that people don't care about you and your pain, when in fact they might, this belief will have a big impact on your emotions, your decisions and behaviors, as well as your physiological state of well-being.

Patient: So, are you saying that I have support?

Therapist: I'm not sure yet, since I don't have enough information. But maybe we can find out how much support you really have by viewing this thought as a hypothesis to test out and have you conduct an experiment to test the accuracy of your thoughts about how people treat you.

Patient: Okay, but how do we do that?

Therapist: Before we move to that process, let's quickly write down the best, worst, and most realistic outcomes you mentioned earlier.

That way we can refer back to these later when you do conduct an
experiment to see if your predictions will hold true.
Patient: Sounds good to me.

Most patients initially believe that their worst-case scenarios are the realistic ones. It is in these cases that behavioral experiments can be implemented
to see if patients worst fears or concerns are indeed realistic and true.

CONDUCT BEHAVIORAL EXPERIMENTS TO TEST
ACCURACY OF AUTOMATIC THOUGHTS

Patients can be encouraged to test out the reality of their automatic
thoughts by conducting behavioral experiments. These tests or experiments are often behavioral in that patients are asked to take some action
to investigate the accuracy of their thoughts. To start this process, the therapist can ask questions such as:

- How could we find out whether this thought is accurate?
- How could we put this thought to the test to see if it is true?

Here are some general guidelines for developing behavioral experiments:

- Encourage the patient to be actively involved in this process.
- Use open-ended questions to help identify possible ways to test the
  accuracy of the patient's automatic thoughts.
- Brainstorm a number of possible experiments.
- Realize that you, as the therapist, are responsible for guiding the
  development of the behavioral experiments. Because some patients
  have been stuck in their negative thinking for some time, they may
  not have the objectivity needed to develop such experiments.
- Behavioral experiments should be individually tailored to the patient
  and to the automatic thought(s) being tested.
- Develop experiments that will test the accuracy of the patient's automatic thoughts. This goal should always be kept in mind when gen-
  erating experiments.
- Develop experiments that are likely to be carried out by the patient.
  Do not develop an experiment that the patient cannot or will not
  carry out. This involves keeping the patient's motivation and ability
  levels in mind. (For example, if the patient has poor social skills, he
  or she may not be successful in testing out thoughts in social situations until competence is developed in this area.)

- Once an experiment has been developed, discuss the plans for implementing this experiment—help the patient to succeed in putting it into action.
- Encourage the patient to document the actual outcomes of the experiment (e.g., journaling, audiotaping interviews).

Here are some examples of behavioral experiments:

- Monitor times when the patient's thoughts are not true, and chart these in a journal entry. In other words, put the "spotlight" on any evidence that the patient's thoughts are inaccurate.
- Have other people (e.g., friend, family member) monitor or record the patient's behaviors (e.g., how often the patient remains inactive; how often the patient pushes himself or herself too hard).
- Have the patient act as if his or her thoughts are not true (e.g., act as if he or she can manage the pain). This requires teaching the patient to play specific roles between therapy sessions.
- Have the patient face his or her fears and take on challenges (e.g., prepare for a medical procedure, then go through with it).
- Interview a person who is going through the same experience (e.g., another person who has chronic pain).
- Interview people who are close to the patient about the topic of concern. (This is especially helpful when the patient makes assumptions about his or her relationships with others, e.g., "No one cares about me or my pain").
- Talk with physicians or other healthcare professionals about the patient's concerns. (This puts the automatic thoughts "out there" with physicians to determine their impressions of the concerns.)
- Collect information about topics of concern (e.g., patient's chronic condition or medical treatment), and generate specific questions to ask doctors at their next visits; obtain books and other materials, including Internet resources, on the topics of concern.
- Try out new strategies (e.g., relaxation to reduce pain, assertiveness training to improve communication) to see if they are effective.

Chronic pain patients need to understand that there may be a number of benefits as well as potential risks involved in conducting a behavioral experiment. In many cases, behavioral experiments expose the inaccuracies of patients' automatic thoughts. By taking risks to collect more information and evidence, patients' worst fears and expectations may prove to be unfounded. If this is the case, patients can begin to alter their thoughts and beliefs about their pain and distress. Behavioral experiments also help patients become "action-oriented" about their problems and provide a structured opportunity to interact more with others (e.g., if they were to interview others; if they were encouraged to attend a social event), instead of isolating themselves—a common occurrence in this patient population. These are just some of the possible benefits associated with this technique.

It is also possible that behavioral experiments indeed confirm patients' worst fears or expectations. In these cases, patients will have the support of their therapists to help them cope with this reality (i.e., that the negative thought is realistic and accurate). When this happens, some patients may be motivated to change, whereas others may become more despondent. Ultimately, patients can choose to hold on tightly to their misery, or they can take steps to deal with their problems, whatever they may be (e.g., their conditions may be chronic, doctors may not have clear-cut diagnoses regarding their pain conditions, they may have to deal with pain for the rest of their lives, some people in their lives may not care about their pain).

> To test the thought "I can't control my pain," Bernice and her therapist decided that she would investigate how other people manage their pain, including their perceived level of control over their pain. The actual test would involve interviewing several people with chronic pain about these experiences. Bernice was asked to select some people who are further along in their treatment or experience of pain, so that she can learn from their experiences. For example, Bernice just recently joined a chronic pain support group. This group would provide the opportunity to test out her negative automatic thought to see if it was accurate or not. Bernice might also find more support in such a group by realizing that she is not alone in her struggles with pain.

> Although this experiment is not a direct test of the hypothesis "I am not in control of my pain," it tests the assumption that no one with chronic pain is in control of his or her pain, which Bernice said at times during the sessions to justify her negative automatic thought. If Bernice finds that other people with chronic pain perceive some control over their pain, then it invalidates her assumption, which may invalidate her original thought, "I am not in control of my pain." She may also learn some new ways to cope with her pain by interviewing others.

Another possible behavioral experiment for the automatic thought "I can't control my pain" involves having patients notice their attempts to cope or manage pain when it occurs. Because patients have had a lot of practice remembering when they cannot control the pain, they need to focus on the situations and times when they actually took steps to try and manage it. Any time that patients notice personal attempts to cope with pain, they can record the situation, their pain levels, and how they coped. This written homework assignment can be reviewed in the next session to see how often patients try to take charge of their pain and what their current success is in coping with their pain.

To prepare patients to conduct behavioral experiments, the specifics of the experiments should be identified. For example, Logan agreed to act as if he is competent and capable over the next week (in contrast to his negative thought, "I can't do anything."). Defining this role will be very important. What will he do differently if he is competent and capable? ("Move slower and with more confidence.") Will he feel differently? ("Confident and comfortable with myself.") What will he say to himself if he is competent and capable? ("I am capable of doing things. I just need to slow down. If I trip again, it is just an accident, not a sign of my character.") How will he handle his pain? ("I will cope with it the best that I can. Slowing down my pace will help prevent accidents.") For behavioral experiments that involve interviews, key questions need to be developed so that patients are testing out their hypotheses. In Bernice's case, the following questions were generated for her interviews with people in group (or elsewhere) who have chronic pain:

- Do you have any control over your pain?
- How much control do you have over your pain, on a scale from 0 to 100, with 0 being *no control at all* and 100 being *total control?*
- How do you control your pain?
- How do you cope with your pain?
- Have you ever thought that you didn't have any control over your pain? If so, how did you deal with that thought?

Patients next prepare to gather information or "evidence." In Logan's case, he agreed to keep a daily journal of his experiences ("collecting data") when he acted as if he was competent and capable. In Bernice's case, she identified a few people she knew she could interview. If patients know other people with chronic pain, then these people can be asked for their help. If not, patients can contact their doctors to ask if they have any patients who would be willing to talk about their pain and their experiences with them. Bernice agreed to "interview" people in the group after getting acquainted with everyone.

Therapists and patients then decide how patients will introduce their experiment if it involves talking with or interviewing others. The therapist might say to Bernice, "How do you want to start the interview? You may want to provide these people with a brief introduction to your topic of interest, without revealing your hypothesis." A neutral introduction might be "I am interested in asking people a few questions about their pain and how they deal with it. I have chronic low back pain. So, I am really interested in how your experiences compare with mine." To keep track of each response to the question, Bernice could either write down people's responses or audiotape their responses with their permission. Audiotaping may be acceptable to people who are familiar with the patients but not for group members.

Once therapists and patients have taken steps to prepare for the the experiment, therapists should ask the patients what, if any, predictions they have about the outcome. Here is Logan's prediction: "Well, if I act like I'm more confident and capable, maybe I won't get into so many accidents . . . like tripping or hurting my body. I might actually feel better about myself too." In Bernice's case, she expected that other people with chronic pain will not have any control over their pain either. These are the hypotheses to be tested.

After the behavioral experiment has been conducted, therapists and patients can explore the outcomes in the following therapy session. Ultimately, any outcome of these behavioral experiments will help patients learn about new information and experiences that can offer further insight. As a result, patients will either modify their thoughts or form a different action plan. Problem solving will be discussed later in the next chapter.

Bernice and her therapist reviewed the outcomes of her behavioral experiment.

Therapist: Well, how did things go this past week? Were you able to complete your interviews?

Patient: Yes, I did. I interviewed three people with chronic pain, like we discussed last week. These were all people I knew from work and from the gym. I didn't feel ready to ask the members of my chronic pain support group yet. But I hope to talk with them about this next week. I was a little nervous about doing this experiment. . . . It was awkward at first. But I told them that I wanted to know how they coped with their pain and how much control they had over their pain. I found out that I wasn't alone in feeling frustrated with this chronic pain. I learned that there were times when all of them wished they could be in "total control" of their pain.

What I learned is that "controlling the pain" is not the issue—managing or coping with pain is. Most of the people still have pain. They just cope with it differently now than they did before. One of them does yoga and meditates regularly; another person found that it took over 2 years to finally find the right medication that worked for her pain; another uses relaxation techniques and enjoys watching sports as a distraction.

One guy said, "It's all about your attitude toward your pain." This really hit me hard because I realize now that I have had a pretty negative attitude about my pain. [pause]

So, I guess what I learned is that the pain might remain with me for a while, maybe even the rest of my life. But if other people can deal with their pain . . . maybe I can too. I can't believe it, but I feel a little better now that I did this exercise.

Therapist: You seem surprised. What has allowed you to feel better?

Patient: I guess realizing that having "total control" over my pain is an ideal that can't be reached . . . realizing that I am not alone in feeling frustrated . . . just feeling hopeful that others have found something that helps them feel better.

Therapist: That's great! Well, we have taken a good look at the thought "I can't control my pain." Now that you have conducted your investigation, how accurate or helpful is this thought or hypothesis?

Patient: Well, no one has total control over pain. So, to expect myself to achieve this goal is not helpful to me. But managing my pain is a realistic goal.

Therapist: How strongly do you believe the original thought "I can't control my pain," on a scale from 0 to 100?

Patient: Zero. It's just not accurate.

Therapist: Okay, you mentioned a number of things you learned from conducting this experiment. Let's write these down now. This will help remind us of what you learned from this experiment in case you get stuck in your negative thinking again. It will also help us construct an alternative, more realistic response to your thought, "I can't control my pain."

The results of these experiments can be written in the Alternative Response column of the Automatic Thought Record or on a separate form (see Figure 8.3). This information will help patients construct alternative, more realistic responses to their original negative automatic thoughts.

CONDUCT ADVANTAGES/DISADVANTAGES ANALYSIS

Some patients hold on tightly to negative automatic thoughts about their pain and life events, despite therapists' efforts to help them evaluate their thoughts. (This is usually a sign of an intermediate or core belief being activated.) Therapists can use an advantages/disadvantages analysis to better understand patients' motivations for holding onto these thoughts

---

FIGURE 8.3 Results of the behavioral experiment

Automatic thought: "I cannot control my pain."
Behavioral experiment: I interviewed several people with chronic pain to see if they think they have control over their pain. If so, I want to know how they control it and cope with it.
Summary of findings:
- Everyone at some point in time said they had thoughts that they could not control their pain.
- It is not an issue of control, it is an issue of pain management—how to cope with it.
- Attitude is important. Don't let the pain convince you that you can't do anything.
- Stay active in some way, by meditating, relaxing, or exercising (with consultation from doctors).
- Some people use hot pads, cold packs, or take medications to cope with their pain, especially when it is really bad.

What have I learned? How do these findings apply to me?
- I realized that I am not that different from other people who experience chronic pain. It is very frustrating at times, especially when I am in a lot of pain, but that doesn't mean that the pain has to consume me—to consume my life.
- I need to start getting more actively involved in coping with my pain.
- This is not an issue of control. It is an issue of dealing with the pain. I can learn to cope with it.

(advantages) as well as the consequences (disadvantages) of doing so. This technique helps patients evaluate the usefulness of their thoughts. How is thinking this way helping me? Hurting me? What is this thought doing for me? Not doing for me?

There are two steps in this technique. The first step is to explore the advantages and disadvantages of believing the negative automatic thought. The second step is to explore either the advantages and disadvantages of changing the negative automatic thought in general (used in the evaluating phase) or the advantages and disadvantages of believing an alternative, more realistic thought (developed during the modification phase). This intervention helps patients realize the costs and benefits of thinking negatively as well as the reasons or the motivations to change them. This will prepare patients for the last step in the cognitive restructuring process: modifying automatic thoughts. Here are some examples of open-ended questions that therapists can use to explore the advantages and disadvantages of patients thinking negatively versus changing their thinking:

- What is the effect of believing this thought?
- What are the advantages of believing this thought?
- What are the disadvantages of believing this thought?
- What could be the effect of changing your thinking?
- What could be the advantages of changing your thinking?
- What could be the disadvantages of changing your thinking?

Here is a therapist–patient dialogue demonstrating the use of advantages/disadvantages analysis.

Therapist: Bernice, what are the advantages of believing that you cannot control your pain?

Patient: I don't think there are any. [pause] I guess it allows me to feel miserable when I want to be.

Therapist: Any other advantages you can think of?

Patient: I guess I might get attention for it, if I said it to other people, like my doctor or my partner.

FIGURE 8.4 Advantages/Disadvantages Analysis Form

Automatic thought:

Advantages of Believing This Thought (benefits, what it does for me)	**Disadvantages of Believing This Thought** (costs, drawbacks)
Advantages of Changing This Thought (letting it go)	**Disadvantages of Changing This Thought** (letting it go)

From "Worksheet Packet," Bala Cynwyd, PA, Beck Institute for Cognitive Therapy and Research. Copyright 1996. Adapted with permission from Judith S. Beck, PhD.

Therapist: What are some other ways that you can get people's attention?

Patient: Probably letting them know that I am feeling frustrated that the pain is still severe and strong off and on throughout the week. Probably telling my doctor that I don't think the medications or the injections are working.

Therapist: How would you feel if you approached support in that way?

Patient: It would be awkward at first, but I would probably feel a lot better in the long run if I tried that out. Sometimes I am not always direct in telling people what I need.

Therapist: Okay, those are some great insights that we can come back to later. Are there any other advantages to holding onto the belief that you can't control your pain?

Patient: No. I think that covers it.

Therapist: What might be some of the disadvantages of believing that you can't control your pain?

Patient: I'm not sure I understand.

Therapist: Are there some costs or drawbacks to thinking this way?

Patient: It really doesn't make me feel better. It makes me feel so anxious and desperate. I guess I really don't want to feel that way. [pause] I wonder if people might think I'm complaining and not take me seriously.

Therapist: Help me understand how that would happen.

Patient: If I said it loud enough and often enough, people might just give up on me and not listen to me anymore.

Therapist: So if you kept saying "I can't control my pain," over and over again, people might tune you out?

Patient: Yes. That does concern me.

Therapist: Any other disadvantages of believing that you cannot control your pain at all?

Patient: Maybe I'm not giving myself credit for my efforts. Remember earlier in the session when you asked me the best thing that could happen if I couldn't control it? Well, I caught myself saying that I am trying to cope. At least I'm trying. I haven't totally given up hope yet, even though I feel like it. So, focusing on what I can't do may prevent me from acknowledging what I can do to cope with this pain. I'm also hoping that, just maybe, this therapy can help me control my pain better. I think that's all that I can think of for now.

Therapist: Okay, well, I've written what you said on this form. Let's review what we've just discussed.

Advantages and Disadvantages of Believing "I cannot control my pain"

<u>Advantages</u>	<u>Disadvantages</u>
It allows me to feel miserable.	It makes me feel anxious and desperate.
	I might be perceived as a complainer.
It might help me get some attention.	I might not be taken seriously.
	I'm not giving myself credit for my efforts.

Therapist: What do you notice as you look at this page so far?
Patient: Gosh, there are clearly more disadvantages here.

Therapist: Yes. Thinking this way makes you feel anxious and desperate, and it doesn't give you credit for your coping efforts. You're also concerned that people may not take you seriously and view you as a complainer if you keep telling people how out of control your pain is.

[Starting the second step of this technique: advantages and disadvantages of letting go of this negative thought.]

Therapist: What would be the advantages of letting go of the thought "I cannot control my pain," of thinking differently about your pain?
Patient: [long pause] Well, if I didn't carry that thought around with me all the time, maybe I would feel better . . . I might feel less anxious and depressed.

Therapist: Any other advantages?
Patient: I might be able to do more things if I wasn't so focused on what I can't do.

Therapist: Anything else?
Patient: No, I think that covers it.

Therapist: What would be the disadvantages of letting go of the thought "I cannot control my pain"? Are there any drawbacks or costs of thinking differently about your pain?
Patient: No. I can't think of any costs of letting it go.

Therapist: Okay. Well, let's take a look at what we just did.

Advantages and Disadvantages of Changing
(Letting Go of) the Thought "I cannot control my pain"

<u>Advantages</u>   <u>Disadvantages</u>

I might feel better (less anxious and depressed)   None
I might be able to focus more on what I can do.
I might be able to accomplish more.

Therapist: What was this exercise like for you?
Patient: This negative thought is not helping me feel better. I'm start-
    ing to realize that now.

Once the advantages/disadvantages analysis is completed, therapists
may decide to go back to review each item under the Advantages (of believing the negative thought) column with the patient to see if there are errors
in these thoughts and if there are other possible ways to get these concerns or needs met directly. Some of that work was demonstrated in the
preceding therapist–patient dialogue. It is also helpful to review each item
in the Disadvantages column as evidence to support the possible benefits
of modifying this thought.

In the next chapter, readers will learn how to modify automatic thoughts
about pain.

9

Modifying Automatic Thoughts About Pain and Implementing Problem-Solving Strategies

As patients go through the process of evaluating their negative automatic thoughts, they begin to realize the unrealistic or unhelpful nature of their thoughts and consider the possibility of changing or modifying them. Therapists can help patients explore and develop alternative ways of viewing their chronic pain and events in their lives. However, identifying alternative thoughts should not immediately follow the identification of an automatic thought. The evaluation process is one of the most difficult steps for patients to learn, but it is through this process that they are eventually able to arrive at alternative, realistic thoughts.

GENERATING AN ALTERNATIVE RESPONSE USING QUESTIONS

After automatic thoughts have been identified and evaluated, the therapist can use a variety of open-ended questions to help the patient develop alternative, realistic thoughts about his or her pain and other life events, including

- Is there an alternative explanation?
- What is another way of thinking about your pain (the situation)?
- What is a more realistic way of viewing your pain (situation)?
- It seems as though this automatic thought does not hold true for you now (or is not helpful for you now) that we have explored it fully. If we were to revise this thought to make it more accurate, what would it be?

- If you notice this thought again, what could you say in response to it, given the information you have now?

Here is a therapist–patient dialogue that demonstrates how alternative, more realistic responses can be developed in session using open-ended questions.

Therapist: Now that we have reviewed all of the evidence, what is another way of thinking about your pain and your ability to cope? Is there an alternative explanation?

Patient: Well, I can't control my pain all of the time, but neither can anyone else. I should just hang in there.

Therapist: Why don't we write this down? So, if that original automatic thought, "I can't control my pain," comes back to you the next time you are really hurting, you could respond by saying "I cannot control my pain all of the time, but neither can anyone else."

Patient: Yes, and I'm not alone in feeling frustrated. I'm learning new pain management techniques. I guess if I start learning some ways to cope better, then I will feel better and more in control.

Therapist: Can you read back your response?

Patient: "Hang in there. I cannot control my pain all of the time, but neither can anyone else. I am not alone in feeling frustrated with my pain. However, I am taking steps to learn new pain management techniques. This will help me feel better."

Therapist: How strongly do you believe in these new, alternative thoughts—on a scale from 0 to 100?

Patient: About 90.

Therapist: Okay . . . and how would you feel if you told yourself these new thoughts, over and over again?

Patient: I would feel a lot better . . . probably more satisfied and . . . happy.

Therapist: How would you rate the intensity of each emotion on that 0 to 100 scale?

Patient: Oh, about 85.

Therapist: Before you reported feeling frustrated and sad when you had the thought of not being in control of your pain. Are those feelings still there?

Patient: Yes, but not as strong.

Therapist: How would you rate those emotions now using that same scale, given this new perspective about your ability to cope with your pain?
Patient: I'm slightly frustrated and sad . . . probably around 35.

Therapist: So, those feelings are less intense for you. How would you rate your pain now?
Patient: Probably a 6.

Therapist: So, even your pain levels dropped a bit—from 8 to 6. That's great! What was it like identifying and exploring your emotions and thoughts about pain and arriving at a new conclusion or perspective about your ability to cope?
Patient: I didn't realize how high a standard I had set for myself about my pain. "Having total control" is not realistic. I also realized how much support I could have and that I am not some freak because I feel pain.

To help the patient remember his or her modified thoughts, it is important that the thoughts be written down in session in the Alternative Response column of the Automatic Thought Record (ATR). In the very last column of the ATR, the patient notes the emotions and pain levels associated with the new thought as well as their intensity. It is also helpful to write down the previous emotions and pain levels when the patient had their original automatic thought. This will help gauge the extent to which these emotions and pain experiences are still felt and at what intensity. Most patients find that changing their thinking helps them feel better (i.e., less emotional distress and pain than before).

The patient also can write down any alternative responses on coping cards. On one side of the index card, the original automatic thought is written down along with the evidence for and against the thought, including the outcomes of any behavioral experiments. On the other side of the card, the alternative response is written down along with the strength of belief rating. These cards can be reviewed on a daily basis. The patient can start by reading the alternative thought. If the patient is having a difficult time believing that thought between sessions, he or she can turn the card over to review all of the evidence that led to the development of this alternative thought. Most patients appreciate carrying these cards with them because they are a reminder of what they have accomplished in session and because the cards encourage them to think more realistically. If the patient is having any difficulties with the coping cards, this could be an agenda item for the next therapy session. Here is Bernice's coping card (alternative thought side):

- I cannot control my pain all of the time, but no one else can either. I am taking steps to learn pain management techniques.
- If I am not satisfied with my medical care, then I can talk with my doctor about it.
- If I want people's attention, I can ask them for what I need instead of feeling helpless.

Bernice's completed ATR and thought evaluation form are provided in Figures 9.1 and 9.2, respectively.

GENERATING ALTERNATIVE RESPONSES BY OFFERING "ADVICE TO A FRIEND"

Another way patients can learn to generate alternative, more realistic thoughts is to ask themselves,

- If a good friend of mine was in this situation and had this negative automatic thought, what would I tell him/her?

This technique helps patients to step outside their pain or their situation for a moment. It is amazing how often patients can readily give helpful and realistic advice to others, whereas they tend to be much harsher in their feedback to themselves. This double standard can be confronted in therapy. The therapist can say, "You have some helpful advice for your friend. How does this advice sound to you? How would it feel if you took your own advice?"

Some patients may not have helpful or supportive advice for their hypothetical friends. In that case, the therapist can explore the potential impact of their feedback: "How do you think your friend would feel if he/she received that advice from you?" Another option is to ask the patient what he or she needs to hear from others. This may help the patient develop meaningful alternative thoughts. As a last resort, the therapist can provide some alternative responses the patient had not considered before.

ADVANTAGES/DISADVANTAGES ANALYSIS

As mentioned earlier, the advantages/disadvantages analysis is used to explore patients' motivations to hold onto their original automatic thoughts rather than changing them. The advantages/disadvantages analysis also allows patients to explore the consequences of believing the old automatic thoughts rather than believing the new alternative thoughts. This second

FIGURE 9.1 Bernice's Automatic Thought Record

SITUATION	AUTOMATIC THOUGHT(S)	EMOTION(S)	PAIN	ALTERNATIVE RESPONSE	OUTCOME
1. Describe the actual event or the experience of pain that led to the unpleasant emotion.	1. What thought(s) and/or image(s) went through your mind? 2. How much did you believe each one at the time? (0–100)	1. What emotion (sad, anxious, angry, etc.) did you feel at the time? 2. How intense (0–100) was the emotion?	1. Where did you experience the pain in your body? 2. How intense (0–10) was the pain? 3. What words would you use to describe the pain (throbbing, burning, aching, tender, etc.)?	1. What cognitive distortion did you make? 2. Use questions at bottom to compose a response to the automatic thought(s). 3. How much do you believe each response? (0–100)	1. How much do you believe each original automatic thought? 2. What emotion(s) do you feel now? How intense (0–100) is the emotion? 3. Describe your pain now. How intense (0–100) is your pain?
Bent over to pick up a sock off the floor and felt a sharp, stabbing pain in my lower back.	I can't stop my pain. 90 I cannot control it. 90 I can't even pick up a sock without hurting. 100 Hottest cognition: I can't control it.	Upset 100 Frustrated 100	Sharp, stabbing pain in my lower back 8	Automatic thought: I cannot control it. 1. Magnification/ minimization; Negative mental filter; all-or-nothing thinking 2. Alternative response: Hang in there. I cannot control my pain all of the time, but neither can anyone else. I am not alone in feeling frustrated with my pain. However, I am taking steps to learn new pain management techniques. Hopefully some of them will help. If I start learning some new ways to cope better with my pain, then I will feel better and more in control. 3. 90	I can't control it. 0 Emotions now: Upset 35 Frustrated 35 Satisfied 85 Happy 85 Pain now: 6

Questions to help you compose an alternative response: (1) What is the evidence that the automatic thought is true? Not true? (2) Is there an alternative explanation? (3) What's the worst that could happen if the automatic thought were true? Could I live with it? What's the best that could happen? What's the most realistic outcome? (4) What's the effect of my believing the automatic thought? What could be the effect of changing my thinking? (5) What should I do about it? (6) If _____ (friend's name) was in this situation and had this thought, what would I tell him/her?

From Judith S. Beck's *Cognitive Therapy: Basics and Beyond.* Copyright 1995 by Judith S. Beck, PhD. Adapted with permission from the Guilford Press.

FIGURE 9.2 Bernice's Thought Evaluation Form

Automatic thought: I cannot control my pain.

What is the evidence that the automatic thought is true?
No matter what I do, the pain is still there.
My doctor said that I will always have this pain.
My medication does not take pain away for very long.

What is the evidence that the automatic thought is not true?
When I push myself too hard, my pain gets worse, so pacing myself
helps some.
I am taking steps to better understand my chronic pain condition.
I am taking medication (which gives me some control), even if it isn't
leading to a pain-free existence.

Is there an alternative explanation?
Hang in there. I cannot control my pain all of the time, but neither can
anyone else. I am not alone in feeling frustrated with my pain. However,
I am taking steps to learn new pain management techniques. Hopefully
some of them will help. If I start learning some new ways to cope better
with my pain, then I will feel better and more in control. (90)

**What is the worst that could happen if the automatic thought were true?
Could I live with it?**
Miserable and unemployed, full of pain and suffering, isolated from
others. I don't know if I could live with it.

What's the best that could happen?
My doctors and family will start to realize what I have been worried
about for so long. They will finally find the right treatment or medication
for me to stop this pain and suffering. People would stop blaming me.

What is the most realistic outcome?
Explore other medications and treatments. They won't find a "miracle
cure." I will continue to be in pain.

**What's the effect of my believing the automatic thought?
(advantages/disadvantages of believing it)**
Advantages: It allows me to feel miserable when I want to be. I guess I
might get attention for it if I said it to other people.
Disadvantages: I will continue to feel anxious and desperate. I might be
perceived as a complainer. I might not be taken seriously.

What could be the effect of changing my thinking? (advantages/disadvantages of changing it)
Advantages: I might feel better. I might be able to focus more on what I can do.
Disadvantages: None.

What should I do about it?
Learn some ways to cope with my pain. Find more support for my chronic pain condition.

If _____ (friend's name) was in this situation, what would I tell him/her?
Hang in there. Pain is not something that you can control. It is something that you have to manage or cope with. I know how much it can hurt to be in pain. I'll be there for you when you need me.

From Judith S. Beck, PhD, *"Worksheet Packet,"* Bala Cywyd, PA, Beck Institute for Cognitive Therapy and Research, Copyright © 1996. Adapted with permission.

type of advantages/disadvantages analysis can be implemented after the new alternative responses have been generated in session (see Figures 9.3 and 9.4). The open-ended questions that therapists and patients can use to carry out this part of the exercise include:

- What would be the advantages of believing this new thought?
- What would be the disadvantages of believing this new thought?

Here is a therapist–patient dialogue that demonstrates the second type of advantages/disadvantages analysis, given that the pros and cons of believing the original automatic thought have been identified earlier in therapy.

Therapist: What would be the advantages of believing this new thought?
Patient: Well, it would help me stop thinking so negatively about my pain. It would also remind me of what I have to look forward to—learning how to cope better.

Therapist: Any other advantages?
Patient: None that I can think of right now.

Therapist: Would there be any disadvantages of believing this new thought?
Patient: No, not at all. I think in the past, I used to be pessimistic, to prepare myself for the worst. Now I'm finding that this strategy isn't working too well.

FIGURE 9.3 Advantages/Disadvantages Analysis

Automatic thought:

Advantages of Believing This Thought (benefits, what it does for me)	Disadvantages of Believing This Thought (costs, drawbacks)

Alternative, more realistic thought:

Advantages of Believing This Thought (benefits, what it does for me)	Disadvantages of Believing This Thought (costs, drawbacks)

From "Worksheet Packet," Bala Cynwyd, PA, Beck Institute for Cognitive Therapy and Research, Copyright © 1996. Adapted with permission from Judith S. Beck, PhD.

ROLE-PLAYS

Therapists can also engage patients in role-plays to teach patients how to "talk back" to their negative automatic thoughts. This exercise helps patients develop alternative, realistic responses to their thoughts in the moment. It is recommended that these role-plays be used after patients understand how to identify, evaluate, and modify automatic thoughts using the ATR.

To begin role-playing, the patient typically plays the role of his or her negative automatic thoughts, and the therapist typically plays the role of the "rational responder" to these thoughts. Sharing negative thoughts in such a way offers the therapist a great deal of information about the nature of these thoughts. When the therapist responds rationally to these thoughts,

FIGURE 9.4 Patient's Final Advantages/Disadvantages Analysis

Automatic thought: "I cannot control my pain."

Advantages of Believing This Thought (benefits, what it does for me)	Disadvantages of Believing This Thought (costs, drawbacks)
It allows me to feel miserable when I want to be.	I will continue to feel anxious and desperate.
I guess I might get attention for it if I said it to other people.	I might be perceived as a complainer.
	I might not be taken seriously.
	I am not giving myself credit for my efforts.

Alternative, more realistic thought: "I cannot control my pain all of the time, but no one else can either."

Advantages of Believing This Thought (benefits, what it does for me)	Disadvantages of Believing This Thought (costs, drawbacks)
It would help me stop thinking so negatively about my pain.	No. (In the past, such a thought would not prepare me for the worst.)
It would remind me of what I have to look forward to— learning how to cope better.	

From "Worksheet Packet," Bala Cynwyd, PA, Beck Institute for Cognitive Therapy and Research, Copyright © 1996. Adapted with permission from Judith S. Beck, PhD.

the patient is given the opportunity to hear some possible alternative responses. After a few minutes of dialogue, the therapist and the patient can switch roles. The therapist plays the role of the automatic thoughts, and the patient becomes the "rational responder." This gives the patient the opportunity to practice developing alternative, more realistic responses "in the moment."

Here is an example of a rational role-play with Logan, the patient who thought he was stupid for hurting his back while getting out of the car.

Therapist: You mentioned earlier that it is hard to respond to your automatic thoughts when they pop up during the day. I'm wondering if you would be interested in working on this today, that is, to respond to your automatic thoughts "in the moment."

Patient: Yes, I think that would help me. I find myself getting stuck in my negative thinking. I would like to know how to cope when that happens.

Therapist: Well, one way to do this is to play it out in session. We call this role-playing. For example, you could play the role of your negative thoughts, because you know them so well. I could play the role of the "rational responder." In other words, I will try to develop realistic responses to each of your negative thoughts. This role-play would take a few minutes to carry out. How does that sound to you? Would you be interested in giving this a try?

Patient: Well, I've never done this before, but I could give it a try.

Therapist: [setting up the roles] Okay, let's give it a try? If at any point you want to stop this role-play, let me know. You're going to play the role of your negative thoughts. You will share these thoughts out loud, so that I can respond to them.

Basically what we are going to do is to debate your automatic thoughts. You give me the reasons your thought is true, and I will try to find evidence to the contrary. Can you think of an automatic thought that has been bothering you this past week?

Patient: I'm still feeling upset about how stupid I was for hurting my back.

Therapist: Okay, we could start with that thought. As new thoughts come up, don't hesitate to share them. Are you ready?

Patient: I think so.

Therapist: Okay, you start first.

Patient: [pause] Well, I've been so stupid lately. I can't believe I hurt myself while getting out of the car last week. How embarrassing!

Therapist: Telling myself I'm stupid is "labeling" myself. This was an accident. It could have happened to anyone. It does not mean that I am stupid.

Patient: Yes, but it was so embarrassing! I was such a "klutz!"

Therapist: There I go again "labeling" myself. I don't remember anyone making fun of me or laughing at me when I hurt my back. If anything, I was my own worst critic.

Patient: It's hard to argue that one.

Therapist: Try to give it your best shot.

Patient: Even though no one was there to witness it, that doesn't mean people wouldn't laugh at me.

Therapist: Well, if someone did laugh, that would be an insensitive thing to do. Would I really value the opinions of someone who is that insensitive?

Patient: I guess I agree with that.

Therapist: Let's stop here for a moment. What was the role-play like for you?

Patient: It was kind of weird . . . kind of awkward at first, because I haven't done this before.

Therapist: Anything you have learned from doing this so far?

Patient: I'm making more out of this situation than what really happened. I realize how much I label . . . how I tend to be hard on myself.

Therapist: Okay, well, those are great insights. To finish this exercise, let's switch roles now. I'm going to play the role of your negative automatic thoughts, and you're going to respond to them. In other words, you are going to generate alternative, more realistic responses to these thoughts. Are you ready?

Patient: Yes. But what if I don't do it right?

Therapist: Don't do what right?

Patient: What if I don't respond right? What if I get stuck?

Therapist: I don't expect you to have "perfect" responses to these thoughts. Just give it a try. Let me know if you get stuck. The point of this exercise is to help you learn some new skills and to take some steps toward dealing with your pain and your thoughts about it.

Patient: I see what you mean. Okay, I'm ready.

Therapist: I'll start. [pause] I can't believe how stupid I am for hurting my back last week.

Patient: Why am I being so hard on myself? Let go of the guilt. Yes, you *were* moving too fast, but that doesn't mean you're a "screw up." It could have happened to anyone.

Therapist: Yes, but it was so embarrassing!

Patient: I was ashamed of myself for hurting my back, but I cannot change what happened. I can survive this. Besides, no one saw me doing it. And even if they did, they would probably help. I don't have to assume that I'm going to be rejected by others.

Therapist: That's a hard one to argue. I want to be liked by others. I don't want this pain to turn people away.

Patient: The people who are sensitive will be there to support me. I do want to be liked. But like we've discussed in therapy, I need to like myself and to be kinder to myself first.

Therapist: Okay, let's stop here. What was the second role-play like for you?

Patient: I was amazed at how I could come up with some responses to those negative thoughts.

Therapist: You did a great job! Remember, the first step is to catch those thoughts in action. The next step is to evaluate how accurate they are. Then, we can develop more realistic responses to those thoughts. The role-play speeds up that process a bit more than filling out an Automatic Thought Record. So, if you're stuck on how to respond to a negative automatic thought, back up and ask yourself those questions we have talked about in session: What error might I be making in my thinking? What is the evidence for and against that thought? Is there another explanation? If a friend was going through the same experience, what would I tell him/her? These questions will help you develop a response to those thoughts.

Patient: Sounds good.

PROBLEM-SOLVING STRATEGIES RELATED TO AUTOMATIC THOUGHTS

Sometimes, chronic pain patients' negative automatic thoughts about their pain and life events are indeed accurate. Here are some examples of negative automatic thoughts that may be accurate for some patients:

- My pain is going to be chronic (long-term in nature).
- No one really cares about my pain (when the patient lacks social support).

- I cannot return to work because of my pain.
- Medical interventions are not easing my pain.

In these situations, problem-solving strategies can help patients learn how to cope with these harsh realities by deciding what they want to do about the problem. There are several steps to this process (J. Beck, 1995).

IDENTIFY THE PROBLEM

The patient begins this process by discussing what he or she perceives to be the problem. The therapist can help sort out whether the patient has located the actual problem or simply a smoke screen for other problems.

BREAK DOWN THE PROBLWM INTO SMALLER STEPS

Once the problem is identified, the next step is to understand the various facets of the problem and to divide it into smaller steps. The purpose of doing this is to help the patient solve problems one small step at a time rather than trying to solve one big problem all at once.

DEVELOP A LIST OF POSSIBLE SOLUTIONS

The next step is to generate as many possible solutions to the problem selected.

TAKE ONE STEP TOWARD A SOLUTION

Once a number of solutions have been generated, the patient can agree to try out one of them. To prepare for this, the therapist and patient can explore ways to carry out a particular solution, to increase the likelihood of success.

EVALUATING THE RESULTS OF THE SOLUTION

Once the patient has taken a step toward solving his or her problems, it is important to review the outcomes of this solution in the following session to see how effective it was. Some patients may need to incorporate several solutions in order to deal with a problem. Each step taken toward solving the problem should be commended.

Occasionally, some solutions may not be effective. In those instances, the therapist should explore with the patient what happened to see if it was the solution itself that did not work or how it was implemented that affected the results. After this discussion, an alternative plan or solution can be created.

UNDERSTAND THE AUTOMATIC THOUGHTS, FEELINGS, BEHAVIORS, AND PAIN LEVELS ASSOCIATED WITH THE PROBLEM AND THE POSSIBLE SOLUTIONS

It is important to explore the patient's thoughts, feelings, behaviors, and pain throughout this problem-solving process. Automatic thoughts about this process can hamper the patient's efforts to solve his or her problems.

EVALUATE AND MODIFY AUTOMATIC THOUGHTS REGARDING THE PROBLEM OR THE POTENTIAL SOLUTIONS

Once these negative thoughts are identified, they can be examined to evaluate their accuracy, validity, and usefulness, with the ultimate goal of developing more realistic views about the problem and possible solutions.

Here is a therapist–patient dialogue that illustrates each step of the problem-solving process. Bernice (the patient) has been feeling discouraged and has had automatic thoughts such as "Nobody cares about my pain" and "Nobody understands what I am going through." When this was examined more closely, Bernice realized she was talking specifically about her partner.

Therapist: If you had to sum up what you perceive as the problem between you and Jonathan, what would that be?

Patient: Jonathan doesn't understand my pain. He has no clue how bad my back hurts. He just assumes that I can do all of the things that I used to before I was injured. And he gets really impatient with me . . . like I'm not living up to his expectations. I just feel like I'm talking to a brick wall. Sometimes I get so angry that I cry! Why doesn't he try to understand? I wish he could try.

Therapist: So, if we were to write down in one sentence what you think the problem is, what would we put down on paper here?

Patient: Definitely, communication problems.

[Identifying the problem.]

Therapist: Now, let's see if we can break this problem down into smaller pieces . . . like pieces of a puzzle. You mentioned several issues related to the communication problems between you and Jonathan. [Breaking down problem into smaller steps]. One, Jonathan doesn't understand your pain. Two, you feel pressure to meet his expectations. And three, Jonathan is not listening to you. Does that get at the heart of what you were telling me?

Patient: Yes, it does.

Therapist: So, which one of those issues do you want to work on first?

Patient: I want to work on Jonathan understanding my pain better. The other two feel a little overwhelming to me.

Therapist: Okay, the next step is to figure out how he can learn to understand your pain better. Let's brainstorm as many solutions as we can for the next few minutes.

[Developing a list of possible solutions]

Patient: Well, I just want to yell at him sometimes. But I know that won't help. [pause] Maybe he could come with me to some of my doctor's appointments so that he can hear what the doctor says. Or he could come with me when I get an epidural shot . . . maybe he won't be so critical if he can see what I have to go through.

Therapist: How can he learn to understand your pain experience?

Patient: Maybe I need to tell him when I'm in pain. I could try to tell him when I can and cannot do certain activities. If I could just get him to listen . . . I wish he wouldn't get so defensive. Maybe I should ignore him when he gets defensive.

Therapist: As we have discussed before, it's hard to change other people's behaviors, including Jonathan's, unless they are motivated to change. *You* are in therapy, Bernice, because *you* want to make some changes. So this should be our area of focus—how *you* can do some different things to positively influence your situation.

Patient: I know. I know. It sure would be easier if he would just change.

Therapist: Okay. Any other solutions that you can think of?

Patient: Maybe I should be careful not to get so upset when he doesn't understand. That might push him away.

Therapist: Anything else?

Patient: No, that's all I can think of for now.

Therapist: Well, Bernice, we have generated some possible solutions. Let's look at the list. Is there one solution you would be willing to try out over the next week?

Patient: Gosh, it would be hard to pick one. I guess maybe having him go to some of my appointments with me.

Therapist: Do you have any appointments scheduled this next week?

Patient: Yes, I do.

Therapist: So, maybe the first step is to ask him to come to a doctor's appointment with you next week, for support. [Agreeing to take one step toward solution] How would you go about doing that?

Patient: Maybe I could explain to him how much it would mean to me if he could come to a doctor's appointment with me. His attendance might help him understand more about my pain condition, without my pushing him to understand. Also, he can ask the doctor any questions he has about my pain.

Therapist: That sounds like a plan. Do you have any feelings or thoughts about putting that plan into action? [Understanding the automatic thoughts, feelings, behaviors, and pain levels associated with the problem and the possible solutions]

Patient: I'm worried that he might say no.

Therapist: So, you're feeling worried and you're thinking "Jonathan will say no."

Patient: Yes. That's it.

Therapist: Could there be any possible errors in this thought?

[Evaluating and modifying automatic thoughts regarding the problem or the potential solutions]

Patient: I might be assuming the worst—that fortune-telling error.

Therapist: Okay, do you have any evidence that your thought may be true?

Patient: In the past, there have been times when Jonathan said no to me . . . not wanting to help me. So I have experienced that in the past.

Therapist: Any other evidence that your thought may be true?

Patient: He just doesn't seem to have time for me. [pause] I think that's about it.

Therapist: Any evidence that Jonathan might agree to go with you to the doctor's office?

Patient: When I was injured, he did come to my doctor's appointments early on.

Therapist: Anything else?

Patient: He might go if I tell him why and if I ask him nicely.

Therapist: Is there another way of looking at this situation now that we have reviewed the evidence so far? Instead of assuming that Jonathan won't go, is there another possible explanation?

Patient: He might go. He might not go. The only way I'll know for sure is if I ask him. Telling him why it is important would certainly help.

Therapist: That's right. Taking this step will be an attempt to helping him understand your pain from the doctor's perspective. That might be good to share with him too. An additional benefit is that while you are in the office, he will also have a chance to hear your perspective—how the pain is affecting you. Feel free to let Jonathan know that this is an opportunity for him to ask the doctor some questions about your condition too.

Patient: Okay, I think this would help a lot.

Therapist: Let's say that after giving your best effort to ask Jonathan to go, he decides not to go. How will you handle that?

Patient: I can handle it. At least asking him to go is a first step. I don't expect miracles. This is going to be a tough nut to crack.

Therapist: If this first step doesn't work, then we can try something else— we could try another one of the solutions that we brainstormed in session today and maybe a new one that comes to your mind later.

Patient: I guess the most important thing to remember is that I will survive it, even if he says no.

Therapist: Great! Do you feel ready to give this solution a try?

Patient: Yes, I think I'm prepared to give it a go.

Therapist: Be aware of any negative thoughts that might interfere with your efforts to take this first step, just like we did in session. Then evaluate those thoughts to see if they are realistic or helpful. If you have trouble with this, we can discuss it next week.

[Next session]

Therapist: Well, Bernice, how have you been doing since our last session? I'm interested in how your first step in problem solving went this past week.

[Evaluating the results of the solution]

Patient: Well, it was earth shattering, but Jonathan did agree to go to my next doctor's appointment. At first he said no. When I explained how isolated and lonely I've been feeling with my pain, and how his presence would help me with the doctor's visit, he seemed more open to this.

Therapist: Well, that's great news. So, how was the appointment?

Patient: Well, it went better than I thought it would. It was really nice to have Jonathan along. He asked the doctor some questions about the pain in my shoulders and back. He also heard the doctor say that my condition was a chronic one given the degenerative disc disease in my back. I told the doctor that the medication does help some, but that I still have a lot of pain. It was good for Jonathan and my doctor to hear that.

Therapist: So, how did you feel about the outcome of this first step? Remember, the ultimate goal is to help Jonathan understand your pain.

Patient: I feel good about this first step. I think it's going to take some time for Jonathan to learn more about my pain. Another step I need to take is to let him know when I'm in pain and how I'm feeling.

Therapist: Yes, that was another solution you identified last week. Is that a step you want to take this week?

Patient: Yes, I think so, but I need some help with this.

In the therapist–patient dialogue above, the problem-solving steps were illustrated. These concrete steps provide the structure patients need to develop and implement their own problem-solving approaches in the future. Bernice was feeling overwhelmed with the communication problems she was having with Jonathan. But when the problem was broken down into smaller steps, it felt more manageable to her than before. Brainstorming ideas, selecting a solution, and putting that solution into action are aspects of the problem-solving process that help patients feel hopeful that their problems can be solved. In Bernice's case, she had some great ideas about how to recruit support from and to feel understood by Jonathan. The outcome was positive, which led to the development of the other solutions to put into action. If the outcome had not been as positive, other solutions could have been developed. In Bernice's case, couples therapy is certainly an option if both parties are willing to work on their relationship and communication issues.

In the next chapter, readers will learn how to identify, evaluate, and modify patients' images about their pain and other life stressors.

10

Eliciting and Modifying Imagery

Although some automatic thoughts come in the form of thoughts or self-talk, others come in the form of images. Images are brief, fleeting "snapshots" or pictures in our minds. They are very dynamic and ever changing, and can vary depending on patients' moods or pain levels. They can be the products of our imagination or our memories. Sometimes we are aware of our mental images; other times we are not. Images, like self talk, can be realistic or unrealistic in nature. They can also have a positive or a negative quality. Images involve a lot of sensory input and can activate strong emotional states in patients.

Chronic pain patients can have very vivid, catastrophic images about their pain and its consequences. There are four general types of images patients have. The first type involves *images of pain itself,* as having a life of its own, for example, imagining a raging fire in the patient's lower back and legs when she experiences burning sensations, or imagining a large knife stuck in the patient's neck when he feels a stabbing sensation in his neck. The second type relates to *images of oneself in pain.* For example, a chronic pain patient may imagine her body as old, feeble, and frail. The third type of image relates to *how people will interact with or relate to them given their pain.* Often chronic pain patients assume that people will shun them, will not care about them or understand their pain, or will reject them, given their pain and its effects on their various life roles. The fourth major type of pain image is of *the future with pain,* usually forecasting doom, gloom, misery, and rejection. For example, the patient may imagine that he will never be able to walk again—"stuck" in a wheelchair—in the future.

Some patients may have very positive, realistic images about the relational aspects of their pain (because they have a great deal of support) while holding very negative, unrealistic images about the pain itself. Other patients may not have any distressing images of the pain, themselves, nor their world, but have negative, unrealistic images of the future with pain (e.g., pain taking over their lives; people will get tired of them and their pain; becoming paralyzed in the future). Some patients may not have any negative images at all. Knowing the extent to which patients have negative images and in what category (or categories) can guide intervention strategies.

Negative images about pain and its consequences are often the targets of therapy intervention. Once images are identified, the goal is to teach patients how to respond to them. Patients learn to take charge of their images by stopping them, redirecting them or changing or responding to images in some way.

Although most images occur spontaneously, therapists can also induce images (1) to help patients cope with their pain, (2) to prepare them for a medical procedure, or (3) to practice using a cognitive therapy technique (Beck, 1995).

Imagery work can have a positive and powerful impact on patients. However, it is not suited for every patient. For some patients, imagery is very symbolic, not only personally but also spiritually. Cultural beliefs may also influence patients' interest and openness to imagery work. For example, dreams and images can play a very important role in many Native American/American Indian cultures. Some patients will be more receptive to imagery work than others depending on how concrete they are— meaning their ability to imagine and how much they value imagination in general. Some patients do not experience images regularly, if at all. Those patients who benefit from imagery work tend to have negative, catastrophic images related to their pain and their lives, can describe their images in some detail, and are receptive to imagery work.

IDENTIFYING IMAGES

Therapists can assess for the different types of images patients may have related to pain. For example:

- Do you have any images about the pain itself? What it looks like? Feels like? Sounds like?
- Do you have any images about yourself when you are in pain? What do you look like in that image? How do you feel? What are you doing in this image?
- Do you have any images about how other people respond to you and your pain? Do you have any images about how people treat you? What do they say about you? About your pain? What are they doing in this image? And how do you respond to them?

- Do you have any images of the future? What will happen to your chronic pain condition 5 years from now? Ten years from now? Do you see pain in your future? How will you cope with your pain in the future?

Images can be also identified in session by asking, "What thoughts or images were running through your mind just then?" especially when patients experience a change in their pain levels or their moods.

Some patients may initially provide a very brief explanation of the image, for example, "I imagined that the pain was taking over my body." The therapist can use follow-up questions to help the patient describe the image: "How does that happen? How does your pain take over your body in this image?" The therapist can also help the patient identify images when he or she is engaged in negative thinking. For example, the patient might say, "I had the thought that 'the pain is taking over me.'" The therapist could follow up with "Do you have an image or picture of how this would happen?"

Once an image is identified, the next step is to help the patient describe the image. If the image just occurred in session, the patient can explore the image in detail in the moment. In other cases, it may be helpful to go back in time to when the image last entered the patient's mind to capture the image more fully. Patients do not have to close their eyes for imagery work. In fact, patients usually leave their eyes open when they are asked to focus on the images or to talk about them.

Patients are asked to describe their images related to pain in some detail before modification of imagery occurs. The exception to this is when the patient has a very distressing or traumatic image. In those cases, the therapist can move immediately to image-stopping efforts.

It is important that the therapist allow enough time in session for the image to be described and modified in the same session. As a general rule, if an image is identified late in the therapy session, it is recommended that it be explored and modified during the next therapy session.

IDENTIFYING NEGATIVE VERBAL AUTOMATIC THOUGHTS WITHIN IMAGES

In addition to identifying and describing the image, therapists can also ask patients about any verbal automatic thoughts that occurred within the image itself. For example, if the patient imagines that her pain is slowly taking over her body, the therapist could ask her, "What emotions are you experiencing in this image?" and "What thoughts are running through your mind as you imagine the pain taking over your body?" This question will help access the "self-talk" or the verbal automatic thoughts associated with that image. The patient responded, "The pain is controlling me. I am out of control." This information is very helpful because it makes the patient aware of the internal dialogue that is occurring in the image and the meaning the patient is giving to the experience within the image itself. It also prepares the therapist in choosing among a variety of techniques to modify images, including responding to verbal automatic thoughts within an image. This will be discussed later in this chapter.

IDENTIFYING BELIEFS RELATED TO IMAGES

As therapists work with patients' images, they may notice patterns or themes to these images. These patterns or themes may serve as clues to the possible underlying beliefs that are activated. For example, a patient who has images of incapacity—of not being able to move or function, of not being able to work, of not being able to complete any household chores—may be struggling with beliefs related to a theme of dysfunction (e.g., I am dysfunctional; if I cannot do anything, then I am a waste). If the patient tends to have images of rejection—of losing friendships because of his chronic pain condition and being stigmatized by his employers and employees— this patient may be distressed by beliefs related to the theme of rejection or unlovability (e.g., I am not liked/loved by others because of my chronic pain condition; people will reject me/make fun of me if they knew about my pain). These beliefs will be discussed in more detail in the next chapter.

JOURNALING IMAGES

Images can also be identified between sessions and should be written down for discussion during the next therapy session. Patients can keep track of any significant negative images they have by using the Automatic Thought Record. In the Automatic Thought column, patients can write down negative images they experience when they are in pain or when they notice a change in their moods. It is also helpful to write down any verbal automatic thoughts or "self-talk" that occurred within the image itself. For example, if the patient imagined that he was being fired from his job, he should write down the details of that image. In addition, he should ask himself, "What thoughts were running through my mind when I was being fired in this image?" By identifying images as well as verbal automatic thoughts within the image, the patient and therapist will be able to work with both types of automatic thoughts—images and verbal automatic thoughts.

MODIFYING IMAGES

STEP ONE: DETERMINE WHETHER IMAGE-DISTRACTION OR IMAGE-MODIFICATION EFFORTS SHOULD BE USED

There are a variety of ways in which images related to pain can be altered or modified. The first step is to determine whether image-distraction or image-modification efforts should be used. This decision is based on how traumatic the patients' images are. If the patient is experiencing a great deal of emotion, particularly fear or anxiety, when focusing on the mental image in session, this is usually an indication that image-distraction or image-stopping techniques should be implemented. (However, when patients are ready to face traumatic or distressing images, they can be slowly exposed to them.) If patients are experiencing some emotion related to the mental image but are not very distressed by the image in session, this is usually an indication that image-modification techniques can be implemented. When in doubt, therapists should ask patients how they are feeling.

Therapist: How are you feeling right now with this image in your mind?

Therapist: I want to help you learn how to cope with images. One way to cope is to learn how to interrupt or stop an image if it is really bothering you. Another way to cope is to learn how to respond to an image—to learn how to change it in some way or to talk back to it.

STEP TWO: INTERVENE FIRST WITH IMAGERY OR WITH VERBAL AUTOMATIC THOUGHTS?

In teaching patients how to cope with or respond to images, therapists typically choose to intervene with imagery techniques first (e.g., having the patient stop the image or change it in some way). However, on occasion, therapists may also choose to evaluate and modify automatic thoughts within the image or associated with the image if it is believed that this work will assist in imagery coping or imagery modification.

TYPES OF IMAGERY TECHNIQUES

The following are types of imagery techniques used in cognitive therapy with the chronic pain population. Keep in mind that using a variety of techniques in sessions typically produces longer-lasting changes in images than if only one technique is used in therapy. The first two techniques, turn-off/down and image interruption/stopping, are imagery distraction techniques, with the goal being to stop the imagery from continuing. The more the patient practices rehearsing or "playing back" negative images about pain, the more real or salient they may become. Therefore, patients need practice in catching their images and distracting themselves when they are able. In general, these techniques are quick fixes and do not promote long-lasting change. However, they are effective in combination with the other imagery techniques mentioned later in this chapter. The second group of imagery techniques—repeating the image, directing the image, practice coping in the image, and jumping ahead in time—can teach patients to respond to their images via imagery substitution or imagery completion (playing out the image). These techniques teach patients that they have control over these images and can change them. Oftentimes, patients imagine the worst possible scenarios but do not carry the images beyond the worst. Imagining getting through the worst and coping with it can lead to significant changes in pain and moods. The last imagery technique, reality testing the image, teaches patients to use questioning techniques to examine the validity and usefulness of their negative images (e.g., evidence for and against the image) as well as to generate alternative, more realistic images. This technique is similar to the evaluation and modification process of "self-talk" or verbal automatic thoughts.

IMAGERY DISTRACTION TECHNIQUES

TURN-OFF OR TURN-DOWN TECHNIQUE

This technique is adapted from Beck, Emery, and Greenberg, (1985), and Beck (1995). While in touch with an image, patients are asked to imagine turning it off, like they would turn a knob or push a button to turn off the television or a videocassette recorder. Turning off could also include imagining the "pain volume" being turned down and off, imagining the curtain falling down to "close the show," and imagining they are leaving the place "in their mind" and coming back to the present. There are a variety of ways patients can learn to "turn off" their images. Using the patient's ideas or resources for turning off the image will certainly provide more meaning and power to the technique. This technique can be used with any image, but it is particularly useful with those that are very distressing to the patient—those images that ignite intense anxiety.

Here is example of a therapist and patient turning off a distressing image. At the beginning of this therapist–patient dialogue, Molly, a

57 year Caucasian woman, remembered the trauma of her car accident. She nearly lost her arm in this accident. Although Molly was able to save her arm, she still has significant tissue and neural damage in that arm. The pain she feels is a daily reminder of her trauma.

Patient: When I think about the car accident, I get in touch with a very vivid image of myself lying there with my arm hanging out of the car. I cannot feel my arm, and I see blood everywhere.

Therapist: What emotions are you in touch with as you lie there in the car?
Patient: I feel really scared.

Therapist: And what thoughts are running through your mind as you lie there in the car?
Patient: Will I die? [She starts crying uncontrollably.]

Therapist: [The therapist pauses for a moment until there is a small break in the crying.] I can see how scared you are in this image—thinking that you might die. But you are here in my office now. You have survived this traumatic event.
Patient: Yes, I have to remember that. But the image keeps popping up in my mind—even when I don't want it to.

Therapist: One way to deal with this image is to learn how to turn it off. You have that kind of control over your images—because they are a product of your mind—your memory and your imagination. It is important for you to learn how to turn off this image, especially when it is distressing to you. So I want you to take a moment now to turn this image off-like you would a television. Or you could imagine that the picture is getting foggy or out of focus. The picture is slowing fading out. [pause] You have now turned it off.
Patient: Yes, it's off now.

Therapist: So, tell me how you were able to turn off or turn down the image.
Patient: What really helped was when I imagined that the picture turned foggy and slowly faded out.

Therapist: Okay, so you learned a new skill—how to turn down or turn off a distressing images.

Later in the therapy process, the therapist and patient can work more directly with the image to help reduce the anxiety associated with it by exposing the patient to this image again and teaching her how to respond to it. This work should be done when the therapist believes the patient has the ability to turn off or stop the images at will and the patient feels motivated to move to this next step. Patients who experience posttraumatic stress as a result of some traumatic event, such as a life-threatening car accident, benefit from exposing themselves to the images they fear and learn how to modify those images in therapy to help them cope better with the memories and images of the event.

Here is an example of using the turn-down, turn-off technique with a less distressing image. Tony, a 75 year old Italian man, has been diagnosed with herniated disks in his neck. In this example, Tony and his therapist are working on turning down and turning off his images of pain.

Therapist: When you are in pain, do you get in touch with any images, Tony? Anything that you see, hear, touch, taste, or smell?

Patient: Well, I do imagine that the pain is like a fire. The flames have different colors . . . hot colors like red, hot pink, and purple. I see the red, purple, and hot pink flames moving around in my neck.

Therapist: Do the colors ever change when your pain subsides?

Patient: Yes, as the pain lessens, I notice cooler colors coming in, like pale blues and purples, light greens, and yellows.

Therapist: Okay, well, now I would like for you to focus on the reds, purples, and hot pink colors in your neck. [pause] Now, imagine that you are slowly turning down these colors, so that they become cooler. Begin to notice the colors becoming paler, more blues and purples, along with light greens and yellows, as you turn down the hot colors.

Another way of handling these images of pain colors is to have patients imagine they are "turning off the colors."

Therapist: Now, imagine that you are turning off the colors of red, purple, and hot pink. Turn off the colors, like you would a television, pressing the "off" switch. The television screen turns black.

Here is another image of "turning off the colors."

Therapist: Imagine that you are putting out the fire in your neck. Put out the fire so that all of the colors are gone. No embers are in sight. The fire is out.

STOPPING THE IMAGE

This technique is adapted from Beck et al.(1985) and Beck (1995). Patients are taught how to interrupt or stop their images. After patients are focused on an image, they are asked to imagine a stop sign in their minds or say, "Stop." Patients can distract themselves by focusing on something else, such as their current surroundings (e.g., the therapy room), or they could substitute another image in its place, for example, an image of a favorite or safe place, a place of total relaxation—where no pain or harm can exist or occur. For patients to substitute other images, they need practice developing these alternative images in session.

Here is an example of a therapist–patient dialogue that demonstrates the image-stopping technique. Benny, a 34 year old Chinese American man, has been working for a delivery service company for the past 10 years. Six months ago, a heavy box landed on his head at work. Since his head injury, he has had severe intermittent headaches and mixed pain in his neck and shoulders.

Patient: Where I worked, there were just tons of boxes . . . heavy boxes. And it was my responsibility to ship them out. One time, a heavy box fell down from a tall stack and landed on my head. I remember feeling the box crushing my head and upper body. I couldn't breathe. I couldn't move. [Patient starts to hyperventilate and becomes very anxious.]

Therapist: Okay, for a moment, I want you to stop this image. Just say, "Stop," out loud, and imagine a stop sign in your mind.
Patient: Stop! [pause]

Therapist: Are you in touch with the image of the stop sign?
Patient: Yes.

Therapist: Now, I want you to focus on breathing in and out, using the abdominal breathing that you learned in session a few weeks ago. Breathe in relaxation, then breathe out. Breathe in 2-3-4, the breathe out 2-3-4. Do you remember the image of the trail in the forest we developed in session a few weeks ago?
Patient: Yes, I remember.

Therapist: Okay, I want you to take a moment and get in touch with that image now. [pause] Are you there?
Patient: Yes, I am standing by the stream right now.

Therapist: Good.

After the patient calms down, the therapist can go back and explore what the process was like for the patient to remember the heavy box landing on his body, to stop the image, then to substitute another, more relaxing image in its place.

Therapist: Tell me what it was like for you to remember the heavy box landing on your body.

Patient: It was very scary. It felt like it was happening all over again. [Pause] At the same time, it is good to remember it because it reminds me of what I have survived. Even though my headaches are horrible at times and my neck and shoulders feel so numb at times, I am still here, you know.

Therapist: That's great. So the meaning you give to your image is that you are a survivor.

Patient: Yes, exactly.

Therapist: What was it like stopping the image of the heavy box landing on your head and switching to the nature scene while doing some deep abdominal breathing?

Patient: I wasn't expecting to feel so anxious when that image came up, but I am glad that you taught me how to stop it. I was able to imagine the stop sign. It was kind of weird saying "Stop" out loud, but I think it helped. Switching to a relaxing image helped too.

Therapist: Okay. Well, remember, when you're experiencing an image of the box falling or of some other traumatic event that is really bothering you, you can interrupt or stop that image by using this same technique in the future. Just imagine the stop sign, say "Stop," then substitute a more relaxing image.

After patients learn image distraction techniques, they can learn to face these images (e.g., exposure therapy) and modify them to reduce their distress. Molly and Benny would benefit from exposure therapy to cope with the memories of their accidents.

IMAGE MODIFICATION TECHNIQUES

Another set of imagery techniques can be used to teach patients about the control they have in responding to or changing their images. This can be accomplished in one of several ways, for example, by repeating an image over and over again—noticing changes in the image with each repetition (repetition technique)—by jumping ahead in time and imagining what their pain or their life will be like in the future (fast forward; jumping ahead in time), by imagining that they are in charge of the image like a director is with a movie project and changing the image in some way (directing an image), and by moving beyond worst-case scenario images and practicing coping in that image.

REWIND AND PLAY BACK: REPEATING THE IMAGE

This technique is adapted from Beck et al. (1985) and Beck (1995). Patients learn that aspects of an image can change each time they repeat an image over and over in their minds. It is also possible for the patients' moods to shift or even for pain levels to change each time an image is repeated. The purpose of this technique is to help patients realize that they have some control over these images—by attending to certain details (selective attention) and by spontaneously changing some aspects of the image.

To start the image-repetition technique, the patient presents a negative image in the therapy session. After the negative image is recalled, the therapist asks the patient to "play back" the image again—like rewinding a videotape and playing it over again—this time remembering as many details of the mental picture as possible.

One analogy to the image-repetition technique is storytelling. When a person tells a story over and over again, most of the main themes in the story remain the same. However, some of the details may be embellished, and other details may be discarded. Another analogy is the editing process in making a movie. Editors review the cuts of a scene and piece them together to make a complete scene. They are also responsible for the scenes flowing smoothly to create the complete picture. During this process, some parts of the scene may be cut, and other parts may be added.

When repeating an image, the patient usually keeps the main themes of the mental picture, but some of the details may change. Like an editor, the patient may spontaneously edit parts of their mental image, without prompting from the therapist.

> Andrea, a 49 year old Native American woman, was diagnosed with peripheral neuropathy related to a low back injury. She had been feeling very vulnerable lately about several incidents that occurred over the past week: a heated argument with her mother, a "bad" appointment with her physician, and worsening pain in her lower legs and feet. When asked which incident she wanted to discuss first, Andrea began talking about her last appointment with her physician. She

recalled an image of that visit which was very disappointing to her because she felt rushed, as though her physician did not care. When the therapist asked Andrea to describe what she saw in the image, Andrea focused on his "rushed pace." In her image, he was shuffling through paperwork, asking questions very quickly with little time for a response, and he exhibited little or no eye contact. After reviewing this mental image in session, the therapist asked Andrea what might be some possible explanations for her doctor's rushed pace. Her physician was normally attentive, so she just assumed he was rushing because he did not want to take time for her—that he did not care about her or the pain. The therapist took note that some of Andrea's possible cognitive errors in her negative automatic thought ("He doesn't care") included personalization, all-or-nothing thinking, and mind reading. However, this information was put aside for the time being because the therapist decided that the image-repetition technique could be used to teach Andrea how she may be selectively attending to certain aspects of the mental picture to confirm her hypothesis that her doctor does not care about her.

Next, Andrea was asked to repeat the image. The therapist said, "Let's repeat this image—like we were rewinding the videotape of this image and playing it back. Try to remember as many of the details of that office visit as you can." This time, Andrea recalled her doctor's "rushed pace"—seeing him shuffle through paperwork, asking questions in a "rapid-fire manner," and noticing his lack of eye contact. She also remembered two different nurses knocking on the door, interrupting the appointment during the process. The therapist asked when these interruptions occurred. One occurred soon after the physician entered the room. The second interruption occurred about 5 minutes later. After describing it, Andrea and her therapist discussed how these two images were similar or different. The patient admitted that the second image included the memory of the nurses interrupting the appointment with questions. Then the therapist explained, "When images are repeated, it is possible that their content changes, and that we may attend to aspects of the images we had not noticed the first time around." Next, the therapist asked if Andrea noticed a change in her moods or her pain levels between the first image and the second. Andrea said she felt a little less frustrated because she remembered the other interruptions.

After the image-repetition technique, the therapist followed up on Andrea's negative automatic thought that her physician does not care when she imagines the visit. The therapist asked Andrea how the interruptions by the nurses may have affected her doctor or the visit. She acknowledged that he seemed more distracted than usual. Would her physician have responded differently to her if he had not been interrupted? If he had not been busy? Maybe. What did Andrea do to deserve this type of treatment? Andrea could not recall anything she did to create distance in her physician–patient relationship. After exploring evidence for and against the thought that he did not care, Andrea came to the conclusion that her physician still cares, but sometimes his "bedside manner" can be affected by interruptions, a busy schedule, and his own fatigue. To handle the situation differently, Andrea could have asked her doctor some questions about her pain that day because it had worsened since the last visit. She could have asked him about his rushed pace to find out what factors were affecting his behavior (instead of assuming it was personal). Andrea and her therapist wrote out a list of questions about her pain to ask during the next office visit. This list will help Andrea remember what to ask during the next office visit and increase the likelihood that she will assert herself with her doctor.

This example illustrates how imagery interventions, automatic thought work, and problem-solving strategies can be integrated to help a patient.

DIRECTING THE IMAGE

This technique is adapted from Beck (1995). Patients can learn to take charge of images by viewing themselves as the directors of their images, like directors of movies or plays. Directors can make suggestions or changes in the cast, the scenery or setting, the ways in which the characters communicate with one another, and so on. Teaching patients that they can change or alter any aspect of their negative, catastrophic images, whether real or imaginary, is very empowering for them.

Here is an example of a therapist explaining the idea to a patient named Lorie. Lorie, a 40 year old Caucasian woman, had a complicated hysterectomy a few years ago. In addition, she had one abdominal surgery to remove scar tissue built up from the hysterectomy. When she feels pain in her lower abdominal cavity, she imagines lobsters pinching her.

Therapist: Images are similar to dreams, movies, television shows, and plays—they all include visual depictions of events and involve our auditory sense. They are also similar in that someone is in charge of their direction and their production. For example, movies, television shows, and theater productions have a director who is responsible for how the individuals act out their parts and a producer who is ultimately responsible for the costs and oversight of the production. Images and dreams are ultimately under your direction and production. For example, did you ever wake up in the middle of a bad dream and go back to sleep so that you could make changes in the dream, making it a better one?

Patient: Yes, that has happened before. It doesn't always work, but I try.

Therapist: Well, that's an example of your taking a "directing role" in your dream.

Patient: I never thought about that before.

Therapist: Okay, why don't we go back to that image we were reviewing earlier in the session? When your pain is really intense in your lower abdomen, you tend to imagine lobsters inside your lower abdomen, pinching your nerves with their claws. Let's take a moment to get in touch with that image again. Now, remember, you are the director of this image. What changes would you like to make to the image? For example, you said the lobsters' claws were very big earlier. Do you want to make them smaller? Do you want the lobsters to do something different? Do you want them to stop pinching you? Do *you* want to do something different in the image?

Patient: I think making the lobsters' claws smaller might help.

Therapist: Okay. Imagine the lobsters' claws becoming smaller and smaller.

Patient: Sometimes when I am in a lot of pain, I imagine a bunch of lobsters coming. I think I will make some of them go away.

Therapist: Imagine that some of the lobsters are leaving. Is there something you can say or do that will make them go away?

Patient: Yes. I told them to leave me alone. I don't want them around.

Therapist: Okay. Is there anything else you would like to change in this image?

Patient: No. I think that helps a lot. My pain is still there, but it doesn't hurt as bad as it did a couple of minutes ago.

Therapist: Great! It is very important that you practice directing this image over the next week to help you cope with your pain.

Here is another example of the "directing the image" technique. Hakeem, a 22 year old African American man, tore the rotator cuff of his left shoulder several times over his 4-year career pitching in minor league baseball. He continues to have chronic pain in his left shoulder despite surgical interventions. He has been unable to continue pitching in the minor league because of his injury. Hakeem recently found out that his contract would not be renewed next year. He is very upset about this and is particularly worried about what his friends and family will think of him now that he will no longer be playing ball on a professional basis.

Therapist: Hakeem, you mentioned being afraid of what your friends will think of you now that your contract has not been renewed.

Patient: Yes, I'm afraid they'll reject me. I just can't handle that possibility.

Therapist: Do you have an image of how your friends may reject you? (Hakeem nods). How do you imagine this happening?

Patient: I imagine telling a group of friends that my contract was not renewed for next year. Then, I notice a few friends just rolling their eyes at me, telling me that I shouldn't have pushed it so hard . . . that if I hadn't rushed back into the game, I would have been okay. Then they tell me that I really let them down. I was the one who was going to make it big. Now that dream is over.

Therapist: What happens next?

Patient: After that, I notice that my friends are not hanging around me anymore. They seem to come up with reasons why they can't come over or get together. Now no one is coming around anymore. I just see myself sitting there at home just miserable and alone.

Therapist: So, in your image, your friends are criticizing you and not getting together with you anymore because you can no longer play ball. I'd like for us to stop this image for a moment. Just freeze-frame it. Now, has any of this happened yet? Have any of your friends criticized you or rejected you yet? [reality testing the image]

Patient: No, it's just like that in my image.

Therapist: Do any of your friends know about your contract not being renewed yet?

Patient: One friend does, but he's keeping it to himself like I asked.

Therapist: And how has he responded to you and your situation?

Patient: He has been very supportive so far. He's bummed out about it like me, but he's still hanging around . . . you know, being there for me.

Therapist: Okay, so up until now your image has not come true. [Reality testing the image ends here.] Let's take a moment now and go back to this image of your friends criticizing you and rejecting you. At this point, I want you to think of yourself as the director of this image, as if you were the director of a movie or a play. You are in charge of this image. You created it, and you can change anything you want about this image. Take a moment now to decide what changes you want to make to this image, and share them with me when you're ready.

Patient: Okay. I'm willing to give this a try. [pause] When my friends tell me that I shouldn't have pushed too hard, you know, rushing back into the game after my injuries, I want to tell them that they probably would have done the same thing if they were in my shoes. I loved baseball so much that I didn't care if I was hurting or not. I wanted to play ball. Maybe it was my fault that I pushed too hard, but I guess I can live with that.

Therapist: Okay, imagine telling your friends those things. What do they say? How do you want them to respond?

Patient: I want them to say, "I know, man. I'm sorry that this happened to you."

Therapist: Imagine your friends saying that to you in your image. [pause] What happens next?

Patient: Well, maybe some of my superficial friends drop off the face of the earth . . . you know, the ones who liked me because I was a minor league player, not because of who I am. A few of my friends stick it out with me, like Jamal, Caryn, and Xavier. They've been friends with me long before I ever entered the minor leagues. I think they may stay true to me as friends even through this difficult time.

Therapist: Okay, let's stop this image for a moment. Did you notice a difference in how you felt emotionally and physically between the first image and the second?

Patient: Yeah. I felt very anxious and down, and my muscles were tense when I imagined everyone rejecting me. I feel more grounded, more relaxed with this second image.

Therapist: Images can have a significant impact on our moods and on our pain levels, just like self-talk does. You did a great job today of directing your image. It's important for you to stay in tune with any images you have and to learn how to respond to them. Remember, you are in charge of your images, and you can change them whenever you want.

Patient: I think I'll give it a try. It reminds me of some visualization I did with a sports psychologist to improve my performance.

Therapist: Great! Athletes are taught to spend time imagining their performance on the field to improve their sport, for example, imagining throwing a strike. While in reality, you may not always throw
a strike as a pitcher, mentally preparing to throw a strike can increase
the likelihood it could happen. The same is true for images about
your pain, your relationships with others, and your future. It is
important to practice directing or changing your images to help
you cope and practice succeeding.

Although this patient spontaneously imagined himself coping in the
image during the "directing the image" intervention, patients can be taught
to practice coping in their images using the technique that follows.

PRACTICE COPING IN THE IMAGE

Practice in coping with the worst, best, and realistic scenarios is a technique adapted from Beck et al. (1985) and Beck (1995). When patients
are in touch with negative, catastrophic images, they typically imagine that
they are not coping very well, if at all, in these images. Therefore, chronic
pain patients need practice imagining how they want to cope, for example, with their pain, their relationships with doctors or medical staff, and
their career goals and financial responsibilities. If patients are "stuck" and
cannot imagine coping, therapists can suggest that they imagine how someone else might cope in that situation; for example, they can bring a con-
sultant into the image or imagine how someone else with pain (or similar
circumstances) would cope.

Coping in Worst-Case Scenarios

Most patients have a great deal of practice imagining the worst-case scenario. However, this is where most patients stop their images. This next
imagery technique teaches patients to carry their images beyond the worst-
case scenario and see what follows—what the outcomes will be. Patients
are asked to focus on how they would like to cope in those situations.

In the following case vignette, Karla, a 65 year old British woman,
imagines that her chronic pain will ultimately lead to total disability.
She fears becoming paralyzed by her pain. This belief was precipitated
by a recent physician appointment when her lower back and legs
became numb following an epidural injection.

Patient: I imagine that I will become totally paralyzed.

Therapist: Let's take a moment to get in touch with this image. Tell me what you see.

Patient: I see myself lying in bed. All of sudden, I can't move anymore. I have no feeling in my back or legs.

Therapist: What else do you see in this image?

Patient: I just look shocked and miserable . . . I'm frowning, my eyes are glued to the tube [television] because I cannot handle my own life . . . my own miserable existence. This then moves to shock—shocked that I cannot move anymore . . . my eyes become very big.

Therapist: Can this image get any worse?

Patient: I look really frail, very thin. I feel like I have no energy, no motivation, and there is no one there to help me.

Therapist: Sounds like you feel depressed and anxious in this image. What thoughts or images are running through your mind, as you lie there paralyzed?

Patient: Oh my, I can't move anymore! What am I going to do? I can't believe how horrible my life really is.

Therapist: Can this image get any worse?

Patient: I imagine that I will be like this for the rest of my life.

Therapist: Okay, take a moment now to imagine this. [long pause] Is there a point when you are able to get up and reengage with life, even if it means that you cannot walk?

Patient: Yes, I see myself using a wheelchair. I'm still able to use my upper body, but I'm paralyzed from my lower back on down to feet. I guess at some point, I accept that this is the way my life is, and I start to engage in life more.

Therapist: Okay, take a moment to imagine what that would be like.

Patient: I'm still working. People actually treat me pretty much the same, despite their initial concerns and worries. I don't want them to pity me. [pause] I can't walk anymore. But my partner is still with me. I can't have sex with my partner like I used to, but we find ways to make each other happy. [pause] I guess I could cope with this reality if I really had to.

Therapist: What was it like to imagine getting beyond the worst and coping with it?

Patient: Well, I remind myself that other people have gone through worse things than I have. You know, if Christopher Reeve [an actor with a severe spinal cord injury] can cope with it, I can too.

In going beyond the worst image, Karla was able to see that she could continue to live a meaningful and productive life even if she became paralyzed.

Occasionally, a patient may get "stuck" trying to move beyond worst-case scenario images. In such cases, it is recommended that the therapist use the fast-forward technique. This technique will be discussed later in this chapter.

Coping in Best-Case Scenarios

After imagining the worst-case scenario, patients could also rehearse imagining the best-case scenario, or the ideal situation, and how they would cope in that image.

Therapist: Karla, now I want you to imagine the best thing that could happen if you felt numbness in your lower back and legs.

Patient: Well, the best thing that could happen is if the numbness would go away. I imagine going back to my doctor and telling her that I had some numbness since the epidural injection, and she reassures me that it is not a permanent condition, but probably a reaction to the injection.

Therapist: Okay. Great. Let's stop here and discuss what it was like to imagine coping in the best possible scenario.

Patient: It was great. I'm not sure how realistic it is, but it sure gives me hope.

Coping in Middle-Ground Scenarios

The last step would be to have patients imagine coping in middle-ground scenario images—images somewhere between the worst- and best-case scenarios.

Therapist: Karla, let's take a moment now to get in touch with what we call a middle-ground image. That image is typically somewhere between the worst and best possible situations.

Patient: Well, based on what we have talked about earlier, I probably won't be permanently paralyzed. I imagine that the numbness will eventually subside. I've noticed that it isn't as bad now as it was earlier today when I had the injection.

Therapist: How does the numbness subside? Can you put an image to this?

Patient: Well, I imagine calling my doctor as we discussed and telling her what sensations I've experienced since the injection. She tells me that the numbness was probably a reaction to the epidural injection. However, if it continues, I should schedule another appointment to see her. This eases my anxiety. I notice the numbness in my lower back and legs less often as the day continues. It will eventually subside.

FAST FORWARD: JUMPING AHEAD IN TIME

This technique is adapted from Beck et al. (1985) and Beck (1995). Most chronic pain patients focus on their chronic pain and its effects on their lives, and they cannot imagine themselves getting through difficult times. Fast-forward or jumping ahead in time is a technique that involves imagining getting through a difficult situation in the near future or imagining what life will be like later in time, for example, 6 months, 1 year, or 10 years from now.

In the next example, jumping ahead in time is used to get a picture of what the patient's life will be like 10 years from now to help the patient become more focused and goal-oriented. The patient, Will, a 37 year old gay Caucasian man, has had neuropathy related to muscular sclerosis for the past several years. He has been feeling "stuck" with his pain, and he does not see much hope for the future. He was asked to imagine waking up 10 years later and to describe what he would like to be doing then.

Therapist: Will, we've been talking today about how stuck you feel with this pain—that it is always going to be in your life, that you cannot imagine what next year will be like. I was wondering if we could do some imagery work together in session today to get you focused on what you would like to see ahead of you, in the future.

Patient: Okay. But I don't have any clue what the future will hold.

Therapist: That's true. There is no way to know for sure what the future is like until you get there. But think back to when you were in school. Do you remember imagining what your life would be like when you finished high school?

Patient: Yep. I had lots of ideas then.

Therapist: Well, this is the same process . . . kind of like daydreaming. I want you to imagine that you are just waking up 10 years from now.

You are now 10 years older. This is what you want your life to be like. Take a moment now to imagine where you are as you wake up. Look around you, and what do you see? You are getting up to eat breakfast. Do you see anyone this morning? You begin to get ready for your day. What are you going to do next? Imagine step by step what a typical day will be like 10 years from now.

Patient: I am waking up to smell the coffee brewing in the kitchen as I lie in bed. I imagine that I am getting ready to go to work. I am looking through the closet, trying to decide what to wear.

Therapist: What will you be wearing to work this morning?

Patient: Comfortable, clean slacks, a pressed white button-down shirt, and brown leather shoes.

Therapist: What happens next?

Patient: I see Dave [partner] as I am coming down the stairs for breakfast. He looks very happy . . . big eyes . . . bright smile. I grab some cereal and coffee.

Therapist: You mentioned Dave looking happy. How are you feeling, emotionally and physically?

Patient: I'm feeling pretty happy.

Therapist: What thoughts or images are running through your mind?

Patient: Well, I feel like I've got my life back on track. I still have this pain and my MS to deal with. But the pain is not as bad as before because I'm taking better care of myself. I'm on a health kick . . . trying to get those "six-pack" abdominal muscles, trying to eat better, seeing my doctor more regularly, and be healthy for Dave and me.

Therapist: Okay, that's great. So taking care of yourself has helped you manage your pain better.

Patient: Yes.

Therapist: Now, you mentioned getting ready to go to work. Let's imagine that you are at work now. Tell me what you will be doing today.

[Future-oriented imagery continues.]

Therapist: Okay, now let's bring this image to a close and discuss what this experience was like for you.

Patient: It really got me focused on the future. I want things to get better in my life.

Therapist: What can you do to start making your life better?

Patient: Well, this is a start. [pause] I need to do whatever I can to manage my pain better and also to manage my life better. I need to work on feeling better about my situation and myself. Maybe some of the skills I'm learning in here will help me.

REALITY-TESTING THE IMAGE

This imagery technique tests the reality of an image, including its validity and utility. This technique is similar to the techniques used with verbal automatic thoughts and core beliefs. There are several steps to this process (Beck, 1995):

1. *Identify negative and unrealistic qualities in images.* Most chronic pain patients are able to identify the catastrophic nature of their images or the unrealistic qualities in their images (e.g., their tendency to minimize their strengths).
2. *Test the validity of images.* Patients can be asked a variety of questions to test the validity of their images. These questions guide patients to the evidence, possible distortions within the image, alternative images, and view images from another's perspective.
   - What is the evidence that this image is true or will come true?
   - What is the evidence that the image is untrue or will not come true?
   - What might be some of the errors or distortions in your image?
   - What are some other possible ways of imagining your pain or this situation?
   - What effect does this image have on you? Your pain? What would be the effect of changing this image?
   - If you were to put one of your closest friends or family members in this image instead of yourself, how would you want this image to turn out for that person? (This is used especially when patients have a difficult time considering other images or coping in the image.)
3. *Compare patients' images to their current situation.* The next step is to reality test the image by comparing it to the patient's current experiences. Does the image match what is really experienced in daily life? Where is the grain of truth in the negative image? Where are the mismatches between negative images and reality? The therapist could ask, "To what extent is this image an accurate reflection of your pain, your circumstances, your relationships? Is this image an accurate depiction of what is happening to you in

your daily life?" Separating out what the patient anticipates (in the images) and what really occurs is an important process.

An earlier example illustrated the use of this technique. Refer back to the case of Hakeem, the minor league pitcher who imagined that his friends would reject him if they knew his contract had expired.

Here is another example of a therapist using the reality testing technique with Karla, the patient who imagined that she would become paralyzed.

Therapist: A moment ago, we were able to get in touch with an image of you becoming totally paralyzed at home.

Patient: Yes. That was a scary image.

Therapist: It would be scary if all of a sudden, your whole body went numb and you felt paralyzed. [Patient nods.] I want us to go back to that image for a moment to see how realistic it is. Has this happened to you before—where your body suddenly went numb and you felt paralyzed? [This intervention is getting at the evidence that this image may be true.]

Patient: Well, the only time that happened was a few hours ago when I received that epidural injection at the doctor's office. My lower back and legs went numb, and I almost fell down when I tried to get up and walk.

Therapist: So, the numbing sensation you experienced in your lower back and legs was the result of the injection.

Patient: Yes.

Therapist: Is there any evidence that your image of being paralyzed may not be accurate?

Patient: Yes. Every once in a while, I feel some numbness in my lower back when I sit too long. When that happens, I usually get up and move around. And like we discussed earlier, the numbing feeling I experienced at the doctor's office didn't just come out of nowhere. It occurred after the injection, and it didn't last forever.

Therapist: So, while you have experienced numbness before, you have not experienced paralysis—that is, not being able to move your body, or parts of your body. In addition, you mentioned that there are things you do to cope with the numbness, for example, standing up after sitting for a while.

Patient: I agree. Sometimes I forget that I do take some control over my pain.

Therapist: Does your physician think you are at risk for paralysis? [looking for more evidence for or against the image of paralysis]
Patient: I've never asked her about this. I've just kept this fear to myself.

Therapist: Well, it may be helpful to ask your physician. She could give you information about whether or not the epidural injections and your pain condition could put you at risk for developing paralysis. This medical information would be important evidence to confirm or disconfirm your image of future paralysis.
Patient: I think you're right. I'll plan to follow through on this. [Behavioral experiment to test out image: Ask doctor about risk of developing paralysis.]

Therapist: Now that we've explored evidence for and against your image, what do you think? Is this image realistic?
Patient: No, it's not. And it doesn't help me either. It just creates more anxiety for me.

Therapist: So, the image is not realistic and it is not useful. [brief pause] What are some other ways of imagining your pain or the numbness in your body?
Patient: Well, I could imagine the numbness in my body and notice that I am still able to move.

Therapist: Okay, take a moment to imagine that. [Therapist implements directing the image technique.]

REALITY TESTING VERBAL AUTOMATIC THOUGHTS WITHIN THE IMAGE

Therapists may decide to test the accuracy or utility of the patient's automatic thoughts that occur within the image itself (Beck, 1995). The process of identifying, evaluating, and modifying automatic thoughts within images is the same as when thoughts are modified in session (without being in touch with an image). However, it should be noted that the image itself may change when patients develop alternative responses to negative thoughts within the image.

In summary, a variety of imagery techniques can be used with chronic pain patients in therapy. Imagery techniques should be chosen based on the purpose of the technique itself (i.e., to interrupt or modify) and on patients' interest and ability to access and work with images. Given the powerful nature of images, it is recommended that the therapist allow time in session for the patient to describe and modify the images.

In the next chapter, readers will learn how to identify, evaluate, and modify patients' beliefs related to pain and distressing events. Many of the techniques to accomplish these tasks are very similar to the ones learned in chapter 9. However, beliefs are more ingrained than automatic thoughts and are typically more resilient to change efforts. Therefore, experiential techniques (e.g., "heart" or "gut" dialogue, imagery) will typically be used to restructure patients' beliefs about their pain and other situations.

11

Identifying Beliefs About Pain

Chronic pain patients have beliefs about their pain as well as about other issues, including their functioning, relationships, work, and life in general. There are two general types of beliefs that are explored in cognitive therapy: core beliefs and intermediate beliefs, both of which are related to automatic thoughts.

Intermediate and core belief work often occur simultaneously in the therapy process. For example, although therapists typically work on the intermediate beliefs first, the underlying core beliefs are also identified during this time. Therefore, throughout this chapter and the next chapter, these two types of beliefs will be discussed together. Any important distinctions in working with one type of belief or another in the identification, evaluation, or modification process will be addressed.

CORE BELIEFS

Most people are not prepared to deal with a chronic pain condition. As a result, patients tend to seek meaning given their chronic pain in a number of ways. They want to understand the etiology of their condition, if unknown, and what can be done to treat it successfully. They want to know why this happened to them—why they deserved this pain in their lives. They are confused as to why they continue to experience pain despite medical intervention. They focus on how their pain has affected their life roles and responsibilities as well as their relationships with others. They wonder what the future holds.

Core beliefs are the basic ideas that people have about their pain, themselves, their relationships with others, their life roles and experiences, and their future. Patients often refer to these beliefs as "facts" or "truths" across a variety of situations despite evidence to the contrary. They often hold onto these beliefs because they "feel" that they are true. Although most core beliefs develop in childhood, some beliefs develop later in life, particularly during traumatic events and significant life changes, such as having chronic pain.

Core beliefs serve as filters through which information is processed. They can actually "drive" what information is attended to or discarded in everyday situations, including the experience of pain. These beliefs are at the foundation of how people think on a daily basis (automatic thoughts). Core beliefs can be positive or negative in nature and have a strong emotional component. When patients are distressed, negative core beliefs are likely to be activated.

PAIN BELIEFS

When people develop negative core beliefs about their pain, they often think of their pain and its consequences in terms of losses, threats, and disappointments. Perceived or actual losses related to pain include loss of abilities, loss of functioning, loss of joy or pleasure, loss of will, loss of freedom, loss of self, and loss of relationships. Examples of pain beliefs centered on loss include "I can't do things the way I used to," "I can't control my pain," "I can't cope with my pain," "The pain reminds me of what I have lost," "This pain is ruining my life," "The pain is sucking the life out of me," and "I don't feel like the same person anymore because of my pain."

Patients may also perceive potential dangers related to their pain and discomfort including, but not limited to, the fear of having unrelieved pain for a long time, the fear of further bodily harm, the potential danger of losing one's career and livelihood as a result of the pain, and fear of the unknown (e.g., no clear-cut diagnosis may affect the treatment of their pain condition). Examples of pain beliefs centered on danger include "Bad things will continue to happen to me," "This pain is overwhelming," "The pain is awful," "The pain never ends," "I don't want to do anything to cause further injury or damage," and "'Not knowing' means 'bad news.'"

Patients may be disappointed about their pain and its treatment. When their expectations are not met, patients often feel very angry and. Examples of pain beliefs in this area include "My doctors are supposed to find a cure," "My doctors should be able to diagnose the problem," "I need relief from this pain," and "I shouldn't have this pain in my life."

These themes of loss, danger, and disappointment are related to how adequate or helpless patients feel about their pain as well as how connected or supported they feel by others given their pain (similar to self-beliefs; see next section). For example, if patients perceive their pain and its consequences in terms of losses, it could be losses related to dysfunction or inadequacy as well as losses related to their social connectedness. When pain is viewed as dangerous or threatening, patients may feel helpless to deal with their pain or focus on the perceived personal and social consequences of their pain (e.g., being rejected, abandoned, or disliked). When patients focus on their disappointments, they are usually upset about the injustices of having the pain itself as well as their disillusionments with pain treatment and/or their relationships with others.

Pain beliefs have been grouped into different categories by different researchers and clinicians in the field of pain management. For example, Tearnan and Lewandowski (1992) have identified eight categories of pain beliefs (as mentioned in chapter 4), including catastrophizing (e.g., "My pain problem is more than I can handle"), fear of reinjury (e.g., "When I do things that increase my pain, I am concerned that I might reinjure myself"), expectation for a cure (e.g., reverse score—"I have accepted that nothing further can be done to eliminate my pain"), blaming self (e.g., "I should be able to control the pain much better than I do"), entitlement (e.g., "I deserve better than to have chronic pain"), future despair (e.g., "I will never enjoy life again as long as I have pain"), social disbelief (e.g., "It bothers me that others might not believe my pain is real"), and lack of medical comprehensiveness (e.g., reverse score—"My doctors have left no stone unturned in their attempts to treat my pain"). He also identified beliefs associated with the perceived consequences of having chronic pain, including social interference (e.g., "When your pain increases sharply, how concerned are you that . . . your pain will negatively affect others"), physical harm (e.g., ". . . you will cause a setback in your healing"), psychological harm (e.g., ". . . you will 'lose your mind'"), pain exacerbation (e.g., ". . . your pain will not settle down"), and productivity interference (e.g., ". . . the rest of the day will be shot").

Jensen, Karoly, and Huger (1996) have also categorized pain beliefs into different groups, including control (e.g., "There are times when I can influence the amount of pain I feel"), disability (e.g., "If my pain continues at its present level, I will be unable to work"), harm (e.g., "The pain I feel is a sign that damage is being done"), emotion (e.g., "Anxiety increases the pain I feel"), medication (e.g., "I will probably always have to take pain medication"), solicitude (seeking attention; e.g., "When I hurt, I want my family to treat me better"), and medical cure (e.g., "A doctor's job is to find pain treatments that work").

These theoretical models can be used to conceptualize pain beliefs.

BELIEFS ABOUT SELF

Chronic pain patients typically have two basic types of core beliefs about themselves given their pain: (1) their adequacy or competence to deal with it (e.g., helpless, inadequate, out of control, vulnerable, useless, incompetent, etc.) and (2) their level of social acceptance or their lovability (e.g., unattractive, social misfit, etc.; Beck, Rush, Shaw, & Emery, 1979; Beck, 1995). Examples of adequacy core beliefs include "I am helpless," "I am useless because I cannot do things like before," "I cannot function with this pain," and "I am a failure." Examples of lovability beliefs include "No one cares about me or my pain," "I am undesirable," and "I am a misfit." Patients may think they are inadequate for a variety of reasons: They continue to experience pain despite medical interventions, they might have physical limitations that impair their functioning in certain life role areas (a.k.a. functional limitations), they may not know how to cope with their pain, or they expect to be pain-free and become disillusioned over time. Furthermore, patients may think that they are unlikable or unlovable as a result of having a chronic pain condition. They may think their physicians won't like them if they complain of unrelieved chronic pain despite medical interventions. They may fear abandonment by bosses, coworkers, family members, and friends if their chronic pain affects their work, leisure, or family roles and activities. They may think they are unattractive because of physical changes related to their chronic pain (e.g., limping, wearing carpal tunnel braces, loss of body part, or weight gain/loss).

Core beliefs of inadequacy can be further classified into themes of worthlessness, helplessness, dysfunction, and unreasonable expectations/demands. Core beliefs of lovability can be further classified into themes of disconnection and social worthlessness. Some of these subcategories (or themes) are based on the early maladaptive schema work of Young (1999). For the list of the prominent negative core beliefs about self, see Figure 11.1. Specific examples of negative core beliefs related to chronic pain are provided under each domain. This list can be given to patients to help them identify their own core beliefs.

BELIEFS ABOUT WORLD

When patients have positive views of others and the world, they tend to believe that the world is safe and fair. When patients have negative views of others and the world, they tend to believe the world is very dangerous, untrusting and unjust, including themes of social inadequacy/helpless,

FIGURE 11.1 Negative Core Beliefs Related to Chronic Pain

Core beliefs are relatively enduring and stable ways of how people make sense of events in their lives. Some of these beliefs develop early in life; others develop following significant traumatic events throughout life. Core beliefs influence people's perceptions of themselves, their physical/medical difficulties (e.g., chronic pain), their relationships, and their perception of the future. Negative core beliefs filter out positive experiences. When people see their world through these beliefs, significant emotional, behavioral, and physiological distress can result. Developing chronic pain is viewed by some people as a significant, traumatic event that can lead to different ways of looking at themselves and the world.

Below is a list of negative core beliefs related to chronic pain. Check those core beliefs that you can identify with at this time in your life. Remember that core beliefs are relatively stable views that you have held, at least since the development of your chronic pain condition, if not before.

Core Beliefs of Inadequacy

<u>Themes of Helplessness</u>

- <u>I am helpless:</u> You tend to believe that you cannot help yourself or that others (e.g., family, friends, doctors, physical therapists, or psychotherapist) cannot help you.
- <u>I am weak/I cannot cope:</u> You tend to believe that you are not emotionally or physically strong enough to handle decisions, concerns, daily situations, and physical problems.
- <u>I am doomed to be pain-ridden:</u> You believe that much of your identity is caught up in your chronic pain. You may assume that your pain will last forever and that it will be overwhelming and unbearable.
- <u>I am needy/dependent:</u> You tend to believe that you cannot physically or emotionally cope or function by yourself—that you need to depend on others to cope. Or you tend to believe that it is not okay to seek out help, so you assume that asking for help is a sign of inadequacy.
- <u>I am vulnerable:</u> You tend to assume that you are vulnerable to catastrophes or crises that could occur at any time, for example, health problems or threats to your physical safety.
- <u>I am out of control (of my pain/my body):</u> You tend to assume that you will lose control of yourself, whether it be your body, your pain, your thoughts, your emotions, your behaviors, or your mind.
- <u>I am powerless:</u> You tend to believe that there is nothing you can do to take charge of your pain or your life. You tend to believe that you have no control over events in life.

- I am trapped: You tend to feel stuck in a no-win situation.
- I am suffering/I am a victim: You tend to focus on your emotional misery or your pain. You focus on how your pain or various life events are negatively affecting your life.

Themes of Worthlessness

- I am useless/not important: You tend to believe that you do not have an important purpose or role in your life or in the lives of others. If you are not able to engage in activities and accomplish tasks like you used to because of your chronic pain or your emotional state, you tend to assume that you have little or no value as a person.
- I am incompetent: You tend to believe that you cannot perform competently in various activities or handle day-to-day responsibilities or decision making.
- I am unworthy/a failure: You believe that you have nothing to contribute to yourself or others—no perceived redeeming qualities. You tend to focus on your mistakes or your shortcomings—on what you haven't done, not on what you have accomplished.
- Others should come first (to be adequate): You tend to focus on others and their needs to the detriment of yourself and your own needs.

Themes of Dysfunction

- I am different/not normal: You tend to believe that you are a totally different person compared with who you were before your chronic pain or your injuries (e.g., "I am not the same person anymore," "I am afraid that I won't be normal," or "I am a freak of nature").
- I am defective/flawed: You tend to believe that you are inwardly defective or flawed because of your chronic pain or other qualities in yourself.
- My body is not functional/I am not functional: You tend to believe that your body has betrayed you and that you will not be able to accomplish or do anything, including physical, sexual, or relational activities.
- I am pitiful: You believe that you are pitied by others and you focus on feeling sorry for yourself—thinking about what you cannot do.
- My body is broken/I am not whole: You believe that you are incomplete in some way, whether it be your physical body, your emotional state, or your spiritual self.
- My body has turned old: You believe that your chronic pain has made your body old and feeble. You view your pain as a reminder of your inability to do things—of your losses. You feel old, beyond your years.
- I am a burden to others/I am imposing on others: You tend to assume that you are an annoyance to other people—that you are unduly burdening them in your efforts to seek out help or support related to your chronic pain or other concerns.

Themes of Inadequacy Related to Unreasonable Expectations/Demands

- <u>I don't measure up/I am not good enough:</u> You tend to have very high expectations of yourself for academic, career, and personal achievements, which interfere with your sense of accomplishment or happiness. Not meeting these expectations results in feelings of shame and self-consciousness.
- <u>I am entitled:</u> You tend to believe you have the right to do and say whatever you want without considering your effect on others.
- <u>I am disrespected:</u> When your needs and wants are not met immediately or in the manner you expected, you believe that people are disrespectful of you.

<u>I am being punished:</u> You tend to assume that your chronic pain is a punishment for some negative qualities in yourself or for the things that you have done in your life (e.g., mistakes, recklessness, or sins).

Core Beliefs of Unlovability

Themes of Disconnection

- <u>I expect to be rejected/abandoned:</u> You tend to assume that people will abandon or reject you, resulting in emotional isolation.
- <u>I cannot trust others:</u> You tend to assume that people intend to hurt or harm you or take advantage of you.
- <u>I am a misfit/I am different:</u> You tend to assume that you are different —feeling like a misfit.
- <u>I am bound to be alone:</u> You tend to assume that being alone and isolated from others is your destiny, given your pain and distress.
- <u>I am emotionally deprived/dissatisfied:</u> You tend to expect that your needs for nurturance, empathy, affection, and care will never be adequately met by others.
- <u>I am discounted by others/My pain is discounted:</u> You tend to assume that people don't value you or believe in you or your pain. You assume that people think your pain is not real.

Themes of Social Worthlessness

- <u>I am unlovable:</u> You tend to believe that you are inherently unlovable.
- <u>I am socially defective:</u> You tend to assume that you are incapable of handling social relationships or social situations because of your pain or your perceived flaws and defects.
- <u>I am unattractive/undesirable:</u> You tend to believe that people will not be attracted to you or desire you. You assume that people won't want to be with you (outwardly defective).

- <u>I am unworthy/inadequate:</u> You have recurrent feelings of shame related to perceived inadequacies in relationships (because of your pain).
- <u>I am a bad person:</u> You tend to believe that you are a bad person who doesn't deserve to be loved or to receive help and support from others.
- <u>I am not good enough:</u> You tend to believe that you will not measure up to other people's expectations in relationships.

Adapted from the core belief list identified in Judith Beck's *Cognitive Therapy: Basics and Beyond.* Adapted with permission by Guilford Press: New York. Copyright 1995 by Judith S. Beck. Also adapted from a schema list, author unknown.

social rejection, social victimization, and entitlement. Themes of social dependency and subjugation are common when patients have negative beliefs about themselves and positive beliefs about others. Examples of negative core beliefs about the world include "No one can help me" (socially helpless), "People need to take care of me (or I won't survive)" (social dependency), "The world is a dangerous place," "People cannot be trusted" (socially vulnerable), "People will reject or abandon me" (social disconnection), "People will be burdened by my pain and suffering," "No one cares about my pain" (social disapproval), "My pain is discounted by others" (disrespected), "Others should come first" (subjugation), "Doctors are punishing me for not fixing my pain" (social victimization), "People don't believe my pain is real" (social disbelief), "People should understand my pain," and "Doctors should fix my pain" (entitlement).

BELIEFS ABOUT FUTURE

Chronic pain patients usually tend to have negative core beliefs about the future given their pain, which relates to their feelings of helplessness and hopelessness. Examples of negative core beliefs about the future include "I am doomed to be pain-ridden," "I am bound to be miserable and alone," "The future looks bleak," and "I have nothing to look forward to in the future."

INTERMEDIATE BELIEFS

Intermediate beliefs include conditional assumptions, rules, and attitudes (Beck, 1995). These beliefs mediate negative automatic thoughts and more basic core beliefs.

Conditional assumptions refer to the negative and positive notions patients have about themselves, their pain, and their lives. These beliefs can be identified as if-then statements: If a certain condition is met, then a certain consequence is assumed or expected. "If the doctors cannot diagnose my pain, then they are punishing me" is an example of a negative conditional assumption (assuming a negative consequence). "If the doctors can diagnose my pain, then there will be a cure" is an example of a positive conditional assumption (assuming a positive outcome).

Rules are another type of intermediate belief. These beliefs are rigid, inflexible ideologies about how people should or must live their lives. These "shoulds" and "musts" exert a great deal of pressure on patients who expect life events to happen in a certain, specific way. When events do not turn out as expected, it may become very upsetting to patients. They may feel disappointment, sadness, guilt, depression, anger, and anxiety, among other emotions. Examples of rules include "The medication should work," "I shouldn't have to live with pain," "The pain should go away," "I must have a diagnosis," "I must receive the full attention of my doctor," "I must be in control of my pain," "Everyone should understand what I am going through," "Bad things should not happen to good people," "That accident should not have happened," "People must believe me," "A good person must work hard and be loved to be important," "I should get my job back," "I should not trust doctors," "I should be in total control of my body," "I must not have pain in my life," and "I must keep working, even if my pain is unbearable."

Attitudes are types of intermediate beliefs that focus on the bad or horrible nature of events. In other words, attitudes tend to be catastrophic in nature. Examples of attitudes include "It's horrible when no one understands my pain," "It is a catastrophe that medical advances are not available to take my pain away," "Life stinks—what's the point," and "I am destined to have a life full of pain."

IDENTIFYING INTERMEDIATE AND CORE BELIEFS

The importance of exploring the negative belief systems of chronic pain patients cannot be underestimated. These belief systems develop over time, whether they begin in childhood or follow injuries/events that lead to chronic pain, and are activated by pain or distress. Ultimately, these negative outlooks on the world (e.g., self-doubt, perceived injustices, and skepticism) can feed destructive and disabling emotions (e.g., depression, shame, blame, anxiety, despair, fear, anger, self-pity, paranoia, guilt, and loneliness, among others), as well as destructive, unhealthy behaviors, which may perpetuate pain and suffering (e.g., increased muscle tension, medical adherence problems, substance abuse, isolation, and vengeful actions, such as energies focused on embittered court-related battles).

EDUCATING PATIENTS ABOUT BELIEFS

Although therapists may discover some of their patients' beliefs early on in the course of therapy, they need to proceed in teaching patients how to deal with automatic thought processes first before delving into belief work. The concepts of core beliefs and intermediate beliefs can be introduced after patients have developed a good mastery of automatic thought restructuring work (i.e., identifying, evaluating, and modifying automatic thoughts). Figure 11.2 can help patients understand the three levels of thought—automatic thoughts, intermediate beliefs, and core beliefs—along with examples of each.

Therapist: So far in therapy, we have focused on relaxation training and automatic thought work. As we can begin to see patterns in our thoughts, this clues us in to deeper beliefs we have about ourselves and about our pain, called core beliefs. These beliefs can develop early in childhood, or they can develop later in life, particularly after a traumatic event such as an injury, an accident, or the development of a chronic pain condition. Just like automatic thoughts, there are positive and negative core beliefs. I often think of core beliefs as lenses or filters through which people view the world. People can have core beliefs about their pain, themselves, their world, and their future. We will talk more about this in a moment. Do you have any questions so far?

Patient: No. That makes some sense to me.

Therapist: Intermediate beliefs are thoughts that fall between automatic thoughts and core beliefs. Intermediate beliefs include your rules about your life, your assumptions, and your attitudes. The rules about life are your "shoulds," for example, how you think your life should be. Assumptions refer to what you expect to happen or assume given certain situations or conditions. One way to catch any negative assumptions is to be aware of your "if-then" statements. For example, if some circumstance occurs, then you anticipate a specific negative outcome. Attitudes are catastrophic beliefs—you anticipate outcomes that are worst-case scenarios. To help you identify attitudes, look for times when you say statements like "It's awful when" or "It is terrible when."

DOWNWARD ARROW TECHNIQUE

This technique involves using a series of open-ended questions to uncover the basic meaning or beliefs underlying patients' negative automatic

---

FIGURE 10.2 Levels of Cognition or Thought

Automatic thoughts: include self-talk and imagery (preconscious)
    Self-talk—"This pain is so unbearable."
    Imagery—Imagining the pain taking over my body.

Intermediate beliefs: rules, conditional assumptions, and attitudes
    Rules (or shoulds)—e.g., "I shouldn't have to deal with this pain."
                                            "I should be pain-free."
                                            "My medicine should work."

    Conditional assumptions—e.g., "If I am hurting, then there is
                                            something very wrong with me."
                                            "If the medicine doesn't work,
                                                then I will suffer." (negative)
                                            "If the medicine does work, then
                                                I will be fine." (positive)
                                            "If I continue to suffer like this,
                                                then I won't be able to work."

    Attitudes—e.g., "It is terrible to be in this much pain."
                        "I can't handle this pain anymore."

**Core Beliefs: underlying beliefs about pain, self, relationships, life
roles, and the future**
    Two basic categories of core beliefs—adequacy and lovability
    1. adequacy—e.g., "I cannot control my pain."
                                ("I am out of control")
                            "I am defective"
                                (full of pain; something is wrong with me).
                            "I am inadequate (as a worker, parent,
                                lover, etc.)."
    2. lovability—e.g., "My doctors don't care about my pain
                                (about me)"
                            "I am a burden to others."
                            ("People don't want to help me.")

---

thoughts (Beck, 1995; Burns, 1989). To begin this process, the therapist asks the patients to assume that his or her automatic thought is true so that the underlying meaning can be explored. The open-ended question that is typically used to start the downward arrow technique is

- If that thought were true, what would it mean?
  Asking this question once may or may not uncover patients' beliefs. The therapist typically follows up with the same question again, or the therapist may use a variant of that question until the underlying belief is identified. Other downward arrow questions are provided below. Some questions are geared toward identifying intermediate beliefs (e.g., attitudes, assumptions of consequences, or rules), whereas other questions are focused on identifying core beliefs.

- If that were true, then what would happen? Then what? (identify consequences)
- If that were true, what would be so awful or horrible about that? (identify attitudes)
- If that were true, what would that mean to you? (beliefs about pain or the event)
- If that were true, what would that say about you? (beliefs about oneself)
- If that were true, what would that say about your pain? (beliefs about pain)
- "If that were true, what would that say about your relationship with?" (beliefs about others)
- If that were true, what would that say about your future? (beliefs about the future)

Ladan, 30-year-old Caucasian woman, has been very concerned about not receiving a clear-cut diagnosis for her severe abdominal pain. The meaning of this event (lack of a clear diagnosis) will be explored here, using the downward arrow technique.

Patient: The doctors haven't diagnosed my condition yet. It is really worrying me. What if I never find out?

Therapist: You're worried that you may never have a diagnosis for your pain. [Patient nods.] If that were true, what would it mean?
Patient: It means I wouldn't get the right treatment.

Therapist: And if that were true, what would that mean?
Patient: That I would be stuck with this pain for the rest of my life. [core belief about pain]

Therapist: Then, what would happen?
Patient: I would be miserable . . . just a blob of nothing. [attitude] Who wants to be around someone who is miserable? [no one wants to; core belief about world]

Therapist: And if no one wants to be around you, then what does that say about you?

Patient: That I am not important or needed. [core belief about self]

Therapist: So, you are afraid that you would be stuck with this pain for the rest of your life . . . just miserable and a "blob of nothing." You would not feel important or needed by others.

Patient: Yep. It sounds pretty horrible, doesn't it? I really feel like I am being punished. [core belief about world] Doctors can't leave me hanging here. [rule] I feel so frustrated and angry at times.

Therapist: Ladan, this is a great example of how ambiguity can lead to uncertainty. People handle uncertainty in a lot of different ways. We try to make sense of events that happen in our lives. You are trying to do just that . . . knowing that your diagnosis is still unclear. Let's take a look at several important statements you made. One is that you think you will be "stuck with your pain for the rest of your life." You also said that you feel like you "are being punished." Another belief you stated was that you "will be a blob of nothing" and that you "will not be important or needed." These all seem to be important beliefs that you hold about yourself, your pain, and your future. Which of these beliefs seems the strongest or the most upsetting to you right now?

Patient: Probably that I am being punished.

Therapist: Okay, well, why don't we explore this belief further?

The downward arrow technique allowed this patient and her therapist to uncover a number of beliefs that are related to her intense pain and distress. When using these downward arrow questions, the therapist did not assume to know how the patient would respond to these questions. This is called guided discovery. Neither therapist nor patient really knows what the outcome of the exploration will be—in other words, what beliefs will be identified. This "nonassuming" stance prevents the therapist from being judgmental about the experiences of the patients. It also makes therapy an exciting process for both parties.

To help delineate the beliefs identified by the downward arrow technique, the therapist can diagram the beliefs that were identified following each downward arrow question. Figure 11.3 is a diagram of the beliefs identified in the previous therapist–patient dialogue.

This type of diagram can be written in session and shared with patients to help them see the beliefs that unfolded.

FIGURE 11.3 Downward Arrow Diagram

(The beliefs identified are highlighted in bold print.)

If it were true that you would never have a diagnosis for your pain, what would that mean?→ **I wouldn't get the right treatment.** (conditional assumption)
And if that were true, what would that mean?→

I would be stuck with this pain for the rest of my life. (core belief about pain)
If so, what will happen?→

I would be miserable . . . just a blob of nothing. (attitude)
Who wants to be around someone who is miserable? (no one wants to; attitude; core belief about world)
And if no one wants to be around you, then what does that say about you?→

I am not important or needed. (core belief about self)
So, you are afraid that you would be stuck with this pain for the rest of your life, that you would be miserable—"a blob of nothing," thus ultimately feeling unloved or unneeded by others.→

I just really feel like I am being punished. (core belief about world)
Doctors can't leave me hanging here. (underlying "should" or "must"; rule)

LISTENING FOR KEY TERMS TO IDENTIFY INTERMEDIATE AND
CORE BELIEFS

Conditional assumptions unfold during downward arrow exercises when the therapist and patient explore the underlying meaning of automatic thoughts. The therapist can also identify any assumptions in the patient's dialogue that occur naturally in session. For example, if the patient said, "No one wants to be around a complainer," the therapist could summarize the cause-and-effect statement: "So, if you complain about your pain, no one will want to be around you. Is that what you assume?"

Conditional assumptions can also be identified when the therapist and patient explore evidence for a particular core belief. For example, evidence for the core belief "I am helpless" may include "Doctors cannot find a cure" and "I have been in pain for so long." From that list of evidence, the therapist and patient generated the following conditional assumptions:

- If the doctors cannot find a cure, then I am helpless.
- If I have to deal with this pain for the rest of my life, then I am helpless.

Listening for the "shoulds" or the "musts" in the patient's dialogue during therapy sessions can help identify the patient's rules. Another way to identify rules is to have the patient list the "shoulds" or "musts" related to his or her automatic thoughts or core beliefs using a sentence completion task, for example, "I should . . . ," "People should . . . ," The world must . . . ," "My pain should . . . ," and "The future should. . . ."

Attitudes can be identified when the patient tends to assume the worst (catastrophize) and make statements in session that begin with "It's horrible," "It's terrible," "It's awful," or "It's a catastrophe." The therapist can also introduce these attitude stems for the patient to complete in session. Another way to tap into attitudes is to introduce the awful, horrible, or catastrophic qualities of the patient's thought processes to see if those attitudes are indeed there. For example, the therapist could say: "As you are talking about your pain, it sounds as if you are not only saying, 'My pain is unbearable" but also "And that is awful, terrible, or catastrophic.' What do you think?"

COGNITIVE CONCEPTUALIZATION DIAGRAM

The Cognitive Conceptualization Diagram worksheet (CCD; Beck, 1995) can be used to chart automatic thoughts, intermediate beliefs, and core beliefs on one page to see how they are related (see Figure 11.4). Although therapists begin to conceptualize their patients' cases from the first time they meet, the worksheet can help patients see the bigger picture of their presenting problems from a cognitive conceptualization perspective. The CCD is typically introduced to patients after the following conditions have been met: (1) the therapist has developed a clear understanding of the patient's problem(s), (2) the patient has mastered the use of the Automatic Thought Record and can readily identify automatic thoughts associated with his or her pain and life events, and (3) the therapist has introduced the concepts of intermediate and core beliefs.

The patient and therapist start filling out the bottom of the worksheet by writing three examples of common distressing or upsetting situations that have been discussed over the course of therapy. Then, the patient's corresponding automatic thoughts, emotions, behaviors, and pain sensations are written down. These three entries typically come from previous Automatic Thought Record entries or recent discussions in therapy sessions. Next, the patient is asked what each of their automatic thoughts

FIGURE 11.4 Cognitive Conceptualization Diagram

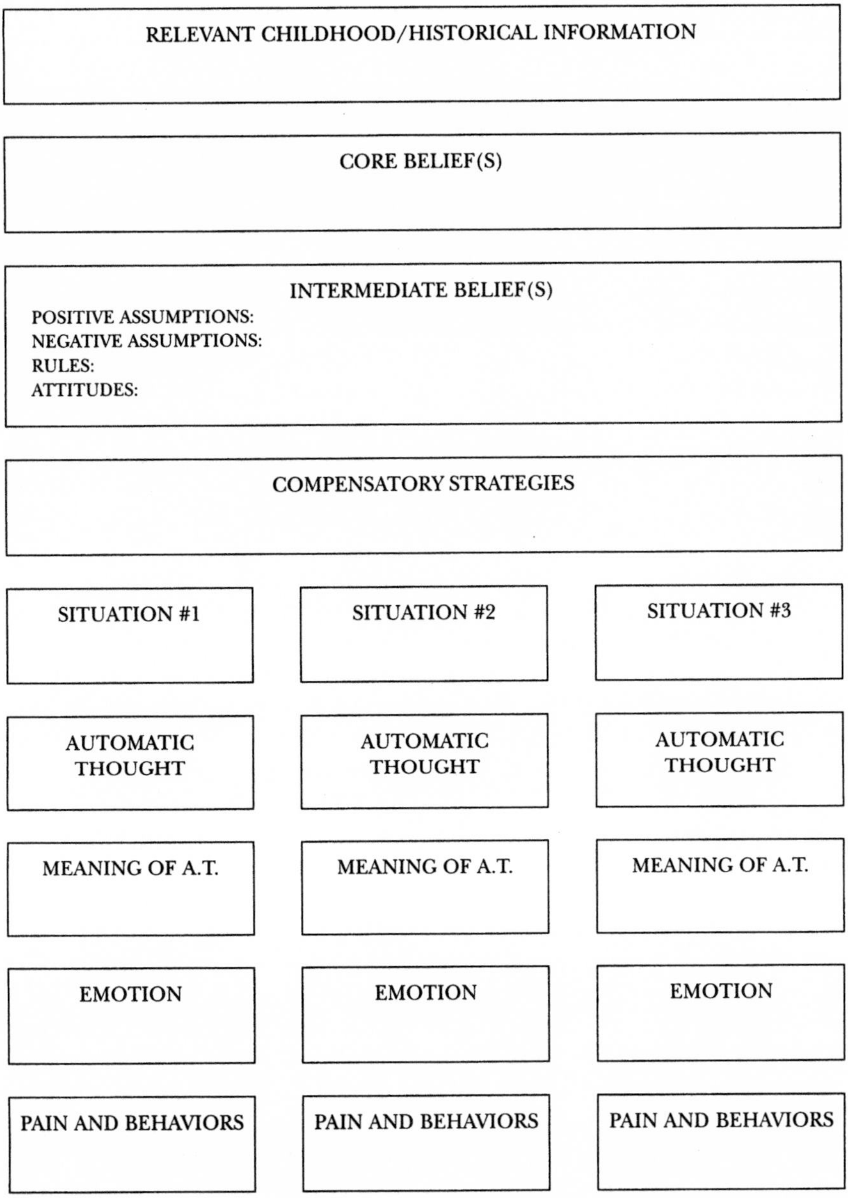

RELEVANT CHILDHOOD/HISTORICAL INFORMATION

CORE BELIEF(S)

INTERMEDIATE BELIEF(S)

POSITIVE ASSUMPTIONS:
NEGATIVE ASSUMPTIONS:
RULES:
ATTITUDES:

COMPENSATORY STRATEGIES

SITUATION #1	SITUATION #2	SITUATION #3
AUTOMATIC THOUGHT	AUTOMATIC THOUGHT	AUTOMATIC THOUGHT
MEANING OF A.T.	MEANING OF A.T.	MEANING OF A.T.
EMOTION	EMOTION	EMOTION
PAIN AND BEHAVIORS	PAIN AND BEHAVIORS	PAIN AND BEHAVIORS

From Judith S. Beck's *Cognitve Therapy: Basics and Beyond.* Copyright 1995 by Judith S. Beck, PhD. Adapted with permission by The Guilford Press: New York.

means (see Meaning of A.T. [Automatic Thought] block) using the downward arrow technique ("If this thought were true, what would it mean?"). Their responses are written down in the section Meaning of A.T. Typically, the underlying meaning of the automatic thought usually identifies a core belief. If that is the case, this same belief will also be written down in the Core Belief(s) section near the top of the worksheet.

Next, the therapist and patient look to find any patterns in the automatic thoughts (Automatic Thought section) or in the meaning that patients' assign to those thoughts (Meaning of A.T. section) to identify any other core beliefs, which are written down in the Core Belief(s) section near the top of the worksheet.

Then, the therapist and patient identify any significant historical events, whether in childhood or adulthood, that may have fostered the development or maintenance of the patient's core beliefs. These events are written down in the Relevant Childhood/Historical Information block.

To identify intermediate beliefs related to the core beliefs, the therapist and patient should start with one core belief and try to identify the rules, the conditional assumptions, and the attitudes connected to that belief before moving on to the next core belief. These rules, assumptions, and attitudes are written down in the section labed Conditional Assumptions, Rules, and Attitudes in the middle of the worksheet.

For example, if one of Logan's core belief is "I am defective," the therapist would ask him what rules for living may be supporting this belief: "What 'shoulds' do you have about your pain or about your life that support this belief?" The therapist can also write down any "shoulds" already identified in therapy that seem to fit with the core belief being discussed. Next, the therapist can help the patient identify the conditional assumptions related to the core belief, using the "if" stem. Negative assumptions are usually identified first. For example, if Logan talks about how he hates being in pain all of the time, the therapist might say, "So, if you are in pain all of the time, then what does that mean?" The patient might say, "Well, then I won't be able to do anything—you know, I'm physically defective." The negative assumption would be written down as "If I am in pain, I won't be able to do anything [physically defective]."

The therapist then inverts the previous "if" stem to uncover the patient's positive assumption, "If you were not in pain all of the time, then what would happen?" The patient responds, "Then I would be physically able to do things." This is a positive assumption because the patient is assuming a positive outcome (i.e., if something happens or some condition is met, a positive result will occur).

Next, the therapist and patient can identify any attitudes that may be related to the core belief. The therapist might say, "When you assume you won't be able to do anything, do you think you might be focusing on the 'horrible' or 'terrible' consequences of your pain?" Logan responds, "Yes. It would be horrible if I couldn't do anything! I used to be a productive citizen in society. Now look at me. I am such a mess. It is awful to be in pain too." Several attitudes were identified here: (1) "It's horrible that I can't do anything," (2) "I am a mess," and (3) "It's awful to be in pain."

It is important to help the patient understand how these intermediate beliefs (rules, conditional assumptions, and attitudes) are connected to their automatic thoughts listed in the three situations. For example, the therapist might summarize the rules, assumptions, and attitudes identified by the patient and ask how these intermediate beliefs might influence how he thinks about his pain and life circumstances on a daily basis. Typically, patients realize in this discussion that rigid rules, attitudes, and negative assumptions are related to their daily negative thinking. The therapist can also help the patient see how the core belief is related to the intermediate beliefs. If the patient assumes a certain outcome, she will be more likely to believe that the outcome is true—in this example, that he is defective (core belief) because he has established a conditional assumption as his reality (e.g., "If I am in pain, I won't be able to do anything"). The rule "I shouldn't be in pain" and the attitudes "It's horrible that I can't do anything," "I am a mess," and "It's awful to be in pain" all feed into the core belief "I am defective." Helping the patient see the connections between the core belief(s) and the intermediate beliefs as well as the relationship between the intermediate belief(s) and the automatic thoughts will prepare the patient to see the connection between the core belief and the automatic thoughts. The therapist and patient can now discuss how the specific core belief identified is a filter that influences daily information processing, (i.e., automatic thoughts) particularly in those situations identified on the form. Here is an example.

Therapist: Logan, your core belief of defectiveness drives your thinking on a day-to-day basis. As you can see in the examples below, your automatic thoughts are focused on what you can't do. The problem with this core belief is that it probably filters out times when you do accomplish things. Can you think of times when you haven't given yourself credit for the small things you can do?

Ineffective or unhealthy behaviors can maintain negative, unrealistic thoughts and beliefs as well as emotions and physiological sensations such as pain. Patients should be encouraged to identify any ineffective coping strategies, also known as compensatory strategies, that are associated with these experiences. Patients try to compensate for their beliefs, thoughts, emotions, or physiology (e.g., pain) in some way. For example, Logan copes with his in defectiveness by isolating himself from others; avoiding physical activities (resulting in muscle deconditioning); idling in the house, focusing on the pain (rather than keeping busy or distracted); and overeating as a way to stuff emotions or the pain. Unfortunately, these overused strategies tend to exacerbate Logan's pain and suffering and maintain his detectiveness belief. These behaviors should be written down in the Compensatory Strategies section of the Cognitive Conceptualization Diagram (see Figure 11.5).

In summary, the Cognitive Conceptualization Diagram helps patients see the relationships among the three levels of thought—automatic thoughts, intermediate beliefs, and core beliefs—and how these thoughts are related to their emotions, behaviors, and pain/physiology. It also makes patients aware of where their core beliefs may have been learned and how they maintain their beliefs (e.g., via compensatory strategies). The information in these diagrams will set the stage for further work on beliefs.

HISTORY OF CORE BELIEFS

It is often helpful to learn how core beliefs developed overtime and how these beliefs were reinforced. The Cognitive Conceptualization diagram can often serve as the impetus for collecting this information. However, historical information related to these core beliefs will emerge at different points in time during therapy, particularly after these beliefs have been identified in session.

> Juan, a 51 year old Hispanic man with complex regional pain, believes he is being punished for being a bad person. His therapist asked him to get in touch with the first time he felt like a bad person. Juan's earliest memory was of his father yelling at him and spanking him for not getting A's in second grade. Juan identified other significant historical events related to his "badness" including his divorce from his wife, his angry temper, and his irregular attendance at mass. In particular, Juan felt that God was punishing him for doing these bad things. He acknowledged that having a strong faith and a commitment to family are important values in his family and in his culture. It is important for the therapist to gain an understanding of the situations or experiences that led to Juan's belief "I am being punished for being bad." The more history to this belief, the more practice Juan has had to think negatively about himself, his pain, and his relationships with others (including God).
>
> Therapists should note the situations that reinforce patients' negative core beliefs, the people associated with these memories, the emotions that surfaced, and the thoughts and beliefs that were activated

FIGURE 11.5 Logan's Cognitive Conceptualization Diagram

RELEVANT CHILDHOOD/HISTORICAL INFORMATION
Parents divorced when young   No medical diagnosis of pain
Few friends during childhood and adulthood   Limited success with medical interventions

CORE BELIEF(S)
My body is defective. (It betrays me.) I am defective.
I am not functional. (I can't do anything.)
I am useless.

INTERMEDIATE BELIEF(S)
POSITIVE ASSUMPTIONS: If I am not in pain, then I am able to do things.
NEGATIVE ASSUMPTIONS: If I am in pain, then I am not able to do anything (physically defective).
RULES: I shouldn't be in pain (all of the time). I should be.
ATTITUDES: It's horrible that I cannot do anything. I am a mess. It's awful to be in pain.

COMPENSATORY STRATEGIES
Lying around the house   Focusing on the pain   Withdrawing from friends
Avoiding physical activities   and family

SITUATION #1	SITUATION #2	SITUATION #3
Sitting at home. Experiencing a dull ache in lower back.	Tries to sweep and mop the floor. Feels "electricity" moving down lower back.	Going for a walk in the park. I tripped on a crack in the sidewalk.

AUTOMATIC THOUGHT	AUTOMATIC THOUGHT	AUTOMATIC THOUGHT
This pain really stinks. I don't have the energy to do anything.	I cannot even mop the floors.	I am clumsy. I can't do anything right.

MEANING OF A.T.	MEANING OF A.T.	MEANING OF A.T.
My body is defective. I am defective.	I am defective. My body is defective (betrays me).	I am not functional. I am useless.

EMOTION	EMOTION	EMOTION
Sad	Angry	Frustrated

PAIN AND BEHAVIORS	PAIN AND BEHAVIORS	PAIN AND BEHAVIORS
Pain: Dull ache in lower back Behaviors: Lying down and avoiding any physical activity	Pain: "Electricity" Behaviors: Stops mopping; lies down; starts eating food	Pain: Sharp, stabbing Behaviors: Sits to rest; then goes home "to hide"

in those situations. Some patients will have a strong history to back up their core belief (starting in childhood). For others, the development of chronic pain or other traumatic events may have triggered new core beliefs later in life. Once therapists have a good understanding of patients' core beliefs and their historical background, then they can move to the evaluation and modification process.

12

Evaluating and Modifying
Beliefs About Pain

Automatic thoughts are more amenable to change than beliefs. As a result, most therapists rely on the Automatic Thought Records, behavioral experiments, and imagery to evaluate and modify automatic thoughts related to pain. Many of the strategies to evaluate and modify beliefs are similar to those used to evaluate and modify automatic thoughts. However, because of the long-standing, global, and rigid nature of negative intermediate and core beliefs, therapists will need to use a variety of intervention strategies to evaluate and modify beliefs regarding pain (e.g., core beliefs worksheets, roleplays, imagery [especially images of past events], cognitive continuum). People are less willing to give up beliefs without a lot of evidence or experiences to the contrary. Throughout the chapter, a patient case will be used to illustrate belief work.

> Austin, a 43 years old Caucasian man, has chronic low back pain as a result of his work as a truck driver—spending long hours sitting behind the wheel. He has been married for 10 years. Austin and his wife have three young children. Since his back surgery, he has been unable to return to work because of the continued pain in his back. Austin has been feeling depressed and reports automatic thoughts including "I cannot work anymore," "No one understands me," and "My livelihood has been taken away from me." "I am useless" was the core belief identified by Austin and his therapist that was related to those automatic thoughts. Austin acknowledged that his fear of survival (his usefulness in providing financially) and his fear of being rejected by his wife for not making money were at the core of his sense of "uselessness."

VIEWING BELIEFS AS IDEAS THAT THEY HAVE LEARNED

The first step in evaluating and modifying beliefs is for patients to learn that beliefs are ideas and not necessarily facts, that they have learned in childhood or in adulthood (especially following a traumatic event or major life change). These beliefs may "feel true" to patients because they usually have a strong historical foundation. Therapists ask patients to suspend their judgment on the accuracy of these beliefs until they have been explored more fully and tested out. Viewing beliefs as ideas (or possibilities) rather than facts will help patients be more objective in examining their beliefs about pain and other life circumstances.

Patient: I feel so useless since my back went out . . . and with all of my back treatments and surgeries. After all, there is not much I can do now with this chronic back pain.

Therapist: Sounds like you're feeling discouraged and down when you believe you're useless. You also sound pretty sure of yourself that this belief is true. Why don't we suspend our judgment for a while about how "useless" you are until we can collect more information? Rather than letting this belief "win" before the race has begun, let's view this belief, "I am useless," as an idea to test out.

Patient: Okay. I'm willing to give it a try.

QUESTIONING

Open-ended questions can help patient evaluate their beliefs (e.g., How do you know your belief is true? What experiences support this belief? What might be some experiences you have had that don't fit with this belief? What is the evidence against this belief?). Questions also help patients develop more accurate, realistic beliefs about their chronic pain, themselves, their world, and their future.

Therapist: You mentioned earlier that at the core of your "uselessness" are your fears of financial survival and personal rejection. Tell me more about that.

Austin: Well, I have always been the primary breadwinner, so I really do believe that I am useless if I cannot provide for my family. That has been a very important role in my life . . . my work. I also do fear what my wife will think about me if I can't work.

Therapist: What does your wife think of you now . . . given the fact that you're not working?

Austin: Well, there has been some stress in our relationship because bills aren't being paid. She thinks I'm doing the best that I can right now and understands that my pain is real and that it is debilitating. However, I have a tough time believing that this will last. I'm just waiting for rejection. I feel that it may be just around the corner.

Therapist: You mentioned stress in your relationship to the point that you anticipate rejection. Has your wife rejected you up to this point in your relationship, considering all of the years you've been together?

Austin: Well, come to think of it, no. Sometimes we call each other names when we argue. There was a time early in our relationship when we considered breaking up, but it wasn't over my work. I guess the pressure I feel to provide financially . . . I don't wish that on anyone, especially my wife. And I don't want this relationship to end because I cannot work and provide for us.

Therapist: Does your wife work?

Austin: Yes. We really need both of our incomes to make ends meet. But I have always made more money.

Therapist: So, up until now, you have shared the financial responsibilities in this relationship. However, you've been the main provider, which seems to be an important aspect of your worth and your identity. What are some of your other "useful" or "valuable" qualities that your wife appreciates?

Austin: Well, I am a loyal and loving person. I care a great deal about people. [Exploring other evidence of his "usefulness"]

From the example above, the therapist used questions to explore the validity or accuracy of the patient's conditional assumption that his wife will reject him if he cannot work. So far, this outcome has not occurred. This issue will be explored further in therapy at some point in time.

The therapist also asked questions to clarify what the patient values as his "useful" qualities. This helps move the patient temporarily away from his negative core belief of uselessness and helps him go "outside the box" of this negative core belief to clarify what he views as his "usefulness." Some patients with chronic pain who have been primarily responsible for the financial welfare of their relationships or of their families tend to put a great deal of their identity into their work and into their breadwinner role. To not be able to work has a variety of different implications, depending on patients' beliefs about work, their livelihood, and their value as human beings.

Therapists do not tell the patient how they should perceive or interpret their pain and its consequences. Through the use of questioning, therapists help patients discover the unrealistic or negative nature of their beliefs
by exploring evidence for and against those beliefs. In addition, therapists'
questions may uncover alternative, more realistic beliefs (e.g., getting the
client to generate reframes). Just getting patients to consider the possibility of their beliefs not being totally accurate or realistic is a small yet important step in the evaluation and modification stage of belief work.

A metaphor that is used to teach patients about alternative explanations ("reframes") for beliefs is to have them look at a picture in the therapy room and then imagine the picture with a different frame on it. The
frame could have a different color, a different texture, or it could even
be made out of a different material. Would the picture look different with
a different frame on it? Would you notice different colors, shapes, and
sizes of the people, places, or objects in the picture? Most patients agree
that the frame "makes" the picture. In the same way, how we frame events
in our lives—the meaning we give to our experiences—determines how
our lives will look to us.

Given that intermediate and core beliefs are more resistant to change
than are automatic thoughts, it is important that the therapist be patient
and not become frustrated when change in belief systems does not come
as quickly as automatic thought work. The therapist also should not push
questioning to the point of interrogating the patient. In keeping with the
collaborative model of therapy, the therapist should choose questions selectively to learn more about the patient and his or her "foundation" of beliefs
(e.g., selective information processing and historical information) or to
evaluate and modify these beliefs. The use of questioning alone may or may
not lead to belief modification. However, combined with other techniques
(e.g., Core Belief worksheet, behavioral experiments, using others as a reference point), questions can lead patients to consider information that they
had previously discarded or discounted, thus loosening the strength or validity of their belief systems. Questioning techniques are among the essential
ingredients for belief work to succeed in therapy. Examples of specific questions will be illustrated under the following techniques.

CORE BELIEF WORKSHEET

The Core Belief Worksheet (see Figure 12.1) helps patients evaluate the
evidence for and against their core beliefs about their chronic pain and
other life issues. It is very similar to exploring evidence for and against
automatic thoughts. However, the main differences are that (1) the ther-

apist and patient are evaluating evidence for and against beliefs that tend to be more ingrained than fleeting thoughts, (2) evidence for and against beliefs tend to include more historical (e.g., lifelong) data and not just data during a moment of distress or crisis,, and (3) patients are taught to refute the evidence supporting their negative beliefs and write alternative explanations for each piece of evidence (otherwise known as reframes) in the Evidence That Supports Old Core Belief With Reframe column.

To start, the core belief that was identified in therapy work is written at the top of the Core Belief Worksheet. The patient is asked how strongly he or she believes the core belief right now on a scale from 0 to 100. Then the patient is asked how much he or she believed that core belief as well as how little he or she believed it over the past week. Next, the patient is asked to provide the information or evidence that supports the core belief. All of this evidence is recorded in the column Evidence That Supports Old Core Belief With Reframe. The therapist should leave plenty of room between each piece of evidence supporting this belief because alternative explanation or "reframes" will be written next to each piece of evidence shortly. Next, each piece of evidence supporting the core belief is reviewed one at a time, and alternative explanations for each piece of evidence are generated.

Then, the therapist asks the patient to provide any information or evidence that the core belief may not be true. Each piece of evidence is written in the column Evidence That Contradicts Old Core Belief and Supports New Belief. Note that a new belief has not yet been developed. So, for the time being, evidence against the core belief is recorded. It is not uncommon to find that patients provide therapists with less information in this category given that they have not had much experience in focusing on or attending to information that contradicts their core beliefs. Therefore, one of the responsibilities of the therapist is to help the patient become aware of information that he or she may have discarded or discounted that serves as evidence against the patient's core beliefs. At this point in therapy, the therapist has heard a number of stories from the patient and is able to provide any information heard in session that could be put down as evidence against the core belief. However, it is still essential for the patient to generate information in the column before the therapist adds evidence to that side of the worksheet.

The therapist then asks the patient to take a look at all of the evidence (both columns) to see if the old core belief needs to be altered or changed to reflect a more accurate reality. A new alternative core belief is generated and written down in the space next to New Belief. Oftentimes, it is a slight modification of the original core belief, not a completely different belief. As a last step, the therapist and patient go back to the column

FIGURE 12.1 Core Belief Worksheet

Old Core Belief:_____
    How much do you believe the old core belief right now?
    (0–100)_____
    *What is the most you believed it this week? (0–100)_____
    *What is the least you believed it this week? (0–100)_____

New Belief:_____
    How much do you believe the new belief right now?
    (0–100)_____

EVIDENCE THAT CONTRADICTS OLD CORE BELIEF AND SUPPORTS NEW BELIEF	EVIDENCE THAT SUPPORTS OLD CORE BELIEF WITH REFRAME

* Should situations related to an increase or decrease in strength of the belief be topics for the agenda?
From Judith S. Beck's *Cognitive Therapy: Basics and Beyond.* Copyright 1995 by Judith S. Beck, PhD. Reprinted with permission by the Guilford Press: New York.

"Evidence That Contradicts Old Core Belief and Supports New Belief to write down any evidence that supports the new belief. These items are recorded in this column.

Restructuring beliefs does not automatically mean that patients will develop brand-new beliefs. In reality, therapists work with patients to slowly "chip away" at these beliefs rather than totally "demolish" them. Because patients are reluctant to give up these beliefs, given the inherent qualities of core beliefs, small changes to these beliefs are more common. For example, if the original core belief is "I cannot trust any doctors to take care of my pain," an alternative, more realistic belief might be "I can trust one or two doctors to take care of my pain, but most of the other doctors I cannot trust" rather than "I can trust any doctor." It is unrealistic for therapists to expect that patients will flip from one extreme to an other in terms of core belief work. Moving from "I cannot trust any doctor" to "I can trust any doctor" is probably not a very common occurrence in core belief restructuring work in one therapy session. Figure 12.2 is an example of a core belief worksheet for Austin.

COGNITIVE CONTINUUM TECHNIQUE

Patients' core beliefs are absolute statements about themselves, their pain, the world around them, or their future, for example, "The pain controls me," "I am a misfit," "No one understands my pain," and "I have nothing to look forward to in the future." One of the main distortions in core beliefs is their all-or-nothing character. To evaluate and modify the all-or-nothing nature of core beliefs related to pain, these beliefs can be put on a continuum of experience rather than viewing pain or other issues from a global, rigid, all-or-nothing point of view.

Patients are asked to rate their core belief on a scale from 0 to 100, with 0 being not at all true and 100 being totally true. Most patients initially rate their core beliefs as being highly true of themselves, usually in the 90 to 100 range. Then, patients are asked to identify the anchors on each end of the continuum with a line drawn between these anchors. For example, some chronic pain patients "feel like" (think they are) failures for not being able to return to work. The term failure could be written on one end of the continuum and the opposite of failure, in this case, success, could be written at the other.

Then, patients are asked to rate their pain, themselves, or their experiences on this continuum. Patients put an X on the line where they see themselves on the dimension of interest. It is not uncommon to find that patients still rate themselves at the negative end of the continuum.

FIGURE 12.2 Austin's Core Belief Worksheet

Old Core Belief: <u>I am useless</u>.

    How much do you believe the old core belief right now? (0–100)   <u>65</u>

    *What is the most you believed it this week? (0–100)   <u>100</u>

    *What is the least you believed it this week? (0–100)   <u>65</u>

New Belief: <u>There is more to me than being a truck driver and making money.</u>
<u>I might have some use (worth) in this world</u>.

    How much do you believe the new belief right now? (0–100)   <u>70</u>

EVIDENCE THAT CONTRADICTS OLD CORE BELIEF AND SUPPORTS NEW BELIEF	EVIDENCE THAT SEEMS TO SUPPORT OLD CORE BELIEF WITH REFRAME
I am a loyal and loving person. I care about people a great deal.	**I cannot work anymore.** I can't drive a truck anymore. That is a given, according to my doctors. However, I can still explore other career options. If my pain prevents me from working in other fields, I can be reminded that there are other people who don't work who have value.
Although I may not be able to work right now, I am able to do small tasks in and around the house. So I am not totally useless. I can help out some.	**My livelihood has been taken away from me.** Because I am not able to financially provide for my family the way I used to, I will have to find some other form of work. Or I will have to accept that I have this disability and find ways to be useful to others. **Men should work and be providers.** That was how I was raised. I can't make myself work and be miserable. My doctor said my condition was severe. **If I can't work, my partner might leave me.** I have to remind myself that my wife thinks I am doing the best I can right now.

* Should situations related to an increase or decrease in strength of the belief be topics for the agenda?

Patients are asked to explain why they rated themselves at that point on the continuum.

Next, patients define the anchors on the continuum by providing examples of behaviors or experiences that represent each anchor concept. The purpose of this part of the exercise is to expand on their definitions of the absolutes for each anchor. Asking questions like "Could it be worse? Could anyone fail worse than this?" and "What does total failure look like? Could anyone else fail more than you have? Is not being able to return to work the worst type of failure possible?" can help to clarify what the negative anchor is. "What does total success look like?" "Could anyone achieve this level of success?" "What would people have to do to achieve total success?" are examples of questions that expand on the definition of this positive anchor. Then, patients are asked to rate themselves again on this continuum given these clarified definitions of the anchors. Many patients learn that they do not rate themselves as negatively as they did before. In other words, they are not on the extremes of the continuum but rather somewhere along the continuum.

Here is an example of how Austin and his therapist evaluated the accuracy of his core belief that "he is useless" in session using the cognitive continuum technique. This is a shortened version of the technique:

Therapist: Before we start testing out this belief, tell me how useless you have been, on a scale from 0 to 100, with 100 being the most useless anyone could ever be. [Putting belief on a continuum]

Austin: Oh, I'd say about 98. There is not much I can do to change my circumstances. I feel like such a cripple.

Therapist: How would you know if someone was totally useless—someone with a score of 100?

Austin: Well, people are totally useless if they didn't work at all, ever again. People have to contribute meaningfully to something . . . like making money, taking care of their partners or families, finding purpose and enjoyment—that is what working does for people.

Therapist: So, are you saying that anyone who is disabled or is retired is useless?

Patient: [pause] Well, not exactly. There are different reasons why people can't work. I'm just saying that I'm useless because I can't work. That doesn't make other people useless.

Therapist: So, how come you're useless but others aren't?

Patient: Probably because I'm being hard on myself and not others.

Therapist: What does that do for you?

Patient: It makes me feel worse.

Therapist: Okay, so if we are defining "totally useless" for everyone, what could we put down here? [points to anchor]
Patient: Not contributing in a meaningful way.

Therapist: Do you have any other ideas about what "totally useless" would look like?
Patient: An example of "total uselessness" is when people just sit around letting life pass them by. People are also totally useless when they don't care about others, just themselves.

Therapist: Okay, anything else? Any images that come to mind when you think of "total uselessness"?
Patient: I get an image of someone who doesn't bathe or take care of himself. I think that's about it.

Therapist: Do you know of anyone personally who would fit this description —of being totally useless—someone who doesn't work at all, doesn't care about others, sits around, doesn't take care of themselves?
Patient: Not really. Some of the homeless people on the streets probably fit the bill.

Therapist: What about the opposite end of the spectrum? What words would you use to define that end?
Patient: I would say, "totally useful."

Therapist: What would "totally useful" look like?
Patient: A person who is totally useful would be working and making money to take care of their partners or their families and would be actively involved with others.

Therapist: Actively involved.
Patient: Yeah. People will get out of their house and participate in meaningful social and community activities. They will have friends and family who love them because they care.

Therapist: Anything else? Any other words or images to describe "totally useful"?
Patient: I think that does it.

Therapist: Okay. Under "totally useful," I'll write "working, making money, actively involved, and loved." Does that sum up what you were saying?
Patient: Yes.

Therapist: Okay, let's look at the figure I drew. This is a line representing a continuum, 0 being totally useful and 100 being totally useless. Underneath the 0 and the 100 are your criteria for these two anchors on the continuum (Figure 12.3). Where would you rate yourself now?

Patient: Well, I am certainly *not* working right now. Don't know if I will ever be. But I do try to take care of myself, at least for right now, you know, taking a bath and stuff. My partner hasn't left me yet. So, maybe I'm at an 80.

FIGURE 12.3 Cognitive Continuum

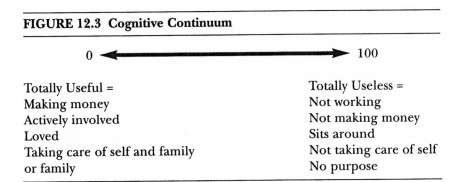

Totally Useful =	Totally Useless =
Making money	Not working
Actively involved	Not making money
Loved	Sits around
Taking care of self and family	Not taking care of self
or family	No purpose

Therapist: Okay, Austin. Now, help me understand how you became more useful, just even in the past few minutes. You went from a 98 to an 80.

Patient: [pause] I guess that I still have friends and family who care and I am still taking steps to take care of myself.

PIE CHARTS

The pie chart technique (Beck, 1995) is similar to the cognitive continuum technique in that it helps patients to graphically display their negative core beliefs to modify their all-or-nothing nature. To represent the "pie," a circle is drawn in the middle of the page and the patient is asked to "cut the pie" into slices representing dimensions of the negative core belief by drawing the slices and writing the content of the slice in the space provided. For example, Bernice's automatic thought, "I cannot cope with my pain," is also one of her negative core beliefs. She could be asked to cut the pie in slices to represent how much control she has in coping with her pain and how much of it is out of her control. Then, she could write down examples of her efforts to cope with the pain in the "slice" representing her control.

Patients can also be asked to draw the slice of the pie representing how much their beliefs are a part of their identity. For example, Austin could be asked to slice the pie in a way that represents how much of him is useless—the pie representing his whole identity. How much of the pie represents "useless"? Are there some pieces of the pie that represent other characteristics? After that, the therapist can ask Austin what ingredients make up his "uselessness." The other slices of the pie could be explored—if any are left—with the goal of identifying other aspects of his personhood. These other "slices" could be discussed, with an emphasis on their "ingredients."

BEHAVIORAL EXPERIMENTS

The nature of designing and conducting behavioral experiments with automatic thoughts or with beliefs is essentially the same, except that beliefs are more resistant to change and typically have more history behind them. Therefore, it will take a series of experiments to modify beliefs. In other words, it takes more evidence to modify beliefs than automatic thoughts.

One of the artistic aspects of therapy is the creativity involved in developing behavioral experiments to test out patients' beliefs. Some patients may have ideas about how to test their beliefs. However, most of them tend to rely on their therapists in developing such experiments. Being collaborative in developing experiments is essential.

Here is an example of a behavioral experiment developed to test the core belief "I am useless."

Therapist: Let's put your belief, "I am useless," to the test. Do you have any ideas how we could put this thought to the test—to find out how useless or useful you really are?

Austin: Well, the reality is I'm not working. I'm used to staying busy in my daily life. Now that I have this horrible back pain, I haven't been able to return to work, so I'm stuck.

Therapist: So, right now, you have viewed "usefulness" as working and making money. Maybe you could interview other people to find out what "useful" means to them—for example, what a useful person looks like, what they do on a typical day, how they spend their time, and so forth. Then, you could interview those same people to find out what "uselessness" means—what a useless person looks like, what they do or not do on a typical day, how they spend their time, and so forth.

Austin: That's sounds appealing to me. I would like to know what others think about this.

Therapist: That's a great plan. I would like to add another part to this. In order to test out whether your belief, "I am useless," is accurate or not, you can also ask the people you interview to rate you on the continuum we developed in session today. Take this sheet of paper with the continuum on it and have three close friends or family members rate your level of uselessness—remember to select people who will be honest with you.

Patient: Gosh, that seems a little scary to me. People may laugh if I show them this. I have never confronted this before directly . . . in this way before.

Therapist: Well, we could see what happens. There are a number of possible outcomes. Maybe, you will discover that people find it silly because it's something you have never asked them about before. Or maybe it will seem silly because they believe in you and your efforts, and do not view you as useless. Maybe they won't find it silly at all. It might help you talk openly with your friends and family about your negative beliefs and feelings about your pain and your physical limitations. What do you think?

Patient: I think I need to do it. This belief has been a core issue for me for some time. When I was growing up, my father was always doing, doing, doing. His concept of success was finding meaningful work and doing it. You know, provide for the family. So I know where this belief started, and I've carried it forward. It sure has motivated me at times in the past. But I find that it's a sore spot for me now— because if I could, I would go back to work. But I can't. The docs have said "no way."

Therapist: This is a common feature of core beliefs: They usually begin early in life and can be activated by a number of circumstances. "I am useful" was a belief you've had about yourself for some time, but now that you're in pain, you cannot return to your truck-driving career. This has activated the opposite belief, "I am useless." [pause] To help you test out the validity of this belief, why don't we have you interview three close friends and family members who can truly speak about your abilities as a person, in other words, your level of usefulness. You can ask them first what it means to be a useful person and a useless person—to search for universal meanings on the topic. You may find that each person has a different definition of it. Then, as part of our behavioral experiment, you will have them rate you on your level of uselessness or usefulness, using this continuum. At least, this would provide us with some outside information to see if your belief is true or not.

Austin: I'm ready to give this a try. I'll ask my partner and maybe my friend Curtis and my mother to help out.

Therapist: Okay. That sounds like a plan. Now, what are your predictions about the outcome of this experiment?

Austin: I think my family and friends will agree with me that worth and work are highly connected. They will probably think I am useless too.

Therapist: Okay, let's write down your predictions. If those predictions come true, how will you handle it?

Austin: I certainly would be hurt, but I have believed this so strongly for so long that it really won't devastate me. In fact, it will probably get this issue out in the open. I haven't really shared with my friends and family how useless I have felt.

Therapist: So you feel that you could cope okay if your family and friends think that you are useless?

Austin: Yes. And maybe I could clarify that I am trying to get better. You know, I am trying to get back up on my feet, so to speak. I mean, the doctors told me that I couldn't work as a trucker anymore, so I've got to face that reality. And now maybe I can face that reality with the people I care about.

Therapist: Well, that sounds like a plan. Do you think you could reach all three of these people over the next week so that you could report back your findings in our next session?

Austin: Yes, I think so.

Therapist: Okay. Remember to suspend your judgment about your level of usefulness until this behavioral experiment is completed. Also, don't share with your friends and family your own ratings of your uselessness or usefulness until after you have completed your interview with them. We don't want to bias their responses. Does that make sense?

Austin: Yes, I agree. I want to hear what they think first.

Therapist: All right. Let's see what happens next week.

[Next session]

Therapist: Well, I know we discussed putting your belief "I am useless" to the test by conducting a behavioral experiment. How did it go?

Austin: Well, I was really nervous about interviewing my friends and family at first. But I knew this was what I needed to do to find out if my thought was true. I was very shocked by what I learned from this. I received so much support . . . more than I ever imagined. And no one thought that I was useless. I couldn't believe it!

Therapist: So no one believed you were useless.

Austin: Yes, well, they totally understand how degraded I feel about not being able to return to work. But no one thought my total worth as a person was centered on my work. They rated me very high on being useful.

Therapist: Where did each of them rate you on the continuum?
Austin: All of them rated me very high on the useful side . . . anywhere from 7 to 10 on the scale. [note: 0 = totally useful, 100 = totally useless].

Therapist: Do you have any idea what led them to that conclusion about you?
Austin: Well it was connected to their ideas about what *useful* and *useless* meant.

Therapist: How did your family members and friends define them?
Austin: Similar to some of my ideas. Work was only one part of the picture. They also identified helping others, giving people a hand, being caring, offering information, and being a guide as important qualities. *Useless* was harder to define for them. My wife said that there is no reality called "useless" because everyone has worth or value.

Therapist: So, what did you learn from this experiment?
Austin: I learned that I have been very critical of myself. My family and friends don't think I'm useless. There is no such thing as being useless, according to my wife. That feedback made me feel better about our relationship.

Therapist: I'm glad to hear that the people you really care about think you are useful. So, when we go back to the original hypothesis, "If I interview my family and friends, they will agree that I am useless," does that prediction hold?
Austin: No. My close friends and family think just the opposite. They view me as useful and acknowledge that work is only one of many roles in my life.

Therapist: So, let's go back to the core belief, "I am useless." How strongly do you believe it now?
Austin: Much less. I rate it about a 40 now.

Therapist: What is another way of thinking about yourself and your life when that core belief "I am useless" pops up in your mind?
Austin: Well, I can remind myself that I do have some value as a person even though I cannot work right now. So, I am not totally useless. I am trying to better my condition and myself. My friends, my wife, and my mom believe in me.

Therapist: And how strongly do you believe that?
Austin: About a 75.

Therapist: Well, let's write this alternative, more realistic belief you just
    developed on a coping card to remind you of this belief when the
    old "I am useless" belief pops up in your mind.

ACTING "AS IF"

Patients can adapt their beliefs by acting "as if" their beliefs were not true.
This is a specific type of behavioral experiment that allows clients the freedom to experience "reality" differently. Most people at some point in time
in their lives have played a role or acted out a part to cope with a situation, whether it be a public speaking situation, a part in a play, a job interview, or a first date.

Acting "as if" means that the patient will learn to act as if his or her
belief was not true. The purposes of pretending or acting are (1) to increase
the patient's range of experiences to handle a situation, and (2) to see
what other emotions, thoughts, behaviors, and physiology emerge if the
patient does something differently.

> For example, Austin, the patient who feels useless, could be asked to
> do a behavioral experiment—to act as if he were useful. To prepare
> for this role, Austin and his therapist could discuss what being useful
> would look like in terms of his behaviors, his feelings, his pain levels
> and how he copes with pain, his thought processes—what would be
> his internal dialogue if he felt useful?—and so on. What kinds of activ-
> ities would he be involved with, who would he be relating to, and what
> would he be doing differently if he believed and acted as if he were
> useful? Austin will be encouraged to just simply observe and note how
> things may feel the same or different for him while he performs this
> experiment over the next week. When he returns for the next session,
> the acting "as if" experiment can be discussed to see what actually
> happened—did his experience of pain change in any way? Did he
> cope differently with his pain when he acted useful? Did he get dif-
> ferent reactions from the people around him? Did he do anything dif-
> ferent than before? What activities did he participate in? How did he
> feel about himself during this week? What thoughts or images ran
> through his mind this week?

Processing this experiment can give the patient insight into what it would mean to try something different—for example, act as if he was useful. This experience can help patients feel better about themselves by thinking and doing the opposite of their beliefs.

It is important for the therapist to understand the meaning of a patient's intermediate and core beliefs, as this will help the therapist and patient develop an effective acting "as if" experiment. For example, two chronic pain patients can have the same negative core belief related to punishment—"I am being punished"—but these beliefs may have different meanings for each patient. Some patients may believe "I am being punished" to mean that God or a higher power is "getting back at them" for their sins. One possible experiment to test this thought may be to act as if the patient's sins have been forgiven, not only by God or a higher power but also by the patient and by others. Other patients may subscribe to "I am being punished" because they believe that they are essentially bad (e.g., Juan). A possible experiment would be for the patient to act as if he or she has some good qualities. Other patients might feel punished by others because they view others as uncaring and insensitive. A behavioral experiment would be to act as if those people's actions are not purposefully malevolent; rather, they just do not understand what the patient is going through.

Usually the acting "as if" experiment involves having the patient believe and act in a manner that is opposite his or her original negative beliefs, but not necessarily the extreme opposite of those original negative beliefs. It is up to the therapist and the patient to decide what will be realistic for the patient to act out. For example, if the patient's belief is "I cannot cope with my pain," to act as if the patient were pain-free would not be getting at the essence of this original negative belief. It would also be an unrealistic exercise because the patient's pain cannot simply disappear. A more appropriate experiment would be to act as if the patient has the ability to cope with the pain—helping the patient to focus on coping efforts and believing in those efforts.

One of the most essential ingredients to this acting "as if" experiment is the patient's commitment to carry out this exercise—to act as if the original belief was not true and to believe and act from a different viewpoint, one that is defined by the therapist and the patient (e.g., acting as if the patient had been forgiven by God or that God is not angry; acting as if the patient were a good person; acting as if everyone was *not* out to "get" the patient).

Here are some other examples of acting "as if" experiments.

Negative Intermediate or Core Belief	*Acting as If . . .*
I have no control over my pain.	I have some control over my pain.
It is not okay to have pain.	I accept my pain as part of my existence and will take action to reduce it if possible.
If I ask for help, then I am a wimp. I should be independent.	It is okay to ask for help.
I am worthless/useless.	I have some worth as a person.
Bad things happen to me.	I am in charge of my destiny.
Nobody cares about me.	The world can be a friendly place. There are people who care about me.

What is acting, and what is real? This is hard to say. The acting "as if" experiments can actually lead to some positive changes in the patient's situation. For example, some patients learn that thinking and behaving as if they have some control over their pain;they may find some real control or more support and understanding. As someone once said, "Attitude is everything." The combination of believing in another possible reality and acting as if that reality were true can lead to positive and meaningful changes in patients' lives. For others, this experience may not be life altering, but it may open patients' minds to different possibilities, which is part of the cognitive restructuring process in belief work.

ADVANTAGES/DISADVANTAGES ANALYSIS OF BELIEFS

When patients identify and evaluate their intermediate and core beliefs, but seem resistant to consider alternative, more realistic beliefs as plausible, there may be underlying motivations for maintaining old beliefs (e.g., keeping the negative beliefs strong and resilient to change) as well as failing to adopt healthy, realistic beliefs. The advantages/disadvantages exercise can clarify what barriers may be interfering with the change process as well as assist in identifying areas that need further exploration in order for belief restructuring to occur.

Below is the advantages/disadvantages analysis for Austin's old core belief, "I am useless," versus Austin's new alterative belief, "I might have some use (worth) in this world.

Advantages and disadvantages of believing "I am useless":

Advantages	Disadvantages
I don't have to expect much from myself.	I get stuck in feeling depressed.
I might get more attention from others.	I am not giving myself credit for what I can do.
	People don't want to hang out with me if I am lost in this madness.
	It makes me want to give up and not even try to do something about my life.

Advantages and disadvantages of believing "I might have some use (worth) in this world":

Advantages	Disadvantages
It might give me more hope.	If I believe this, then I may disappoint my family and myself.
People might treat me differently if I believed in myself.	It doesn't fit with what I learned growing up—I've got to make money and do something meaningful to be useful.

This intervention helped Austin and his therapist identify his stuck points in changing his belief. The one piece of evidence that Austin had to address in more detail was his family of origin rules about making money and doing something meaningful, before he was able to accept the alternative belief. This will be addressed in the next rational emotive role-play. Readers are referred to chapter 8 for more information on this advantages/disadvantages technique.

ROLE-PLAYS

As mentioned in chapter 9, role-plays are used to modify automatic thoughts. Role-plays are also used to (1) modify beliefs about pain and other life issues in the here-and-now and (2) teach patients communication skills and how to relate better to others. Because most chronic pain patients who enter therapy have given their negative beliefs a lot of "air time" in their minds, it is important for patients to learn how to articulate alternative beliefs that can be more realistic and helpful. Although it is common to hear patients talk about their beliefs in session, role-plays allow therapists and patients to hear how these beliefs come out in the patients' own words in session. This provides valuable information for therapists to prepare counterpoints or counterarguments to these beliefs in the moment.

Patients often have difficulty letting go of their negative core beliefs because these beliefs have a strong emotional component, for example, "My head knows it's not true, but my heart/emotions believe it so strongly." Therefore, most role-plays in belief work involve "head vs. heart" dialogues.

There are several steps in facilitating role-plays in session. The therapist starts by explaining that the purpose of role-plays is to help evaluate and modify a specific belief. Next, the therapist prepares the patient for the roles they will play. The patient is usually asked to role-play old beliefs first (e.g., "I am useless") or their "heart/emotions/gut" side. The therapist will either role-play the counterargument (e.g., point out inaccuracies/distortions if role-playing is done before alternative beliefs have been developed) or the viewpoints of the alternative, more realistic core beliefs (e.g., "I am useful"), otherwise known as the "rational/head" side. The next step is to begin the role-play. To help the patient start, the therapist could encourage the patient to get in touch with his or her emotions related to negative core belief about pain or to think back to a recent time when the negative core belief was activating before he or she starts speaking from the old negative beliefs. The role-play is discussed after the patient and therapist have had the chance to explore these viewpoints and emotions in some detail.

The second part of the role-play is very critical, as the patient needs practice speaking from the counterpoint position or from the alternative belief viewpoint. At the end of the role-play, the therapist and patient discuss what the experience was like for the patient and what the patient learned from doing the role-play.

In the following dialogue, Austin and his therapist evaluate his belief of "uselessness" using a role-play.

Therapist: As we discussed in our session last week, what distresses you
   most about your chronic pain is your belief that your pain signifies
   uselessness—your uselessness. I was wondering if we could explore
   this more in session today, with a different twist. This time instead
   of talking about it, we could have the core belief talk out loud in
   session, so we can learn how to talk back to it.
Patient: How are we going to do that?

Therapist: Well, we can do a role-play. One of us can "act out" the core belief by speaking from that perspective—that you are useless. The other person will present arguments that this belief is not true. They will "act out" the other side—the side of you that believes that you have some use or worth in this world. Would you be willing to give this a try?

Patient: Okay. Sounds good.

Therapist: Since you have had a lot of practice viewing yourself and your pain through the "lens" that you are useless, how about if you start and speak from that perspective"? I, on the other hand, will present arguments why you are useful. Are you ready?

Patient: Yes.

Therapist: Take a moment to get in touch with how useless you think you are and all of the feelings and all of the experiences that related to this. If you feel stuck, think of a recent time when you felt useless. When you're ready, just begin explaining to me why you are totally useless. Remember, you are talking to me—I am the side of you that believes that you are useful.

Patient: Let me tell you how totally useless I am. I cannot work anymore. Being a truck driver was my whole life. I really enjoyed getting out there on the road, getting the cargo to its location, meeting new people along the way, the wide open road . . . how freeing. Without work, I'm useless. I have nothing meaningful to contribute. [pause]

Therapist: Just because I can't work as a truck driver doesn't mean I am useless. [using *I* instead of *you* to make it more immediate and personal] I haven't given myself time to explore other possible careers. You know, the average person changes careers at least three times during his or her lifetime.

Patient: I don't think I'll ever be able to work again—not as a truck driver or anything.

Therapist: It's possible that I might not ever be able to work as a truck driver. But that doesn't necessarily mean I can never work again. If working means that much to me, maybe it's time to consider a different line of work.

Patient: What's the point? My manhood has been stripped of me because of my pain and suffering. I cannot work behind the wheel without pain, and I cannot have sex with this pain. I feel like an invalid.

Therapist: It really stinks. I wish I didn't have this pain in my back, but it isn't always so severe. There are times when I can manage it. Maybe I can find ways to work and have sex without the intensity of pain I have been having. I *am* still a man. Maybe I have put so much of my identity into my work that I have forgotten the other parts of me—the many parts of my manhood.

Patient: I just want to know why I was dealt such a bad hand in life! I can't take care of my family like I did before. I'm so ashamed.

Therapist: I am ashamed of myself because of my "shoulds"—because of my rules about how my life should be. I didn't ask for this accident to happen to me. I didn't will it to happen. It just happened. Blaming myself for something that was out of my control is not fair to me or to the other people around me. Maybe I cannot provide financially like I did before. What can I do about it? Maybe if I find another career, I can get myself back on track as a provider. Then again, I may not be able to find work that accommodates my pain. I need to remember that there are other ways that I can "provide" for my partner and others: by showing them love, by listening to them and helping them, by letting them into my world so that they can understand my pain, and by taking care of myself and feeling better about myself. I need to think about how I can contribute to myself and to others.

Patient: [Pause] I really don't know what to say next. I liked what you said.

Therapist: Thanks. Before we switch roles, let's discuss what the experience was like for you so far.

Patient: It's amazing what comes out when I focus on my uselessness. I didn't realize how negative it could get.

Therapist: What feelings did you get in touch with when speaking from the useless belief?

Patient: Despair, shame, anger, depression.

Therapist: What were some of the main themes you heard when speaking from this side?

Patient: It makes me want to give up, feeling hopelessness, feeling out of control.

Therapist: Good. I also heard several other themes that we may want to address further after the role-play. One is thinking that you have lost your manhood; this seems to be related to your perception that you cannot work, provide for your family, or enjoy sex with your wife. Another important theme is feeling like you've been dealt a bad hand in life.

Patient: Yep. I think that sums it up.

Therapist: What did you hear from this side—the "useful" side?

Patient: Well, you made me aware that it is up to me how I define myself. Maybe I've put too much emphasis on my work role as a big part of my identity. But I had forgotten about other ways of contributing—like caring for others and giving to others. You also made me aware of the possible reality that there may be another line of work that I could do. I had not seriously considered that before.

Therapist: Okay! Sounds like you learned a lot from this role-play. Why don't we switch roles now? This will help you practice speaking from the side of you that believes you have something to offer, that you are useful. And I will start speaking from the useless side. Are you ready to switch roles?

Patient: Okay.

Therapist: Please take your time to develop your arguments or to explain your points. I don't want you to feel rushed in any way with this part of the role-play because you haven't had much practice speaking from this side.

Patient: Okay.

Therapist: Okay, here we go. Well, what's the point of trying? I'm totally useless.

Patient: You are not totally useless. You've been a productive person all of your life. This is a difficult transition right now. It's a real bummer sometimes, but you can handle it.

Therapist: But I don't know how to handle my life now. I feel so useless.

Patient: You're trying to sort out what you want to do with your career right now. The pain in your back is legit. It's hard to sit for long periods, but maybe you can start redirecting your focus on what you can do.

Therapist: I feel like I have been stripped of my manhood. It's horrible.

Patient: You are still a man. Your wife still loves you, even though sex is not as enjoyable right now with the pain. Maybe you can learn other positions that will work better. Besides, who says being a man is all about work and sex? There's more to life than you have been giving yourself credit for.

In this role-play, Austin was able to access his feelings and identify his arguments for being "useless." At the same time, he was able to assimilate some new information about his potential worth as a person when he listened the "useful" side, which gave more credibility to his alternative belief,

"I have some worth/use in this world." Patients often mention role playing and imagery work as some of the most significant events in therapy. In the next section, imagery interventions in belief work will be described.

THE USE OF IMAGERY TO EVALUATE AND
MODIFY NEGATIVE CORE BELIEFS.

As mentioned in Chapter 10, imagery techniques can be used to identify nagetive core beliefs related to pain. They can also be used to evaluate and modify negative core beliefs. In this next example, Austin was asked to get in touch with images of times when he felt useless. Then, he was encouraged to change the image in some way (directing the image).

Patient: I noticed having a lot of dreams about my dad last week. On one of my dreams, he is pointing his finger at me, with that stern look on his face, telling me how useless I was. It brought back a flood of emotions for me, because he used to do that to me when I was a child.

Therapist: Would you be willing to work with that image in session today?
Paitent: Yes, I think I need to. In fact, I have it in my mind right now.

Therapist: Tell me what you see and what is happening in this image.
Patient: My dad just got home from a hard day at work. He looks really tired and worn out. I accidentally dropped a model airplane toy right in front of him. It broke into small pieces. He got up from the sofa and pointed his finger at me. With a stern look on his face, and yelled, "You useless piece of shit." Then, he started spanking me. I was so scared of him. He was really hurting me. (Patient starts to cry.) I was angry at him. He shouldn't have done that to me.

Therapist: I am so sorry that he hurt you and put you down. (Pause) How old are you in his image?
Patient: I am about 10 years old.

Therapist: So, your 10-year-old self feels scared and angry. What thoughts are running through your mind when he hits you and yells at you?
Patient: My dad is so mean. I hate him for hurting me.

Therapist: What does your 10-year-old self need right now?
Patient: I want someone to protect me and tell me I'm okay.

Therapist: Who do you want to come into the image? Do you want to bring your older self into the image, or someone else?

Patient: I think I would like my grown-up self to come into the image.

Therapist: Okay, bring your 43-year-old self into the image and tell me what is happening. Remember, you are the director of this image.

Patient: I am telling my younger self that it is okay. I am telling him, "You're a good kid. I know you didn't mean to break that toy." I pick him up and give him a big hug and tell him that I will protect him.

Therapist: How does the 10-year-old self feel?

Patient: He feels loved . . . worthy . . . useful.

Therapist: Is there anything else you would like to do in this image?

Patient: No, I think I will stop here.

Therapist: Okay. What was it like to get in touch with this image?

Patient: It was actually very healing for me. I have been waiting all of my life for my dad to love me . . . to make me feel worthwhile. He died 2 years ago. He never said he was sorry. He never had time for me. Work was more important to him than anything else, including me. (Pause.) I guess this exercise taught me that my grown-up self can protect and care for my 10-year-old self. I need to be kinder to myself.

Therapist: I am glad you were able to be compassionate and caring toward your younger self. This is what we have been working on in therapy—speaking more from the side of you that feels useful and worthwhile. I believe that is your compassionate self.

This imagery intervention was a pivotal moment in Austin's therapy. He learned that he could nurture and protect himself, even if his dad didn't. It also helped Austin differentiate his rules for living (e.g., "It is not okay to put people down." "Treat people with love and respect," and "Don't let work interfere with your family life.") from his dad's rules, which gave Austin a greater sense of identity and worth than ever before.

PART IV

PSYCHOSOCIAL STRESSORS TO ADDRESS

13

Managing Medical Care

Chronic pain patients can experience a number of stressors related to their medical care, including the demands of treatment, treatment adherence problems, managing their relationships with physicians and staff, and dealing with unrelieved pain despite medical and pharmacological intervention. Some of these medical stressors will be reviewed along with case examples of intervention strategies.

COPING WITH TREATMENT DEMANDS

It is not uncommon for chronic pain patients to experience a great deal of anxiety about medical treatments for pain. They may fear that the medical procedures or treatments will hurt, will not work, or will cause something bad to happen. Many of these expectancies or assumptions are related to the patients' limited knowledge or information about the medical procedure or treatment itself; some have no clear understanding of what to expect.

COLLECTING INFORMATION ABOUT TREATMENTS

One very helpful intervention is to have patients collect as much information about the utility of diagnostic, medical, or surgical procedures as they can by having them consult with their physicians, talk with other patients who have had the procedure, check web sites for information (realizing that this information alone may not be totally accurate), read articles or books about the treatment, and seek out a second opinion from another professional. Patients who are more assertive with their physicians and take an active role in collecting information are also more likely to make informed decisions. This intervention will be demonstrated in the next therapist–patient dialogue.

ADDRESSING FEELINGS AND EXAMINING NEGATIVE THOUGHTS ASSOCIATED WITH MEDICAL TREATMENT/PROCEDURE

Another possible intervention strategy is to reflect the patients' feelings about their medical treatment/procedure and explore their automatic thoughts about it.

> As mentioned earlier, Karla is the patient who feared epidural injections given her misinterpretation of the sensations in her body as well as her catastrophic expectations regarding the epidural treatment. Epidural injections involve placing cortisone into the epidural space between the disc and the spinal column. Its purpose is to decrease the swelling in or around a herniated disc. (It is an outpatient procedure.)
>
> During therapy, Karla presented with a great deal of anxiety and dread regarding her upcoming third epidural injection given the fact that she experienced numbness in her back and legs following the second injection. When she was at the physician's office, she actually fell to the floor as she was getting up from her chair after the second injection as a result of the numbness in her legs. Karla interpreted this episode as an indication of possible paralysis.
>
> In this next therapist–patient dialogue, Karla's feelings and negative thoughts will be addressed. In addition, she will be encouraged to collect more information about epidural injections.

Therapist: Karla, what leads you to the conclusion that you will become paralyzed?

Patient: The numbness in my lower back and legs really scared me during the second epidural, especially when I fell in the doctor's office. I was very frightened by those sensations.

Therapist: It sounds like you weren't expecting the numbness to occur, so it was scary to you.

Patient: Yes, it was.

Therapist: Before you received the epidural, did your physician explain some common symptoms during and following the injection?

Patient: Well, she said I would probably feel a little prick at first when the needle was inserted. I really don't remember anything else she said after that because I was so anxious about the needle.

Therapist: That is okay. Do you have any other information or evidence that supports your thought "I will be paralyzed after the third injection"?

Patient: Well, the first time I had the epidural, everything went fine. The second time, I fell to the ground. That was very scary for me. Now I fear that it will be worse if I have another injection.

Therapist: So, if you fell during the second epidural, you anticipate that it will be worse the next time, that is, not being able to move at all, being paralyzed.

Patient: Exactly.

Therapist: Did your physician discuss the potential side effects of the epidural injection procedure with you?

Patient: I'm sure she did, but I can't really remember it now.

Therapist: If you were to collect more information on the possible side effects of this injection, you may be able to find out if paralysis is a potential side effect. This would allow us to put your thought to the test, to see if it is accurate or not. Would this information help clarify what you could anticipate?

Patient: Yes, I think it would.

Therapist: Is there any evidence that you won't be paralyzed if you receive another epidural injection?

Patient: Well, despite all of my worrying about it, it hasn't happened yet.

Therapist: That's very true. You haven't become paralyzed yet. How do you explain this?

Patient: I don't really know for sure. Maybe getting answers to some of those questions we discussed a moment ago might help me understand why it hasn't happened yet.

Therapist: I agree. Let's write those questions down on paper so that you can be prepared to talk with your physician about them. What questions do you want to ask your doctor?

Patient: Like you said, what are the common symptoms and side effects involved with epidural injections?

Therapist: Anything else you want to know?

Patient: Was the numbness I experienced during the second epidural injection a normal reaction?

Therapist: Okay. Anything else?

Patient: Will I become paralyzed?

Therapist: These all sound like great questions. Let's write those down. If you have any other questions, add them to the list. Do you think these are questions you can ask your doctor?

Patient: Yes, I do.

Therapist: Okay, I want to switch gears for a moment. If we looked at our list of cognitive distortions, do you think there may be some errors in the thought "I will be paralyzed"?

Patient: Well, I may be doing some all-or-nothing thinking. You know, being paralyzed or being totally well, with nothing in between those two extremes.

Therapist: Okay. Let's write that down. [pause] What about assuming the worst or "jumping to conclusions"? Do you think that might fit as a possible type of cognitive error?

Patient: Yes. I think I expect the worst. Like looking into a crystal ball.

Therapist: It does not sound like a good fortune-telling experience to me.

Patient: [laughs] Yes, I could use a good fortune.

Therapist: Any other errors that you see on the list that fit for the thought "I will become paralyzed"?

Patient: No, not that I can see.

Therapist: Okay. I just noticed another error on the list that might fit— emotional reasoning. You feel so scared and worried about the possibility of this happening that you assume it will come true. If you feel it emotionally, you expect it to happen. Your emotions are riding so high that it's driving your negative thinking here.

Patient: I had never really thought about that before, but I think I do reason with my emotions a lot. I view myself as an intuitive person, and I tend to put a lot of weight on my emotions. This can help me sometimes, and it can hurt me other times.

Therapist: I think emotions are an important cue for us to be in tune with in order to identify our thoughts. However, when we reason with our emotions, we tend to focus on the evidence that drives the emotions rather than looking at the other information out there. Does that make sense?

Patient: Yes, it does. I get the sense that my fear of paralysis may not be realistic. It is probably driven more by my fear of the numbness— I don't want it to take over my body. I also don't want to lose my ability to move and to do things.

Therapist: I think it is important to differentiate between temporary physiological sensations and permanent sensations. You fell because you lost some feeling in your lower back and legs. However, this was a temporary state, not a permanent loss of feeling or a permanent loss of mobility, right?

Patient: Yes. You're right. My fear tends to focus on the negative part of the epidural at that moment.

Therapist: Let's move beyond your fear for a moment to see what actually happened. What was the final outcome of your second epidural?
Patient: It did help ease my lower back pain and leg pain for a while. I did get feeling back into my lower back and my legs within a few hours.

Therapist: And did the numbness take over your body?
Patient: No, it didn't.

Therapist: Okay. This will be important information for us to remember when your negative thought pops up again. As we look back on this part of the session, what do you remember?
Patient: I assumed that I would be paralyzed if I continued more epidural treatments. However, my evidence is based on my feelings of fears rather than on facts. I tend to expect the worst.

Therapist: That's a great summary. We also wrote down some questions for you to ask your doctor so that you can collect more information about the symptoms commonly experienced during an epidural injection and about the typical side effects. You can also let your physician know how anxious you have felt about the third treatment because you anticipate becoming paralyzed. By putting your thought out there "on the table," your physician can help you clarify whether your thought has some truth to it or not. It is important for you to have a clear understanding of the risks of this procedure.
Patient: Sounds good. I'm ready to give this a try.

Therapist: In the meantime, when your thought, "I will become paralyzed," comes to your awareness, how can you respond to it?
Patient: I need to remember that I haven't become paralyzed yet and that I don't have enough information to know whether this is realistic or not.

Therapist: Great!

Karla did indeed consult with her doctor and found to her surprise that numbness, or loss of sensation in the lower part of her body, is a potential side effect of epidural injections. She also learned that paralysis was possible a side effect of epidurals. However, the likelihood of paralysis is relatively rare. Infections, headaches, and a sudden drop in blood pressure are among some of the other side effects of epidural injections. Karla shared her concerns about the numbness and her fear of paralysis with her physician, who provided her with the information and the support to go ahead with the third epidural injection. This injection went smoothly with no problems, which provided further evidence that her thought, "I will be paralyzed," was unrealistic and inaccurate. (Note: Some patient may decide to forego this procedure given the minimal risk of paralysis. In those cases, patients and physicians can explore other treatment options.)

PREPARING FOR SURGERY

Many patients are often scared about the idea of having surgery. Although their physicians may have discussed with them the benefits and costs of surgery, they may not have weighed the benefits and risks themselves. This exploration (the advantages and disadvantages of having or not having surgery) can be done in session to help patients make a decision and to discuss concerns about their upcoming surgery in more detail with their physicians.

For patients who plan to pursue surgical intervention, they may meet some roadblocks in having the surgery itself, such as health problems (e.g., obesity), financial concerns, and overwhelming anxiety. For example, some chronic pain patients are requested by their physicians to lose weight before having surgery.

> Goutam, a 30 year old Asian Indian man, was 5'4" and weighed 250 pounds. He had gained over 80 pounds in the past 2 years since his work-related back injury. The doctors wanted to perform surgery on his back (herniated disks at L4–5) but would not consider it until Goutan focused on lose weight first. Goutam started on a crash diet and ate only one meal a day so that he could lose weight as quickly as possible. However, Goutam was unable to maintain his one-meal-a-day diet plan and would often binge on fattening foods later in the evenings. Goutam was stubborn and unwilling to pursue outside help for his weight problem because he wanted to do it on his own. His therapist asked, "What gets in the way of doing something healthy for yourself? Any thoughts that interfere with your goal of losing weight?" Goutam reported feeling depressed, thinking that he was a failure for gaining weight: "I am a fat tub of goop." After some discussion, Goutam came to the conclusion that his weight loss plan had not been successful. His therapist pointed out that although his dieting plan failed, he was not a failure. Telling himself he was a failure added more pressure and reinforced his binge-eating habits. Dieting in moderation was possible only after Goutam was willing to experiment with another approach to dieting that was actually safer for him. He agreed to par-

ticipate in a certified weight loss program and a low-impact exercise program (designed by his physical therapist). Goutam and his therapist developed a coping card, which he reads on a daily basis: "It is important for me to lose weight so that my back can heal. And if I do need back surgery, I will be ready for this treatment. I can lose pounds by eating sensibly and by conditioning my body through low-impact exercise. It is important to take small steps to lose weight."

About 8 months later, Goutam had lost the pounds he needed to schedule his back surgery. This was a great accomplishment.

TREATMENT ADHERENCE PROBLEMS

Some patients have difficulty following through with medical recommendations or treatment for a variety of reasons: (1) they do not understand the rationale for the treatment, (2) they do not trust their physicians, (3) they believe they will get better on their own, (4) they do not consider the consequences of not following physicians' recommendations, (5) they do not want to comprise their schedules or lifestyles, (6) they assume to know what is best for them, (7) they fear embarrassment if they use visible, physical aids (e.g., wheelchairs, crutches, or hand braces), and (8) they do not believe they can be cured. It is imperative that therapists explore some of these potential "roadblocks" to treatment adherence.

As mentioned, one possible reason why patients do not follow through with physicians' recommendations is their fear of embarrassment in using devices to cope with chronic pain. For example, devices such as orthopedic back or neck pillows, wristbands for carpal tunnel, slings, and knee braces are often visible reminders of pain and their injuries. Even the use of medication in public can trigger feelings of embarrassment for patients because people may ask them about it. Examples of negative thoughts and beliefs include, "People will think I look silly and laugh at me," "It's so inconvenient to wear/use it," "People will feel sorry for me, and I don't want pity," "I am unattractive when I wear it/use the device," "It reminds me of my pain and how hopeless my condition is," and "I don't want to attract [negative] attention to myself or my injuries/pain."

Josie, a 46 year old Latino woman was diagnosed with bilateral carpal tunnel disease. Her doctor recommended that she wear hand braces on a daily basis. Josie recently returned to work at the post office; her job there involved sorting and typing. However, she did not wear her hand braces regularly. She would sometimes wear them to therapy sessions. When her therapist pointed out this observation, Josie reported feeling self-conscious about wearing the braces. It was embarrassing to wear them because she thought the braces looked ugly and attracted people's attention (e.g., staring, laughter). The underlying belief being activated was of dysfunction ("I am dysfunctional"). Josie's therapist asked her what was so ugly about the braces. Josie responded that she did not like the color because it did not match her skin and because it was boring. In addition, the brace covered a lot of her hand and upper arm. Josie was encouraged to check medical supply offices as well as a seamstress in town (who made a variety of colorful wrist-bands) to see if there were other hand brace options in terms of color and size. Next, her therapist asked how often people gave her nega-tive attention when she wore the braces. Josie responded that she really did not know for sure. A behavioral experiment was devised to see how people would respond to the braces in general (positive, neu-tral, and negative responses). Josie was agreeable to wearing the braces every day over the next week to assess how often she received nega-tive attention (and by whom). She was encouraged to observe behav-iors and collect information. She kept a journal to track her findings. As much as possible, Josie was asked not to make judgments about people's comments or behavior.

Next, Josie and her therapist reviewed the advantages and disad-vantages of wearing the braces as well as the advantages and disad-vantages of not wearing the braces. Overall, Josie realized that even though some people make fun of her hand braces and even though the braces can be cumbersome at times, the main advantage of wear-ing them was to reduce the pain experienced in her hands, with the ultimate goal of delaying the need for further surgery. Josie and her therapist discussed ways in which she could be more assertive with people who are inquisitive about her braces. Examples of assertive tac-tics included "I wear these braces because I have carpal tunnel syn-drome in both hands" and "They help reduce the pain in my wrists when I work with my hands."

Josie made contact with the seamstress in town, who designed a col-orful brace to fit her upper arms, wrists, and hands. Because the new brace would not be ready for 2 weeks, Josie wore her original hand braces every day as part of the behavioral experiment. She learned that not very many people paid attention to them. A few people asked her questions about the braces, and two people stared at her. They were acquaintances or people she had never met before. Here is a continuation of the session.

Therapist: What types of questions did people ask you?
Patient: They asked me about the braces, like "Why do you wear them? What are they for?" I kept my response short like we talked about

last week. I told them I have carpal tunnel and that I wear them to reduce the pain in my wrists.

Therapist: How did you feel about those interactions?

Patient: I felt less self-conscious because I had a planned response. The last session really helped me with that.

Therapist: I'm wondering if you also felt less self-conscious because of the meaning you gave to their questions and actions. For example, last week, you assumed that people were picking on you or making fun of you because you were weird or dysfunctional in some way. Does that explanation still hold true?

Patient: I don't think so. A couple of people did stare at me, but for the most part, people either ignored my hand braces or they asked me questions.

Therapist: So, when people ask you questions, they were not picking on you or viewing you as dysfunctional. They were just interested in learning more about your hand braces. [This alternative response will be written down later on a coping card.]

Patient: Exactly.

Therapist: What I have noticed so far in our session today is that you haven't personalized people's questions about your braces or their stares. You haven't interpreted their questions or stares as a sign of weirdness or dysfunction in yourself. Instead, you focused on the fact that their stares or questions were about your braces. That's a big switch for you since our last session.

Patient: I guess it comes down to whose opinion I really care about. I didn't know these people, so I was less invested in what they thought of me.

Therapist: Great! What else helped you take questions or stares less personally?

Patient: I guess looking at all the evidence made a difference. It helped a lot when you told me to view my thoughts as hunches or hypotheses and not necessarily as facts. So, I had to look for the evidence. I also remembered what you said about observing people's responses, rather than judging them. That made a difference too. [Therapist wrote down "observe people's responses . . . don't judge them" on a coping card.]

Therapist: Great!

Patient: And another thing: While some people might think that my hand braces are strange, that doesn't necessary mean that I am weird. They were probably more interested in my hand brace's than they were about me. [Another alternative response to write down on a coping card.]

Therapist: Okay. Let's be sure to write those ideas down on coping cards so that you can remember these thoughts.

During this part of the session, Josie learned that people sometimes ask questions because they are truly interested in her hand braces, not just because they are trying to pick on her or point out her differences. Josie and her therapist acknowledged that there may be times when people might tease her about the hand braces or laugh at her, but that does not make her weird or dysfunctional. It is a reflection of their character, not hers. Josie and her therapist role-played ways to handle such scenarios. Instead of feeling demoralized, she now felt empowered to handle people's comments and questions, whether they are curious or rude.

She learned how to put some of the basic principles of cognitive therapy into action in her daily life: (1) be aware of a shift in her emotions and identify her negative thoughts or images, (2) view her thoughts as hunches or hypotheses instead of facts, (3) test out the accuracy of her thoughts by exploring the evidence for and against her thoughts, and (4) observe people's comments and reactions rather than judging them during the behavioral experiment. This last step seemed very helpful to Josie because she did not jump to any conclusions about people's intentions or her worth.

RELATIONSHIPS WITH PHYSICIANS AND MEDICAL STAFF

Chronic pain patients' relationships with their physicians, medical staff, and other health care professionals can have a major impact on treatment adherence issues as well as on their beliefs about their pain and physical health. In general, most therapists help patients manage their impressions and expectations of their relationships with their physicians (e.g., primary care physician, orthopedic doctor, neurologist, neurosurgeon, or chiropractor) and medical staff as well as improve these relationships. Some patients are concerned about (1) what their physicians think of them (e.g., "My doctor thinks I'm a basket case," "My doctor doesn't believe that my pain is real," and "My doctor might think I am a bad patient because of my cancellations due to transportation difficulties"); (2) the quality of the relationship, including their physicians' intentions toward or feelings about them as patients ("My doctor doesn't care about me or my pain,"

"She doesn't take the time to listen to my concerns"); and (3) communications with their physicians. Some patients do not have the basic communication skills needed to be assertive with their medical doctors regarding treatment issues. For example, some patients are very angry or upset about the nature of their medical care in general (e.g., believe their physician is not treating their pain aggressively enough) and tend to be either passive (e.g., "I'll just do what the doctor says even though I don't agree with it") or aggressive (e.g., "I feel like I am pushed in and out of doctors' offices all day," and "Doctors are just out to make a buck"). (Some physicians may not treat patients' pain aggressively [e.g., fail to prescribe opioids when it is needed] due to their fears of being sued.) Other patients have the skills necessary to communicate their concerns to their physician; however, they fear that the relationship may be threatened if they are more assertive (e.g., "My doctor will become angry with me if I ask questions").

MANAGING PATIENTS' IMPRESSIONS OF THEIR RELATIONSHIP WITH THEIR PHYSICIANS

Frequently, chronic pain patients can misperceive their physicians' intentions during office visits. These patients are particularly sensitive to potential rejection and may, perceive long waits or short, abrupt visits as a rejection by their physician.

> Lorena, a 60 year old Native American patient, was particularly concerned about a recent appointment with her neurologist regarding her fibromyalgia pain. She recalled feeling depressed about her pain, telling her physician how much the pain she was in and how hopeless she feels about the pain. She felt self-conscious when she started crying in his office. Her thought was "My doctor probably thinks I am a complainer. He may think I am a basket case." The emotion connected to this thought was fear. Lorena's therapist asked if her physician made those judgments about her. She acknowledged they were her own words. Was she a complainer? The only time Lorena "complained" was when she was hurting a great deal or when she was distressed. It was during those times she really needed his help. Lorena's therapist had never observed her complaining, so she wanted to see Lorena complain, like she did in the physician's office. Lorena agreed to role play this situation in session. It became apparent to her therapist that Lorena was actually fairly assertive. In the following therapist–patient dialogue, Lorena and her therapist explore the thought that she is a basket case.

Patient: A basket case is someone who cries a lot. A basket case is some-one who is not in control of her emotions.

Therapist: So, anyone who cries a lot and is not in control of her emo-tions is a basket case.
Patient: Well, not everyone. I was raised to keep my emotions hidden.

Therapist: When is it okay for you to share your emotions in public?
Patient: If someone dies or if you are suffering from a severe illness, then it is okay to cry.

Therapist: So would your family or members of your tribe label you a basket case for crying in front of your doctor?
Patient: When I was younger, I might have been shamed for crying in public, but I am an elder of my tribe now and people respect me.

Therapist: So if another family member or tribal member cried in the doctor's office because of their pain and suffering and came to you for guidance, as an elder, what would you tell him or her?
Patient: I would tell them that their spirit needed to release those tears of pain.

Therapist: How would you feel if you accepted these words of guidance for yourself?
Patient: I probably need to. I have been so strong for others. I need to be strong for me.

Therapist: It takes a lot of courage and trust to cry in front of your doc-tor. You are still a strong person.
Patient: Thank you.

Therapist: I want to come back to your fears of what your doctor might think of you.

Therapist: You label yourself as a basket case for crying. [labeling error] How do you know that your doctor thinks you are a basket case? [pointing out mind-reading error]
Patient: Well, I guess I really don't know for sure, except that I cried.

Therapist: Do you think he has seen other patients cry?
Patient: I'm sure he has.

Therapist: So, are those people basket cases too?
Patient: No. I would think that if a person cries, they are really upset about something.

Therapist: So when you cried, what were you upset about?
Patient: I am just so tired of hurting. My pain hurts so much.

Therapist: Do you think your doctor understood that?
Patient: I think so.

Therapist: So, maybe your words and your tears communicated what you wanted to say—that unrelieved pain hurts a lot. Does that sound crazy to you?
Patient: No, when I step back from the situation, I can see what you are saying.

> When reviewing evidence that she is a "basket case" (the cognitive errors were labeling and mind reading), Lorena laughed, stating that she did not have any evidence except that she cried in her doctor's office. In addition, she commented that the label *basket case* sounded silly even though it felt real to her (this is emotional reasoning). Lorena and her therapist discussed how the labels *complainer* and *basket case* are vague words that do not describe what she said or did—they are perceived judgments of her character. Her therapist suggested that Lorena conduct a behavioral experiment to test out her negative thoughts that her physician viewed her as a complainer and as a "basket case" by asking him about this during the the next office visit ("Did you think I was a complainer or a basket case when I cried in your office last month?"). The therapist and patient collaboratively identified any potential barriers to conducting the behavioral experiment ("What if the doctor does not have time to talk?" "What if I 'chicken out'?"). Once those barriers were addressed and resolved, the therapist asked Lorena to predict the outcome of the experiment. Lorena's prediction was that the doctor would tell her she complained too much but that she was not a basket case.
>
> A few sessions later, Lorena reported that the behavioral experiment was a success. Lorena's physician normalized her crying. He did not view Lorena as a complainer or as a basket case. This behavioral experiment was an important intervention for Lorena because it encouraged her to test out her thoughts rather than make assumptions without evidence. It not only enhanced Lorena's relationship with her physician but it also enhanced Lorena's perceptions about her self. Lorena's alternative thoughts were "I am not a basket case. It's okay to cry in front of my doctor. He understands that my pain hurts. He is trying to help me."

ANGER REGARDING MISTREATMENT BY DOCTORS

Some chronic pain patients have difficulty coping with their anger regarding past medical treatment, especially when their physicians did not believe their pain was real. As a result, they may harbor negative feelings regarding past mistreatment despite the fact that they may now receive adequate treatment by their current physician. Examples of patients' thoughts and beliefs regarding mistreatment include "Why didn't someone help me when I was really hurting?" and "Why didn't they believe me?" Some patients become so distrustful of their physicians because of past negative experiences that they become paranoid regarding future mistreatment.

Zelda, a 42 year old Caucasian woman, was injured in a work-related accident and was diagnosed 2 years later with herniated disks in her lower back. Zelda reported that her first physician viewed her as a malingering patient because her verbal report of excruciating pain did not match the clinical findings. In addition, she lost her job because of her inability to carry out the tasks required because of her pain. According to Zelda, her employers made only limited attempts to locate alternative work options within the company. As a result of these events, Zelda became very distrustful of others and spent much of her time in therapy venting intense anger and frustration for being mistreated. Zelda commented, "I can't handle things. My employers are trying to destroy me, and my doctors probably think I'm crazy. I am annoyed that I am being treated this way. I am stupid to think I would be treated differently. I'm such a fool." She interpreted every medical evaluation or appointment as another "hurdle" to deal with. Her attorney's infrequent contact was perceived as a "violation of trust." Although Zelda had a very reasonable desire to be treated fairly and being taken care of by her physicans, her sense of entitlement (constant "shoulds") and her rage were interfering with her medical and legal care. Her anger and frustration put professionals and acquaintances on the defensive. As a result, some physicians refused to work with her.

Zelda's therapist pointed out how her anger had taken on a life of its own. It was driven not simply by the events that occurred, but by the meaning she has given to these events—that she has been mistreated or wronged. Zelda agreed that her anger was spinning out of control because she was focused on the injustices that led up to this point. As a result, Zelda was losing sight of the fact that she did have a physician now who was supportive and caring. This physician found medical evidence to confirm a physical basis for her pain. She also had an attorney who was trying to obtain the medical evaluations necessary to prepare for her court date. She knew her attorney had a good reputation in the community. These people were not the same as those she had worked with, when she was first injured. If she is going to be angry, she needed to clarify who she is really anger at— that is, her employers and her first physicians who evaluated her following the work-related injury, and maybe even herself.

Zelda and her therapist discussed the importance of "parking her emotions." Zelda said it felt good to vent her anger and identify the mistreatment issues of the past. However, the problem with her anger was that it kept her stuck in the past and fixated on counterattacks, and it alienated professionals involved in her case. Zelda learned that there were positive as well as negative consequences of remaining "stuck" in her anger. Her therapist reframed the anger as cancer that was destroying hopefulness.

Imagery was particularly helpful in getting Zelda to "park her anger" (i.e., putting it in a box, leaving it in the car before she walked into the office building, etc.). Zelda learned to cope with her anger by sharing it in session with her therapist who would listen (and would not retaliate), which helped her to feel heard and validated. The Automatic Thought Records helped her keep track of the negative thoughts and beliefs fueling her anger. Every "should" was changed to a desire or hope. Whenever "mistreatment" beliefs were activated, she was asked about other possible explanations for people's behavior. When actual mistreatment occurred, Zelda and her therapist incorporated problem-solving strategies to cope (e.g., document incidents in a diary, give feedback in an assertive way, contact her attorney to explore options). Once she was able to step outside her anger, she was able to see that many of her interpretations of other people's behavior were inaccurate. She learned ways to be more assertive when communicating her frustration or anger.

Graded task assignments helped reduce her tendency to feel overwhelmed and hopeless about her case and about her recovery. Examples of "small steps" included meeting with her physician regularly, attending recommended medical evaluations with other physicians, meeting with her attorney to clarify concerns regarding her legal case, and continuing the job search. These were all important steps in her recovery, with the end goals of coping with her pain, settling her case, finding a new career, and "putting the past behind her."

All of these interventions helped Zelda release her pent-up hostility and allowed her to feel more centered and relaxed, which also helped her pain.

DEALING WITH UNRELIEVED PAIN DESPITE INTERVENTION

Some patients become disillusioned with the medical profession when their physicians cannot diagnose their pain condition or adequately treat it. Many patients want the pain to stop, but for some patients, no medical intervention to date has been effective in alleviating the pain. This is a source of great frustration and disappointment. Despite this, some patients are afraid to discuss these realities with their physicians. As a result, they continue to suffer with severe, debilitating pain with no end in sight.

To get the best medical care possible, patients can learn to take responsibility for their part in the physician–patient relationship, which is to educate their physicians about their symptoms, to explain any potential problems, including pain response, side effects, and other physical and emotional responses/reactions to the treatments, and to discuss any concerns about their treatment. In therapy, patients learn to ask questions about their condition, to inquire about medical procedures and laboratory tests, to explore medical treatment options with their doctor, to seek second opinions if necessary, and to learn how to obtain prescriptions refills from medical staff when necessary.

> Don, a 28 year old Asian man, has chronic pain in his right arm and hand. He often has questions about his medical care but has been afraid to talk with his physician about them. For example, why is there no physical evidence for his chronic pain? What is his diagnosis? Why hasn't any medical intervention (e.g., prescribed medications, physical therapy, occupational therapy) fixed his pain? Why does he still suffer with this pain? His typical negative automatic thoughts were "I think about asking my doctor some questions, but I can't read his reactions. He might disapprove of my questions." The beliefs underlying these thoughts were "Asking questions is disrespectful to doctors" and "I am a bad patient if I do." Loyalty and respect were important personal, family, and cultural values for Don. He did not want to jeopardize his relationship with his physician. Here is a therapist–patient dialogue that explains his dilemma and how this was handled in session.

Patient: Well, I felt really bad about the last office visit with my doctor. I was thinking about asking him some questions, but I was afraid he would disapprove.

Therapist: What questions or concerns have you been holding back?
Patient: So far, the medical and physical treatments haven't worked, and I am so tired of being in pain. I want to stop the occupational therapy and try another approach. I want to know if there are any other treatment options we can explore. I am afraid that I'm not getting better. Not having a clear diagnosis has made me very worried.

Therapist: Those are reasonable concerns to share with your doctor. How do you know that he would disapprove of these questions?
Patient: I don't want to tell him how to do his job. I really don't have much of a chance to talk with him anyone. He always seems so busy, and oftentimes our visits are only for 10 minutes. Once I get up the nerve to ask a question or to make a comment, the office visit is over.

Therapist: "So, it sounds like you have two assumptions: (1) your comments or questions might offend him and (2) your doctor is too busy to listen to you. What do you anticipate would happen if you expressed your concerns to him?

Patient: He would probably think my questions are disrespectful, and he would become upset with me.

Therapist: Usually physicians provide some opportunities for patients to ask questions or share concerns during the appointments. Has he done that regularly?

Patient: Yes. When he provides that structure, I do ask some questions.

Therapist: How has your doctor responded to your questions and comments so far?

Patient: So far, so good.

Therapist: So, we really don't have any evidence that your doctor has been "put off" or offended when you ask questions. It just feels as though he might. Is that right?

Patient: Yes.

Therapist: This is what we call emotional reasoning. When you reason with your emotions, you assume that the consequence or outcome will come true because of the way you feel: If I feel it, it must be true.

Patient: Yes, I see what you mean. But it feels so real.

Therapist: It feels so real because you have convinced yourself that your doctor will react negatively to you if you "rock the boat" or disagree with him. It is important to remember that our feelings are not facts. However, if we made decisions based simply on our feelings without collecting important information, we might not make the best decisions for ourselves. You, as a patient, are a consumer of services, and you have the right to ask questions about your medical treatments, and you have a right to let yur doctor know how your body is responding to these treatments as well as your concerns. I know I just shared a lot with you just now. What did you hear me say?

Patient: Well, feelings are not facts . . . that I have a right to ask questions and make comments because I am a consumer of services . . . and that all questions have some purpose.

Therapist: That's right. Another error you may be making is what we call "mind reading." You assume you know how your doctor will respond to you. Although we would like to be able to anticipate how he will respond, we won't know until you ask. In fact, so far, he has not been upset or offended by your questions and comments.

Patient: This is true.

Therapist: Is it possible that your doctor may have a different reaction to your questions or comments, other than being offended?

Patient: Since he has been supportive so far, he might want to know how I'm really doing. In fact, he's tried to ask me questions about how I'm doing. I guess I just don't want to be perceived as a bad patient.

Therapist: So, a bad patient asks questions about his medical treatment.

Patient: Well, no. I guess it's okay to ask questions when you are uncertain about your treatment. [pause] I see what you're saying. I'm labeling myself as a bad patient for asking questions when I realize that it is okay for other patients to ask questions of their doctors.

Therapist: All right. I would like you to fill in the blank: It's okay for me to ask my doctor questions about my medical treatment because . . .

Patient: It's okay to ask questions because sometimes I don't understand the medical jargon my doctor uses.

Therapist: Anything else? It's okay for me to ask my doctor questions or to share my concerns because . . .

Patient: Because I am a consumer of medical services. I have a right to know why a certain treatment is recommended over another and why a certain treatment is not working.

Therapist: How strongly do you believe those statements, on a scale from 0 to 100 percent?

Patient: Oh, about 80.

Therapist: It is also okay for patients to ask questions or share their concerns because they might be disappointed in medical treatment outcomes. They may want to discuss other treatment options too.

Patient: Yes, I guess that's the hardest part, expressing my disappointment and being able to discuss other treatment options with my doctor. My parents taught me to be respectful of others.

Therapist: So, what would be the worst thing that could happen if you expressed your interest in pursuing other options besides occupational therapy.

Patient: Well, he might get mad at me and say that I'm not being compliant.

Therapist: Anything else?

Patient: He might think I am a bad patient for questioning his treatment plan for me.

Therapist: What would be the best thing that could happen.

Patient: Well, he might be willing to discuss other treatment options with me. We might find a better solution to my pain.

Therapist: What do you realistically anticipate will happen if you share your concerns?
Patient: I'm not really sure.

Therapist: It might be worthwhile to test out your assumption that asking questions of your doctor will result in offending him and being perceived as a bad patient. Maybe we could develop a behavioral experiment to test out this belief, so that we know whether indeed this belief is accurate or not. How would you feel about doing this?
Patient: Well, I'm a little scared, but I'd be open to trying it out.

Therapist: Okay, let's sit down and write out the important questions or comments you would like to share with your doctor during the next visit. We can focus on ways to show respect for your doctor and still discuss treatment options with him. Then we can clarify your prediction, so that we can compare it with the actual outcome of the visit.
Patient: Sounds great.

Don and his therapist role-played ways he can communicate these concerns without offending his physician. Then he tried it out with several family member and friends to get their feedback first. Overall, they did not view his concerns as offensive. After this test, he was able to put it into action. Don reported being relieved when his physician was agreeable to exploring other treatment options. In fact, he was put on some different pain medications, which seemed to help his pain. So, by sharing his concerns, Don was able to be an active participant in his own treatment, which made a difference in his perception of his pain and in his overall health. Don was able to maintain his family and cultural values of respect and loyalty, while at the same time, letting his physician know his body's response to occupational therapy and exploring the treatment options available to him.

14

Family, Friends, and Lifestyle Issues

Not only do chronic pain patients have to cope with their pain, they also have to deal with a variety of other personal, social, and environmental stressors related to their pain. Chronic pain often results in physical limitations, which can affect various life roles. Occupational, financial, legal, and family problems can develop as a result of chronic pain. For example, some patients may not be able to return to work, which results in financial hardships. Other patients are involved in legal cases related to their injuries, which may affect their livelihood. Patients can also experience difficulties in their relationships with partners/spouses, other family members such as children or parents, and friends. In this chapter, psychosocial stressors related to family, friends, and lifestyle issues will be highlighted, along with brief case examples based on actual patient cases. In the next chapter, occupational, financial, and legal stressors will be discussed.

FAMILY STRESSORS

CHANGE IN FAMILY ROLES

When patients develop a chronic pain condition, they may go through a series of losses, including physical limitations, unemployment, financial problems (e.g., Mims, 1989), divorce, loss of identity, and loss of meaning in their lives. With the onset and continuation of chronic pain, it is very likely that patients' pain can affect their roles in their families. For example, if patients were the breadwinners in their families and are not able to return to work over time, their sense of identity can be negatively affected. Or they may have been in the role of homemaker and can no longer perform the chores necessary to keep the house organized and to clean, feed the family, and take care of the children. This can be devastating.

"I've lost my family."

In some cases, changes in family roles can lead to relationship difficulties and, ultimately, separation or divorce.

Nate, a 45 year old Greek man, presented with chronic pain problems (i.e., herniated discs in neck and lower back), severe depression, and hopelessness. He was a divorced middle-aged man with four children. As the noncustodial parent, Nate saw his children infrequently, only on weekends, which was upsetting to him. He was very depressed, lonely, and hopeless and spent much of his time watching television. According to Nate, the consequences of his pain (physical impairment, permanent disability, inability to return to work) drove his wife to divorce him a few years ago because he could not longer provide financially for the family. Therefore, he made a strong association between his experience of chronic pain and his subsequent losses: his divorce, his termination from work, and his limited opportunities to visit with his children. His negative core beliefs included: (1) I am a stranger to my family, (2) I have lost my family, and (3) I am unlovable.

Negative memories and images related to the divorce, his job loss, and chronic pain were the particular foci of therapy with Nate. He wanted his wife and children back in his life. When family memories came to mind, he often focused on what he had lost. It hurt him to remember the times when they were a happy family. "Those times are lost now." His therapist empathized and directed Nate to discuss memories he has made with his children since the divorce. This seemed to move Nate in session and helped him to realize that although they are not all together again, he still can have good times with his children and create new memories. Nate and his therapist discussed the nature of his weekend visits with his children and ways to maximize quality time with them. Scheduling activities on the weekends and increasing his resources in conversational strategies (i.e., assertiveness training) did enhance his time with his children. Emphasis was placed on enjoying time with his children instead of obsessing on when they would be leaving and reducing his tendency to put his children "in the middle" (i.e., not asking the children about their mother and how she disciplines them during their time together). He was still very proud of his relationships with his children and how his children have coped with the divorce so far. By the end of therapy, Nate was able to move beyond some of his grief about his divorce. His depression remitted, and his relationships with his children improved.

SPOUSE/PARTNER ISSUES

Pain can have a rippling effect on patients' relationships with their part-
ners/spouses, particularly in the areas of support and intimacy. In fact,
social support problems can have a negative impact on patients' pain and
emotions (less perceived support, more pain and distress; e.g., Feldman
et al., 1999; Jamison & Virts, 1990; Saarijarvi, Rytokoski, & Karppi, 1990).
In addition, chronic pain can have a negative impact on sexual and emotional intimacy with partners/spouses. The following points illustrate some
of these problems and how they can be resolved.

Social disbelief—"My family doesn't believe my pain is real."

Chronic pain patients may have been productive, hardworking individuals, but they may not be able to carry out previous life roles or significant
tasks because of their pain. This can lead some family members to make
negative assumptions about patients that may be inaccurate, such as, "She's
lazy," "Why can't he get back to work?" "She cannot help around the house
like she used to," "He obviously doesn't have the same motivation and
drive." These family messages create meaning about chronic pain. In these
examples, the patients' pain is minimized or invalidated (e.g., "not real"),
resulting in negative assumptions of their character. Therapists should try
to understand the meaning of pain and other chronic illnesses in patients'
families by exploring not only their immediate families' perceptions but
also their family and cultural histories to see how meanings of pain may
be transmitted across generations (see Seaburn, Lorenz, & Kaplan, 1992,
for more information). As part of this process, it may be important to
identify significant chronic conditions among family members across
generations.

If patients are at odds with family members about the validity of their
pain and suffering, this can be a major stressor, particularly if they value
their family members' opinions of them. If patients feel unsupported or
misunderstood, they can be empowered to convey these feelings to their
family (e.g., "That hurt my feelings") and to explain their experiences.
For example, if family members label them as "lazy" or "unmotivated,"
patients can tell them that their pain makes them feel fatigued or tired.
It is not an issue of drive.

Therapy can provide the context in which family members and friends
can learn to understand patients' experience of pain and the realistic
aspects of having chronic pain, thus promoting empathy. At times, it is
helpful to have these individuals attend psychotherapy sessions with patients
to educate them about pain, to clarify misunderstandings, to build better

lines of communication, and to establish realistic expectations for what the patient can do in terms of school, work, chores, household responsibilities, and/or social activities. Chapter 16 demonstrates how therapists can help patients communicate with family members and to ask for the support they need.

Concern about social disregard—"My partner doesn't care about my pain."

Sometimes patients assume that their partners or spouses are not supportive or do not care about their pain because of their own negative information-processing biases, for example, engaging in mind reading (assuming to know what their partners or spouses think or feel) or overgeneralizing (assuming that one negative interaction is an indication or reflection of no support in that relationship).

> Fred, a 28 year old Caucasian man, had chronic migraine headaches and felt depressed and anxious about his relationship with his wife. He believed that she did not care about his pain. Further exploration revealed that his belief was centered on his wife's frustrations. When asked to provide examples of situations when his wife became frustrated, he recalled times when they had to leave parties or social events early because of his pain, or when she wanted to do something but he was not up to it because of the pain. His therapist wondered if perhaps his wife was frustrated because she wanted to do things together like they used to or because she felt frustrated because she wanted the pain to go away. Was her frustration a sign of disinterest or rejection of his pain, or was it a sign of grief or of helplessness about the effects of the pain on their activities? These comments and questions opened Fred's mind to the possibility that perhaps she was upset about the pain and how it affected their relationship. As a behavioral experiment, he talked with his wife about the frustration he noticed in her over the past few months. He discovered that she was not angry with him; she was frustrated at times with the pain, especially when it interfered with their activities. She missed doing more things together. She wished she could make the pain go away. She apologized for her frustration, which made Fred feel a lot better. His alternative explanation for her frustration was "My wife does get frustrated at times when she sees me in pain, but that doesn't mean she doesn't care; it may mean that she wants me to feel better—to get well—or it may mean that she is discouraged because we couldn't do something together because I wasn't feeling good that day. In any case, I need to check out my perceptions with her. This will help me cope better, and it will improve our relationship."

Sexual problems

Many patients struggle with physical and emotional limitations in being sexually active with their partners or spouses. Some feel guilty for not being able to perform sexually. Other patients fear reinjury if they engage in sexual activity. Typical thoughts and beliefs regarding sexuality include "I am afraid that I may never be able to have sex again without experiencing excruciating pain," "If I really love my partner, I should have sex with him/her even if it means aggravating my medical condition," "Why did this happen to me? I can't enjoy sex. I feel isolated," "I am disinterested in sex because of my pain," "My whole body has turned old," and "I am not attractive."

"I may never be able to have sex again without experiencing excruciating pain."

Some patients worry about their ability to handle their pain during sex or lovemaking activities with their spouses/partners. The first step is for therapists to ask questions about the patients' experience of pain when engaging in sexual activity, for example, "How often do you experience pain when engaging in sexual activity?" "How long does the pain typically last?" "Tell me about the pain and what do you think contributes to it?" and "Do you experience any enjoyment or pleasure when having sex/making love?"

A number of factors may influence patients' pain levels when having sex including their activity schedule that day (pushing themselves too hard), their perception that they must continually meet their partner's expectations, their motivation or desire to be sexually intimate, the positions used during sexual intercourse, the amount of effort put into the act of sex itself, and the time of day when having sex (typically, patients report more intense pain in the evening). Once these significant factors have been identified, the patient can conduct behavioral experiments to assess whether some modifications in thinking patterns or behaviors may result in different and more positive experiences with sexual intimacy. Patients are encouraged to consult their physicians regarding the impact of sexual activity on their pain and to obtain recommendations regarding ways to enhance their sexual gratification (e.g., appropriate sexual positions given pain) in healthy ways.

"I should have sex to appease my partner."

Some patients tend to give into their partners' sexual requests despite the fact that they are in a lot of pain. By doing so, they appease their partners but end up experiencing more pain, resulting in feelings of depression, guilt, and dissatisfaction. Patients often think, "If I really love my partner, I should have sex with him/her even if it means aggravating my pain." Although it is admirable that they love their partners/spouses enough to be in more pain for their partners'/spouses' pleasure, can they experience sexual pleasure and gratification as well? This is an important goal: to find ways of having sex that is enjoyable and safe for both parties. Which aspects of their sexual experience are painful, and which ones are not? Certain sexual positions may ease their pain and discomfort, whereas other positions may worsen it. Exploring alternative avenues to sexuality is important. Patients tend to assume that sexual intercourse is the only avenue, when in fact there may be other possible modes of expression, including kissing, touching, fondling, and oral sex. Or patients can learn to use a variety of sexual positions that may ease their pain or discomfort. Patients are usually urged to consult with their physicians regarding the best sexual positions to alleviate pain.

It may be helpful for patients' partners to attend psychotherapy sessions with them to explore their sexual relationship as a couple's issue. Patients tend to assume that their partners have high expectations about their sexual relationship, when in fact many partners are open to making adjustments in sexual expression for the benefit of the patient's medical well-being (although this is not always the case). Open communication is encouraged between patients and their partners. For example, if a particular posture is uncomfortable, the patients can learn to assert themselves and educate their partners on certain positions that are more comfortable than others.

PARENTING ISSUES

Chronic pain patients are concerned about the impact of their pain on their ability to be good parents, especially regarding discipline and relationship issues. Patients who have young children, in particular, may have difficulties coping with the physical demands of the parent role. Typical parental difficulties include setting physical limits, maintaining appropriate disciplinary methods, and coping with an already low tolerance given their pain. Examples of negative thoughts and beliefs regarding parenting include "My children won't help me," "My children should know my pain," "I am a burden to my children," and "I am not a good parent."

"My child/children won't help me."

Some patients believe that their children do not want to help them. In one case, Zoe, a 33 year old Caucasian woman, was having difficulty getting her son to follow through with his chores. In the past, she would complete her son's chores if he did not finish them. As a full-time homemaker, she had reasoned that her son was too busy with school and extracurricular activities to complete his chores, so it was okay to let chores slide "this time." The patient commented, "It was *my* job anyway." Given her chronic pain condition (temporomandibular joint pain and three herniated disks in the lower back), she could no longer complete physically demanding chores. New rules needed to be established in the home. But Zoe also needed to modify her thinking about the purpose of the chores (e.g., her son will complete certain chores, not only because she could not do them right now, but because completion of chores teaches children important lessons about responsibility and time management). A useful strategy to reinforce new house rules was to have the patient develop a new disciplinary system using index cards to give to her son, listing the chore on one side of the card and on the other side detailing a list of specific activities necessary to complete the chore to her satisfaction (E. Christophersen, personal communication, August, 1992). In addition, certain times were identified for her son to complete the chores. If her son did not follow through on a chore, he lost privileges, such as not being able to watch television or make phone calls to friends, until the chores were finished. By developing consistent rules regarding chores, there was less of an opportunity for conflict and bickering. These strategies helped Zoe feel stronger as a parent and a person. It also improved her relationship with her son.

"They should know my pain."

Some patients assume that their children do not understand their pain and suffering; otherwise, they would be more compliant. However, these patients may have unrealistic expectations of their children, for example, assuming that their children can "read their minds and understand their suffering" (jumping to conclusions). In many cases, parents with chronic pain may not have fully explained their experience of pain to their children. Or, if they have, they do not remind their children about the effects of their pain on their level of involvement and participation in activities and responsibilities. Educating family members, friends, coworkers, and others regarding their experience of pain can enhance others' sensitivity to their suffering.

Lucinda, a 43 year old Latino Woman, was diagnosed with fibromyalgia a few years ago. One of her biggest psychosocial stressors was her relationship with her children. She strongly believed that her children should understand her pain.

Patient: I am so tired of my kids acting out and not following through. They should know my pain.

Therapist: It sounds like you have two rules: (1) your kids should not act out or be defiant and (2) they should know your pain.

Patient: They know I have pain in different parts of my body, even though they can't pronounce the word *fibromyalgia.*

Therapist: Do they know how this pain affects you?

Patient: They should! Can't they see the pain and agony on my face and my movements?

Therapist: I don't know. Have you asked them about this?

Patient: Not really. I just get so disgusted with them.

Therapist: When you expect them to know your pain, are you assuming that they can read your mind?

Patient: Yes, I probably am. They may not know what I'm going through.

Therapist: And what thoughts run through your mind when you feel disgusted with them?

Patient: They are punishing me.

Therapist: What leads you to that conclusion?

Patient: They don't listen to me. They don't consider what my limits are and how the pain is affecting me.

Therapist: Any other experiences that support this belief that your kids are punishing you?

Patient: No, that sums it up.

Therapist: Are there times when your kids do care? Are there times when they don't punish you?

Patient: Sometimes they are sweet and will do things for me, especially at night, when my pain is the worst.

Therapist: Your kids are 7 and 3 years old, right?

Patient: Yes.

Therapist: Kids at this stage of development "act out" as a way to test their parents, and they need to be reminded of the rules in your family. Kids at this stage are also very concrete in their thinking. They aren't little adults. They may not give much thought to how their behavior affects you and your pain. That involves more abstract thinking. Does this make sense? [Patient nods.] You may perceive their "acting out" behavior as personal—being directed toward you and your pain—when in fact, they might have done these things anyway because they are kids. [personalization error]

Patient: I hadn't thought about that before. That is probably true.

Therapist: So being consistent about the rules in your house and providing your children with consequences when they "act out" will be important. You can also remind them what you expect of them, but they will learn more from your actions than what you say. So keep your messages short, for example, "Please share your toys, "No hitting," and "Mom hurts right now."

When Lucinda tried to keep an open mind and not to assume that her children knew her pain, she felt less frustrated with them. She talked with them more about her experiences, including her pain. She also practiced not taking their "acting out" behaviors personally, which helped her feel more relaxed and in control. Establishing family rules was an important task for this family. Once her children knew the rules and knew their mother would reinforce those rules, fewer behavioral problems occurred.

"If I can't lift children, I can't be a good parent."

Some patients doubt their ability to raise children or be good parents in the future because of their pain.

When Tara, a 20 year old Caucasian woman, first entered therapy, she anticipated getting married and quitting her job as a full-time babysitter to become a homemaker and parent. When her orthopedic surgeon recommended that she avoid lifting objects over 20 pounds for the next several months, given her lower back problems, this activated significant anxiety regarding her role as a wife and as a mother in the future. Her assumption was that "If I can't lift children now, then I can't be a good parent in the future, so why even get married?"

Tara and her therapist created a list of what she could and could not do now, which disputed her belief, "I cannot be a good parent." The following list is an example of the identified activities this patient could engage in as well as her current physical limitations regarding childcare activities and babysitting.

<u>What I can do right now with children</u>
  Read stories
  Let young children sit in my lap
  Take short walks with the children
  Change infants' and toddlers' diapers or their clothes (when the child
    is compliant)
  Feed them
  Give baths in the sink

<u>What I can't do right now with children</u>
  Lift or carry children
  Crawling or roughhousing
  Chase after children
  Change diapers or clothes when the child is moving a lot (noncom-
    pliant)
  Give baths in the bathtub

> When Tara and her therapist discussed the "criteria" for "good moth-
> ers," carrying and lifting children constituted only one of many impor-
> tant qualities. Possible coping strategies were explored
> (problem-solving), such as holding a child on her lap while she is
> seated, having the child sit next to her, showing affection in her voice
> and touch, and receiving help from others if needed in order to hold
> or lift a baby. Although these strategies would not be as gratifying as
> lifting or carrying children herself, she realized that these were some
> realistic strategies.

The other important consideration in this particular case was that Tara's
surgeon's recommendations not to lift were for the next 6 months, not
necessarily for the rest of her life. Therefore, to prevent overgeneralizing
and catastrophizing, Tara was encouraged to remind herself of this. Over
time, if she follows her surgeon's recommendations, her back condition
may improve. Through physical therapy, Tara learned how to lift objects
and children correctly to avoid aggravating her lower back pain condition. Over time, her back condition did improve, and Tara was able to lift
the children she cared, but with great care and attention paid to her back.

"I am a burden to my children."

> Chronic pain patients often feel that their children view them as a
> burden and are resentful. Dee, a 51 year old African American woman
> and a single parent of three children, came into therapy with pre-

senting issues of severe depression and anxiety related to her low back pain (2 herniated discs) resulting from a work accident. At the crux of her depression, Dee's core belief was "I am a burden to my children" (I am helpless). Prior to her accident, Dee had always worked very hard to raise her children following her divorce. After her injury, Dee felt that she had lost control over her life and could not be helped. Of utmost concern to Dee was how her children felt about her. She tended to assume that her children were bitter about having to "pick up the pieces" and perform much of the household chores. In her words, she was a burden. Dee was willing to test out this core belief by interviewing her children individually to find out if indeed she was a burden. Dee predicted that all three children would view her as such. Dee decided to tape record the interviews. To Dee's surprise, all three of her children disagreed with her assumption and did not view her as a burden. In fact, her children reported that they understood her chronic condition and the limits she had to set on certain household chores, and they were happy to complete the chores. In addition, Dee's children commented on her good qualities and their hopes that she will feel less depressed over time as she continues in therapy. The therapist asked Dee how strongly she believed her children's feedback. She said, "One hundred percent." Dee realized from this exercise that her assumption of being a burden was unfounded and inaccurate. An alternative, more realistic response to the assumption "I am a burden" was identified: "Although I cannot perform the household duties I used to be able to do, that doesn't mean I am a burden to my children. My children have told me that I have good qualities and important things to offer them. I need to focus on what I can do instead of focusing on my perceived deficits. I need to accept their help as a sign of their responsibility, not a sign of my being weak or helpless."

FRIENDS AND SOCIAL SUPPORT

Chronic pain patients have a tendency to isolate themselves as a result of their pain and negative moods. They experience significantly higher levels of social isolation compared to people without chronic pain (e.g., Trief et al., 1987). Social withdrawal and physical limitations (e.g., participation in physical activities) can negatively affect their relationships with friends and family and significantly reduce opportunities for support.

Therapists must work with patients to break patterns of social isolation and withdrawal. One of the main goals in this area is to enhance or reestablish patients' connections with others by increasing patients' level of support and evaluating and modifying patients' and others' misperceptions in their interpersonal relationships.

On the one hand, chronic pain patients want to feel accepted and understood by others. On the other hand, many of these individuals do not want to be viewed as "disabled," weird, weak, or incompetent. Although there is a desire for social support, there is also a concern about being overly dependent on others. As a result, chronic pain patients experience a great deal of ambivalence in their relationships with friends and acquaintances.

Examples of typical thoughts and beliefs regarding friendships include "I shouldn't depend on others," "I'm a freak [because of my pain], so people will make fun of me," "People don't care about me. No one calls anymore," "People don't realize that I am suffering," "I don't want to burden people with my problems," "I don't want people to think I'm a complainer," and "I feel like I am imposing [if I visit, if I need help]."

"I shouldn't depend on others."

Patients who value independence and autonomous activities often have a difficult time adjusting to the physical limitations associated with chronic pain. Many of these patients push themselves too hard to maintain their previous lifestyles, despite the consequences this may have on their health. They do this because they want to remain as autonomous as possible. These patients view asking for help as a sign of weakness. In order to "fit in," they may try to minimize their pain and discomfort and their emotional suffering, which often only exacerbates their personal, social, and occupational problems.

> Marlene, 83, suffered from degenerative disk disease and rheumatoid arthritis but valued her independence. However, over the past year, Marlene has been feeling very tired and weak as a result of her pain and "old age." As a result, Marlene has become more restricted to the point that it is difficult for her to get in and out of the bathtub, to make meals for herself, and to go for daily walks. She has become more depressed and anxious about her physical limitations. Her friends and family members became very concerned about her because they are afraid she will injure herself if she tries to do too much on her own. One of Marlene's biggest problems is her stubbornness about being independent. She does not want to depend on others, because if she does, she will be a "failure" (core belief). If she asks for help, she is "one step closer to being put in a nursing facility." When Marlene and her therapist explore her rule "I should not depend on others," Marlene acknowledges that she was raised to be a very independent

person. To seek out help was a sign of weakness. When her therapist mentions that her friends and children are worried and want to help, she immediately rejects the idea because "they have lives of their own now. They don't need to be bothered by me." Earlier, Marlene had mentioned a time in her life when she cared for her father and mother in their later years. She recalled how much it meant for her to help them. They appreciated her help too. When her therapist reminds Marlene of this memory and asks her how this relates to her children's interest in helping her, she begins to cry. She realizes that she is denying the people she loves the opportunity to help her and to connect with her. It is something that they want to do—not to pity her, but to help her so that she can live as independently as possible at home. A few months ago, Marlene hired a woman to clean her house twice a week. Did this make Marlene a failure? No. So, when her friends or children help her out, does that mean she is a failure? No. Marlene comes to the conclusion that seeking help does not equal dependency or loss of freedom. Once she was able to change her rule, she was able to accept help from others as a sign of love rather than a sign of weakness or failure. Her new rule is "It makes me feel good when I can do things on my own. But it's okay to receive help from others when I need it. It doesn't mean I am a failure or that I am totally dependent."

"I'm a freak, so people will make fun of me."

Chronic pain patients often feel that they are a source of ridicule. Jean, a 47 year old Native American worman, was particularly distraught over her unstable gait following knee surgery. She feared that other people, including her friends, would make fun of her. In one situation, Jean encountered a woman and a boy in the grocery store who made a rude comment about her gait ("Look mom, she walks really funny"). Jean was very hurt and thought, "I am just going to have to stay home and rot." Her underlying belief was that she was a "freak, like Frankenstein, so of course, people will make fun of me." As this grocery store encounter was discussed, it was clear that the woman and her child were being rude to Jean. However, Jean had options about how she could have handled that situation: (1) she could have internalized it as a sign that she was a freak, (2) she could have told them that she did not appreciate their comment and felt empowered, or (3) she could have ignored them and not personalized their comment. Her therapist said, "So, one way of looking at the situation is to view yourself as a freak and to isolate yourself. What might be some other ways of viewing their comments?" Jean responded,

"They were mean and insensitive." Here was the alternative response Jean and her therapist created in session after reviewing all the evidence: "They don't understand what I've been going through. I am walking as best as I can. I don't have to let strangers' comments get the best of me." This new belief helped reduce Jean's level of anger.

Jean and her therapist discussed how often people teased her because of the way she walked. Jean indicated that most of the time, people were very friendly and accepting of her in public situations despite her difficulties in walking. In fact, Jean could only identify a couple of times when people were rude to her. In looking at the bigger picture, Jean realized that she was not a "freak" or a "victim" who needed to avoid people in order to avoid ridicule. This realization allowed her to be more spontaneous and less paranoid regarding her interactions with others. In addition, she learned that she was still able to survive even those worst-case encounters of being ridiculed. As a result of this intervention, Jean's anxiety regarding ridicule was lessened and she felt more confident in handling people's comments. For example, she could respond by saying, "I just had knee surgery."

LIFESTYLE ISSUES

Some chronic pain patients experience significant changes in their overall lifestyle. For example, they may no longer be able to engage in previously enjoyed activities such as hobbies, sports, and home activities. Even their sleeping behavior may be significantly affected as a result of their pain. Some patients avoid places or events that remind them of how they became injured, for example, avoiding the intersection where the car accident occurred. Other patients may avoid people because they do not want to explain their condition to everyone. They do not want people to feel sorry for them or to pity them. Still others may take on a "sick role" in order to receive secondary gains.

FEAR OF DRIVING A CAR

It is not uncommon for patients who were injured as a result of a motor vehicle accident to develop panic attacks when driving or riding in a car following the accident. Cognitive and behavioral interventions can be used with these patients to reduce their overall level of anxiety and hypervigilance when traveling in a car. Some of these interventions include implementation of deep breathing techniques, distraction techniques (e.g., looking in the rearview mirror for only 2 or 3 seconds at a time when a car is approaching from the rear), imagery exposure techniques (facing memories of the accident), identifying and modifying catastrophic thoughts regarding safety, and emphasizing approach behaviors (e.g., contracting to drive their car three times this week—graded exposures to the feared stimuli). More realistic coping statements when driving or riding in a car can be developed collaboratively in therapy. Here are some examples of coping statements used by patients who have a fear of driving: "The car behind me will stop in time, so it won't hit me," "God is watching over me," "The more I drive, the more I will experience success in coping with my fears," and "I am going to be fine."

It is important to teach patients the progression of symptoms (physiological, cognitive, and affective) that emerge when they experience a panic attack. Some of these symptoms can be processed in the following manner: The chronic pain patient is walking toward her car and thinking, "I can't drive my car. I might get into another accident." Following that automatic thought, the patient first begins to notice her shallow breathing ("What is happen to me?"), then attends to her racing heart rate ("I am not in control of these symptoms"), then becomes aware of her sweaty palms ("You see, you're a wreck. You can't drive"), and finally becomes tearful and heads back into the house. It is important for patients to know their symptoms so they can understand the strong connections between their fear of driving, their corresponding physiological sensations, and their prominent catastrophic thinking regarding their ability to drive and cope with their feelings.

Following this process, therapists can help patients realize that they do indeed have control over their fear and over their physiological sensations. Cognitive-behavioral procedures that promote patients' sense of mastery and control over their anxiety (regarding driving, in this case) include cognitive restructuring techniques, panic inductions (having the patient bring on panic attacks in session by recreating the symptoms using deep, shallow breathing for 2 minutes), and repeated exposures to the feared stimulus (driving a car).

SECONDARY GAINS OR THE "SICK ROLE"

Some chronic pain patients develop a sick role as a result of their chronic pain in order to receive secondary gains such as attention and sympathy (from family, friends, doctors, coworkers, and bosses), dependency, and exemption from responsibilities. Although many chronic pain patients who come to therapy feel depressed, anxious, or angry, patients who develop a sick role may regularly complain about how horrible their lives are to others, or they may purposely use pain behaviors for some personal gain.

Therapists should find out how partners and spouses respond to patients' complaints and pain behaviors. According to Romano and associates (Romano, Jensen, Turner, Good, & Hops, 2000, p. 416), "solicitous behaviors are those that tend to encourage a sick role, for example, by discouraging activity or by expressing concern or sympathy for the patient's pain problem." Attentiveness and solicitation from spouses and partners have been associated with increased pain severity as well as pain behaviors in chronic pain patients (e.g., see review in Turk, Kerns, & Rosenberg, 1992). If partners or spouses provide most of their attention when patients are in pain, then they are reinforcing the patients' pain. Therefore, it is recommended that partners and spouses try to ignore patients' physical demonstrations of pain or their pain complaints, so as not to reinforce these pain behaviors. In addition, patients should be encouraged to stay involved in activities—to participate in life. However, this does not mean that partners or spouses should criticize, put down, or express hostility toward patients when they are in pain, because this can be psychologically damaging to them. In fact, negative behaviors by partners and spouses (e.g., criticism, irritation; Romano et al., 2000) have been associated with psychological problems among chronic pain patients (e.g., Schwartz, Slater, & Birchler, 1996; Turk et al., 1992). We still do not have a clear understanding of the impact of partners' or spouses' negative behaviors on patients' experience of pain (e.g., pain intensity, pain behaviors, and disability) because the research findings have been mixed in this area (e.g., Faucett & Levine, 1991; Kerns, Haythornthwaite, Southwick, & Giller, 1990; Romano et al., 2000; Schwartz et al., 1996; Summers et al., 1991; Turk et al., 1992).

Although some patients develop a "sick role" to seek secondary gains, most chronic pain patients, in the authors' experience, do not. Therapists should be aware of the "payoffs" of having chronic pain. If the benefits outweigh the costs, then patients are probably gaining from their chronic pain status. For some patients, having chronic pain provides them with excuses not to get well, not to move on with life, not to work, to seek potential financial rewards, or to use their pain to get what they want.

One common myth that must be dispelled is that patients who have personal or work-related injuries are faking their pain and are just trying to manipulate the legal system to make some quick money. Just because patients seek compensation for their injuries does not mean that they are seeking secondary gains or engaging in "sick role" behaviors. If patients are diagnosed as not being able to work due their chronic pain conditions or due to chronic psychological distress, then these claims are clearly necessary and legitimate in order for patients to receive some financial compensation for their disabilities. (Most patients do not receive enough disability monies to pay the bills. They typically receive less than $1,000 a month.) As a general rule, it is best for therapists to assume that patients are *not* seeking secondary gains or pursuing a sick role until there is significant evidence to suggest this is the case.

If the therapist notices a significant lack of improvement in a patient's pain management, mood states, relationships with others, or other life roles over time, this may be an indication that other psychosocial factors may be influencing the patient's problems, including social support problems and secondary gains. The therapist should clarify the extent to which these factors may be reinforcing the patient's problems. If the patient seeks secondary gains, he or she needs to be confronted about this. Then the therapist and patient can explore other ways of getting his or her needs met without unnecessary dependency.

The problem with sick role behaviors and secondary gain issues is that they create more suffering for patients and those around them in the long run. Supportive people in patients' lives become disillusioned and cannot tell real cries for help from those that are made up. Taking care of someone who is constantly complaining about his or her pain can become very stressful. In addition, professionals, friends, and family members may become less invested in their patients' care if they think they are being used or taken advantage of.

15

Occupational, Financial, and Legal Difficulties

Chronic pain patients can also experience personal and environmental stresses related to their occupational and financial status, as well as legal issues. Although it is impossible to fully describe all of the possible stressors in these areas, some examples will illustrate the types of problems patients encounter.

OCCUPATIONAL DIFFICULTIES

One of the most significant stressors for the chronic pain population stems from the impact of pain on employment. In fact, one billion lost workdays every year have been attributed to chronic pain (Miller, 1993). Patients may not be able to perform the main duties of their work, which can result in light-duty work (significant reduction in hours), demotion within their field (change in responsibilities), job loss, or early retirement. Some patients apply for disability benefits.

Despite many of the stereotypes in our society, many chronic pain patients want to return to work and feel very frustrated, anxious, and depressed about this loss in occupational status, resulting in self-esteem and financial problems. Examples of automatic thoughts among chronic pain related to work include "I put my whole life into my work." "If I can't go back, I will be devastated," "I am not going to allow myself to be sick," "I may never be able to work again," "I don't know where I'm going," and "What will people at work think of me?"

Patients who are not able to return to their line of work may benefit from some career counseling to explore options within their field or to consider other careers. Vocational rehabilitation counselors and career counselors can provide many of these services.

The following sections offer suggestions for helping patients to cope with occupational stressors.

FEAR OF LOSING ONE'S JOB

Some chronic pain patients believe that if they are not in control of their bodies, they are not in control of their lives in general. The possibility or actuality of losing one's job can heighten a patient's sense of uncontrollability. For patients who have placed a great deal of emphasis on their work performance (e.g., "I put my whole life into my work"), there is a tendency to view job loss as a catastrophe (e.g., "If I can't go back, I will be devastated"). Keisha, a 43 year old African Woman (see chapter 2), is afraid of losing her job as an architect. Keisha and her therapist explore her view that losing her job would be a catastrophe.

Therapist: You were saying that you would be devastated if you could not return to work. Tell me more about this.

Patient: Well, I have invested so much of my life in my work as an architect. If I didn't return to work, I wouldn't be able to provide for my family, and I would be miserable.

Therapist: If that were true, then what would happen?

Patient: Then my family would be destitute. I would become depressed and lose hope.

Therapist: On a scale from 0 to 100, how strongly do you believe that your family would become destitute?

Patient: Oh, about 95.

Therapist: Okay, let's discuss how your family would become destitute if you lost this job. [exploring evidence for negative thought]

Patient: Well, losing my job would be a loss of $80,000 a year.

Therapist: And if you lose $80,000 a year, then what would happen?

Patient: We wouldn't be able to pay our bills, and we might lose our house.

Therapist: Okay, but you also mentioned earlier that your husband works. How would that factor play a role in your family's welfare?

Patient: Well, I guess we could barely get by on my husband's salary, but it would not be satisfying.

Therapist: So, there is some evidence that your loss of salary would have a significant impact on your family's welfare. Is there any other evidence that your family will become destitute?

Patient: No. That's the main issue.

Therapist: Okay, what evidence do you have that your family will not become destitute?

Patient: Well, like you said, my husband does earn an income. Maybe I could pursued another career.

Therapist: Would it be possible for you to find another career that is meaningful or enjoyable?

Patient: I guess it's possible. I just had always planned to work in this field until I retired, so I never considered other possibilities. If I could find another career that would be rewarding both monetarily and personally, I might not be so depressed or miserable.

Therapist: So the evidence against the belief that your family will become destitute is that you still might be able to contribute to the financial well-being of your family by pursuing another career, but also realizing that your husband contributes to the family's financial resources.

Patient: Yes, I'm beginning to see that.

Therapist: How strongly do you believe that you may actually be able to contribute to your family's well-being in the future by pursuing another career?

Patient: I'm not sure yet, but I sure have more hope now than I did a moment ago. The whole idea of considering a career move is a new one for me.

Therapist: What might be another way of thinking about your current situation?

Patient: Well, I haven't lost my job yet, even though I can't return to work right now. And even if I couldn't maintain the same level of performance in my work, that doesn't mean that I couldn't perform other jobs in the company. Maybe I can spend some time planning other career alternatives in case I do lose my job.

Therapist: How strong are these new beliefs about your career situation, on a scale of 0 to 100?

Patient: About a 70.

Therapist: And what feelings do you have about this new perspective on your career?

Patient: I actually feel more optimistic and hopeful.

RELATIONSHIP PROBLEMS WITH COWORKERS AND EMPLOYERS

Another change in a person's occupational role as a result of their pain or physical impairment may be his or her relationships with coworkers, managers, and employers. Some patients report significant distress in their relationships with coworkers if the patients return to work but have been assigned to different responsibilities or lighter duty. One patient recalled a coworker yelling at him: "Move out of my way. I'm going to my real job." In that situation, the patient thought, "Why is he treating me that way? I'm being punished." Esther, a 25 year old Caucasian woman, reported that a coworker teased her and said, "You move like a turtle." This event activated her core belief "I am pitiful. People can see that." She was very hurt by her coworker's comments. Cognitive restructuring and assertiveness training are specific techniques that can help patients improve their relationships with coworkers and bosses. However, the reality is that some relationships may be permanently severed, particularly if patients seek legal recourse against their employer for financial compensation for injuries. This reality needs to be discussed openly with patients.

Here is an example of how cognitive restructuring techniques and assertiveness training can be used to improve relationships with coworkers and employers.

Therapist: Esther, you mentioned earlier that you felt hurt when your coworker teased you, saying "You moved like a turtle." What thoughts or images were running through your mind when she said that?

Patient: My first thought was, "How rude! She has no right to say that to me."

Therapist: [clarifying her thought] So you were saying to yourself, "She shouldn't have said that to me. It was rude." [Therapist identifies the implicit "should" in her thought.]

Patient: Yes, exactly. She has no idea of what I am going through with this pain. I do move slowly, but that is the best I can do.

Therapist: So, when your coworker referred to you as a "turtle," what did that mean to you? Patient: That she was insensitive and that she didn't care about me.

Therapist: And what does her turtle label say about you?

Patient: [pause] It means that I am slow. I am pitiful.

Therapist: So, what really drives your feelings of hurt is not only what she said to you, but also the meaning you have given her words . . . that she doesn't care about you and that you are pitiful.

Patient: Yes. That's true.

Therapist: Okay, let's go back for a moment to that memory of your coworker calling you a turtle. What happened after she said that?

Patient: Nothing. She just walked away. I was so shocked by her comment that I was tongue-tied.

Therapist: That's very common. Sometimes it's hard to find the words to say in moments of shock. Now that you are beyond the shock, is there something you wanted to say to her after she made that comment?

Patient: Yes. But I don't have the words.

Therapist: How about this? Let's not worry about how it sounds. Just say anything that comes to your mind. Then we can work together to "tweak" it or modify it.

Patient: Okay, here goes. That's not a very nice thing to say. That's very rude of you. I do move slowly, but I am doing the best that I can given my pain.

Therapist: Anything else?

Patient: Nope. I think that covers it.

Therapist: So the main message that you want to communicate is that you were hurt by her comments and to clarify why you move slowly.

Patient: Yes, exactly.

Therapist: The second part sounds great. The first part needs some work. While your coworker may have been rude, pointing that out may put her on the defensive. It is what we can a "you" statement, for example, "you are rude." Another strategy is to address your feelings directly instead of pointing out what she did wrong. For example, "Hey, that hurts my feelings [when you call me a turtle]." Another option is to skip the first part and go straight to your explanation: "I do move slowly, but I am doing the best that I can given my pain." What do you think about these options?

Patient: I want to tell her off, but it probably would be rude of me to call her rude. I think I would prefer to go straight to the message, that I am doing the best that I can.

Therapist: That sounds good. I know that the moment when she put you down has passed. However, you can choose to tell her your message now or wait for another opportunity with this particular coworker or with someone else when it arises. What is important is that you feel that you have the words to communicate the essence of your message—that you are doing the best that you can.

Patient: I feel better knowing that I can use that message if I feel people are giving me a hard time at work. The reality is that I am not that close to this particular coworker anyway. So I'm not as concerned about her caring about me as much as I am about being respected.

Therapist: That sounds great. And the best way to be respected is to stand up for yourself, to communicate your main messages, and to do so in a respectful way.

Patient: I feel better already. Even saying what I wanted to say in here makes a big difference.

Therapist: Great! I'm also wondering if this message, "I am doing the best that I can," would be a great reminder to yourself when you start assuming that you are defective.

Patient: Good point. I agree. I cannot change the way that I walk right now. And while that may be unusual to some people, I am doing the best that I can.

Therapist: Let's write that down on a coping card (see Figure 15.1).

FIGURE 15.1 Coping Card

Belief: I am pitiful (because my coworker said I move slow like a turtle).

Alternative belief: I cannot change the way that I walk right now. And while that may be unusual to some people, I am doing the best that I can.

If _____ (coworker) brings up the issue again of "moving slow like a turtle," I can do one of several things:

- Use humor to lighten the conversation and let her know this doesn't bother me: "Yeah, well, remember the turtle beat the hare!"
- Let her know the comment hurt/offended me: "I realize that it might be uncomfortable for you to see me in pain. However, I didn't appreciate you making fun of me. I am trying to get around the best I can."
- Ignore her comments. (She is just trying to get the best of me. She is not worth the energy.)

CHANGE IN WORK RESPONSIBILITIES DUE TO FUNCTIONAL LIMITATIONS

Some patients, particularly those with acute pain, may be put on light duty at work until their condition improves; some are unable to return to work even months or years after their injury or following the onset of long-standing pain. Others can return to work but require a change in responsibilities given their physical limitations. These can be difficult realities for patients to face. For example, a construction worker may not be able to operate heavy equipment after being injured. However, that worker may be able to handle lighter duties assuming these activities are manageable given the injury and are acceptable to his or her employer. As mandated by the Americans with Disabilities Act, employers must provide reasonable accommodations to their employees with disabilities, including physical disabilities. Light-duty activities may allow employees to continue in their line of work temporarily until they recover from their illness or injury. It is also possible that employees are given other jobs within the same organization to accommodate their chronic pain and physical limitations. If patients are not satisfied with these job changes, they can choose to pursue other work, whether it is with the same employer or a new one. For some patients, these changes in work responsibilities can be very dissatisfying, particularly if they affect the nature of their work and what they enjoyed about the job. Patients can learn how to assert themselves with their employers about the nature of their work, what can be realistically accomplished given their pain, and how to seek reasonable accommodations to help them complete their work tasks and responsibilities.

Some patients may deny their physical limitations and return to work, engaging in the same tasks as before, without requesting any accommodations whatsoever. They may push themselves too hard physically (e.g., sitting for long periods without breaks, lifting heavy boxes or equipment), resulting in more pain and potential injury. The therapist can work with the patient, the patient's physician and other healthcare professionals, including physical therapists, occupational therapists, and vocational rehabilitation counselors, to determine what are realistic and reasonable working activities and behaviors for the patient. It is understandable that most patients want to keep their jobs. The goal is to do so while maintaining physical health and well-being.

Actual Job Loss and Unemployment

As mentioned earlier, some patients fear the possibility of losing their job. The reality is that this possibility does exist. If employers cannot accommodate the work responsibilities to the patients' physical abilities, then the employers can rightfully let them go or fire them. Or patients may choose to quit their jobs because of performance problems or dissatisfaction with work due to their pain.

Job loss and subsequent unemployment can be a very degrading experience for patients, particularly those who have maintained a good track record of hard work. If they are laid off, patients can be encouraged to file for unemployment to receive some financial benefits while they continue to look for new jobs.

Many patients assume that there is only one career that is right for them and to switch to a different career would be a catastrophe. This may be the first time that patients have had to reevaluate their career role after having served a number of years in one field. Therapists can help patients evaluate their present and future abilities as well as their interests in pursuing similar or alternative career goals.

In terms of career exploration, it is important for patients to learn more about themselves, including their vocational interests, their work values, and their perceived abilities and talents. They also need to learn more about the world of work, including information about the occupations that are available and congruent with their strengths (e.g., vocational interests, work values, and talents). A variety of self-assessment devices can be used by qualified career counselors and vocational rehabilitation counselors, including interest assessments (e.g., Strong Interest Inventory, Kuder Interest Inventory, Holland's Self-Directed Search, Holland's Vocational Interest Inventory, DISCOVER, and SIGI), work value assessments (e.g., Missouri Occupational Card Sort, DISCOVER, and SIGI), and ability assessments (aptitude tests, e.g., specific work performance tests, perceived abilities via DISCOVER and SIGI computer programs). There are also a number of resources available in career resource centers and libraries for patients to collect more information about other occupations, including the Occupational Outlook Handbook, DISCOVER, SIGI, and state vo-tech career search software packages. For those patients with computers, the Internet can provide a wealth of information about different occupations. Patients can also conduct informational interviews with different companies (employers or employees) to learn more about possible careers of interest. Shadowing professionals in different careers can give patients hands-on insights into what a typical day would be like in that profession.

FINANCIAL DIFFICULTIES

Another critical issue for chronic pain patients is coping with financial difficulties, particularly significant financial losses. If they cannot return to work, these patients may begin to experience significant financial hardship as they wait for disability claims to be processed and verified as well as for their legal cases to be settled and awarded. Even if patients are not involved in a personal injury claim or work injury case, the amount of healthcare bills associated with their chronic pain condition can soar over

time. Some patients are uninsured or have poor insurance benefits, resulting in still further financial hardships. Some third party payers question
the need for pain management services or may not cover them at all. It is
not uncommon for chronic pain patients to experience a number of negative thoughts about their financial difficulties. Examples include "Why
is this happening to me?" "I am being punished," "I cannot provide for
my family [and I should]," "Where are my compensation checks?" "I am
afraid that I will lose my house," "Will my employer force me to retire?"
"Will I lose my job?" and "If I cannot meet my financial obligations, I will
lose everything." Some of these thoughts may be realistic in nature. When
they are, problem-solving strategies are recommended. If these thoughts
are unrealistic and catastrophic, then the goal is to help patients evaluate
and modify these thoughts so that they do not feel overwhelmed.

Some chronic pain patients are concerned about their ability to pay
bills and maintain adequate credit ratings given their situation (whether
it be job loss or extensive health care costs). Some patients are barely able
to pay their bills and thus have to contend with billing agents. This can
be a demoralizing experience for individuals who used to provide adequately for their families. For those patients who are unable to pay their
bills on time due to financial strain, they may need some assistance in how
to handle bill collectors. In general, patients should be referred to financial counseling services in their community. An attorney can provide some
recommendations on how to handle these financial concerns, particularly
if they are related to court settlements.

> Xavier, a 45 year old Latino man, was injured both of his knees in a
> work-related accident. Given the significant damage to his knees, he
> was not able to return to work. Severe financial hardship was all Xavier
> could see in his future until his case would be settled in court. Frequent
> phone calls from bill collectors tended to trigger his depression and
> anxiety about his finances. Xavier's thoughts about his financial situa-
> tion included "I'm in deep trouble financially, with no end in sight,"
> "These bill collectors don't want to hear that I'm waiting for a check,
> or that I haven't worked in 14 months. They don't want to hear it, and
> I'm tired of explaining it," "It bothers me that I don't have any control
> over what goes on day-to-day," and "I feel lost, like there's no solution."
> Xavier had a real problem, but he was making it even worse by
> obsessing about his financial situation when he was sitting at home
> alone with unstructured time. Xavier admitted that he thought about
> his financial situation all of the time. When the advantages and dis-
> advantages of obsessing about his financial situation were explored,
> he realized the negative impact of his obsessive thoughts on his moods
> and his pain levels. His therapist asked him how much time he needed

on a weekly basis to focus on his financial situation in order to organize his financial affairs and to cope in general. Xavier and his therapist agreed that spending more than 1 hour a day thinking about his financial situation would only exacerbate the anxiety and depression he was experiencing.

One helpful homework assignment was to allot a half hour a day to worry and journal about his worries regarding his financial situation and any other concerns (activity scheduling; see chapter 5). When the worrying time was over, Xavier and his therapist contracted that Xavier would plan to do something pleasurable and enjoyable for at least a half hour after his scheduled worry time (increasing pleasurable activities; see chapter 5).

Cognitive restructuring was also emphasized in helping Xavier cope with his negative thoughts about his finances. For example, one of Xavier's most distressing negative automatic thoughts was "I don't have control over my financial situation." When this thought was discussed in some detail, Xavier realized that he did have some control over his financial situation. For example, he stayed in regular contact with the attorney who was handling his financial matters, he made what payments he could, particularly to his mortgage company, and he budgeted his money for basic expenses (e.g., food, clothing, and shelter). It was true that his lifestyle had to be adapted given his chronic knee pain and limited financial resources; however, he was taking steps to gain some control over his finances until his case was settled in court. Focusing on his future settlement and talking with his attorney helped Xavier stay focused and he felt less hopeless about his situation.

Xavier was still distressed about the phone calls from bill collectors. One solution was to ask his attorney to write letters of protection to these collectors. These letters legally assure the collectors that they will get paid out of Xavier's settlement following the court case. By consulting with his attorney and requesting that letters of protection be sent to bill collectors, Xavier put this "heavy load" of responsibility back on his attorney, who was able to handle such matters.

However, Xavier was responsible for how he handled phone conversations with bill collectors and, in particular, how much he was going to allow those phone calls to bother him. Xavier and his therapist role-played ways in which he could be assertive with bill collectors on the phone. Xavier learned to keep the phone conversation short by informing the collectors that he was currently involved in a work injury court case and that they should contact his attorney regarding bill collection matters, then giving them his attorney's name and phone number. Another helpful intervention was to encourage Xavier to screen his phone calls, particularly setting limits on how often he checked the machine for messages.

LEGAL DIFFICULTIES

Patients who are injured as a result of motor vehicle or work-related accidents are often involved in the legal system to seek appropriate compensation for their injuries and suffering. Therapists can help patients cope with potential legal differences that may occur such as clarifying what their rights are, dealing with the legal system, improving their relationships with attorneys, and dealing with anxieties associated with court dates and events.

RECOMMENDATIONS FOR ATTORNEYS

There may be times when patients ask therapists for specific referrals to attorneys in their community because they want to pursue legal services. Therapists should avoid making such recommendations or referrals because of the liability issues that could result if patients are dissatisfied with therapists' recommendations. However, therapists can encourage patients to talk with other people who have sought legal assistance in such cases about their recommendations for good attorneys. Word of mouth seems to be one of the best ways to find the most reputable professionals in any field.

PERSONAL INJURY, WORKERS' COMPENSATION, AND MALPRACTICE CASES

The two most common types of court cases for chronic pain patients are personal injury and workers' compensation. When patients are injured in car accidents or on personal property, they typically are involved in personal injury court cases to seek compensation for their injuries or suffering. When patients are injured at their work sites, they may be involved in workers' compensation court cases to pursue compensation for their injuries, suffering, and salary losses. On rare occasions, patients may sue their physicians and other medical staff for medical malpractice.

BEING INFORMED ABOUT LEGAL RIGHTS, ATTORNEY SERVICES AND FEES, AND THE LEGAL PROCESS

Patients need to discuss with their attorneys what their legal rights are as well as realistic expectations regarding their cases, including but not limited to: options for the recovery of financial losses or job losses, the advantages and disadvantages of pursuing legal action, what the process of pursuing a legal case will be like, the length of typical cases, the likelihood of winning their case given the information provided, and how much of a settlement or award is typical in these types of cases. In addition, patients need to know how much time their attorneys and staff will invest in their case, how much input patients will have in the process, how to handle their financial situation in the meantime, how often they can realistically consult with their attorneys about their case, and what percentage their attorneys and staff will receive from the final settlement if one is awarded. Being informed of their rights, attorney services and fees, and the legal process will help patients feel more in control of their legal care.

KNOWING THEIR RIGHTS: THE AMERICANS WITH DISABILITIES ACT

Patients should become familiar with the Americans with Disabilities Act (ADA, 1990), especially if they are currently employed or were employed just prior to their injuries/diagnosis of pain condition. Signed into law in 1990, this act prohibits discrimination against people with disabilities and provides equal opportunities for people with physical, learning, and emotional disabilities in the domains of employment/work (e.g., requires reasonable accommodations in the workplace unless undue hardship), public service and public transportation (accessible transport), public accommodations (e.g., goods, services, and facilities), and telecommunications (e.g., relay services, intra- and interstate services). Disabilities, in this law, are defined as physical or mental impairments that significantly limit one or more major life activities, that are recorded, and/or that are regarded as an impairment. (Note: Disabilities do not include diagnoses such as current alcohol and drug use, compulsive gambling, kleptomania, and gender identity disorders, among others.) One important aspect of the law has to do with reasonable accommodations in the workplace. Employers with 15 or more employees should provide equal opportunities to recruit, hire, employ, promote, and train qualified (i.e., can perform essential functions of the job) people with disabilities. Employers with fewer than 15 employees or employers that can demonstrate such accommodations would result in "undue hardship" (significant difficulties or expenses to the employer) are exempt. Information about the ADA may be pertinent to patients with chronic pain. Patients can learn more about the ADA from resources such as the local library, the Internet, and their attorneys.

RELATIONSHIPS WITH ATTORNEYS

Sometimes, chronic pain patients become frustrated in their relationships with their attorneys and legal staff. These frustrations arise because of the sometimes lengthy process of their cases, patients' perceptions that their attorneys do not really care about them or do not believe their pain is real, and patients' assumptions that their attorneys are not working hard enough on their case or are taking advantage of them. Many cases can take months to years before a settlement is reached or a verdict is offered. In addition, there is no guarantee of such a financial settlement or award. Therefore, litigation for chronic pain patients can be very frustrating, especially if they are depending on the settlement money to survive. Patients are encouraged to talk with their attorneys and other patients to understand the typical nature and process of court cases such as theirs. Focusing on the aspects of their cases that they can control is of utmost importance. Examples include completing medical evaluations, psychological evaluations, and necessary paperwork for the attorneys, filing a report of the accident and the injuries that resulted, attending appointments with their attorneys, and following up to obtain necessary reports (e.g., medical and psychological) for their legal file. Although it is the attorney's responsibility to collect the necessary documentation to support their client's case, patients can follow-up with their physicians and therapists to see if the reports were indeed sent to their attorneys' office.

For those patients who question the work habits of their attorneys, they need to understand that their case is one of many being handled by their attorneys. They may become frustrated when they do not have regular communications with their attorneys. They may need to find out what is reasonable to expect from their attorneys in terms of the time they have for clients' questions and how timely the attorneys' responses will be. Many patients may find that they will have more communication with the attorney's paralegal or legal secretary than with the attorneys themselves.

If patients are truly dissatisfied with their relationship with their attorney, these areas of dissatisfaction can be identified in therapy, in hopes that the patient can communicate these concerns directly to their attorney in an assertive, brief manner. Ultimately, patients can explore the benefits and costs of obtaining a second opinion regarding their case or pursuing legal services from other attorneys, or whether this is even possible depending on how far along they are in the legal process. Some attorneys are better than others, with regards to relationship-building skills with clients, their timeliness in communications, their efforts and abilities to adequately represent their clients, and their personal investment in cases. Therefore, it is possible that some attorneys may not care about their clients or make much time for them. Therapists can explore how patients want their relationships with their attorneys to be and to see if these are realistic expectations. Some patients can benefit from learning how to be more assertive with their attorneys with regard to their case, instead of assuming that everything is being handled in an adequate manner.

PART V

ASSERTIVENESS

16

Assertiveness Training

Assertiveness training is an important component of cognitive therapy with chronic pain patients. These patients need to learn how to communicate directly with a variety of people (e.g., partners/spouses, children, parents, physicians, nurses, physical therapists, and attorneys) about their pain, their emotions and thoughts, and their wants and needs. This direct communication style—assertiveness—will help patients cope better with their pain and improve their relationships with others, if they can learn how to share their needs and wants without offending or hurting other people in the process. Having chronic pain can make some patients feel very uneasy or irritable in social situations, particularly if they perceive themselves as being misunderstood or unappreciated by others. Therefore, it is important for patients to learn how to communicate their experience of pain as well as their feelings and thoughts with others in order to feel understood and to gain support.

Here is an example of a therapist–patient dialogue in which the therapist introduces the idea of assertiveness training to a patient.

Therapist: As we have been talking, something that came to mind for me is your need for people to understand you and know what you are going through with this pain—not only people who you are close to, like your family and friends, but also people with whom you will interact with on a regular basis, like your medical doctor and her staff.

Patient: Yes, it's just been a struggle for me to get people to understand what I'm going through. I get so depressed that I withdraw from others, when I really should reach out. But when I do, I feel rejected.

Therapist: We discussed this earlier, and it sounds like you have had some experiences when people did turn away from you and other times when you gave up on them.

Patient: That's true. This pain is just so unbearable at times, which makes me so frustrated. It affects my relationships with others and what I want to say.

Therapist: One thing we could work on today is to teach you how to communicate your wants and needs in an open, direct manner, without blaming others, hurting others, or putting them on the defensive. This is what we call assertive communication.

Patient: That would probably help me a lot.

In assertiveness training, patients are taught how to

1. Listen to what others are saying and encourage them to talk.
2. Summarize what they hear that person saying (reflective listening).
3. State their own opinions, feelings, needs, and wants using "I" statements (e.g., " I feel _____ when you _____ I would appreciate it if _____ ").

During this process of communication, patients are asked to

1. Keep an open mind when listening to others (not assume or judging others).
2. Take responsibility for their thoughts and feelings (use "I" statements).
3. Avoid blaming others (avoid "why" and "you" statements).
4. Focus on their main messages when sharing their thoughts and feelings with others.
5. Be concrete and specific when offering feedback.
6. Be aware that everyone has rights.
7. Gauge the frequency and timing of their communications.

LISTEN

An important first step in the assertiveness training process is teaching people how to be better listeners. Listening is a skill that involves paying attention to what the other person is saying. It also involves using a variety of communication skills. Some of these skills include nonverbal techniques such as open body posture (e.g., arms to one's side when standing, not sitting with legs crossed), head nods, and open facial expressions (e.g., eye contact, relaxed jaw and mouth), and respecting the other person's space. Listening skills also involve verbal techniques including summary statements, paraphrases, encouragers, and reflections of feeling. Patients are initially taught to listen to others and to encourage people to talk.

ENCOURAGERS

Encouragers are the sounds people make to indicate that they are listening, including "uh-huh," "um-hum," and "hmm." These brief utterances let the other person know that the listener is paying attention to him or her and what is being said. Patients are discouraged from using "okay" or "right" as minimal encouragers unless they agree with the other person's comments. Head nods also convey attentiveness and encouragement to talk.

PARAPHRASES

Paraphrases essentially put the other person's words into one's own words. Examples of paraphrases include "You really want to know my pain" in response to "I don't understand what you are going through—help me here" and "You are really concerned about my well-being. I appreciate you telling me this," in response to "I am really worried about your health; I have been holding this back for a while. I think we should talk about it."

REFLECTIONS OF FEELINGS

Reflections of feeling are statements of the emotions that the listener hears in the other person's communication. Patients can be taught to identify the emotions present in the other person by being aware of the words used as well as any facial expressions and body language. Reflections of feeling statements typically start with "Sounds like you are feeling _____." Examples of reflections of feeling include "Sounds like you are angry that we don't spend more time together," "I sense that you are frustrated when I complain about my pain," and "Sounds like you are worried about me." It is recommended that patients use this particular technique sparingly, primarily when they want to acknowledge the feelings of others.

After patients listen to others and encourage them to talk, they are asked to summarize what others say before stating their own feelings or opinions on the subject of interest.

SUMMARY STATEMENTS

Summaries include the key points of the other person's communication. An example of a summary statement is "Let me be sure I understand what you have just said. You are concerned that we have not been spending time together for past few months. Is that correct?" After clarification that the summary is accurate, the person can share his or her own thoughts and feelings about this matter.

SHARE THOUGHTS AND FEELINGS USING "I" STATEMENTS

When patients want to share their thoughts or perceptions with others, they can start with the following "I" statements: "I have been thinking about _____," "I have been concerned about _____," and "I think *we* should _____."

Examples of sharing one's thoughts or perceptions include "I have been thinking about how much my pain has affected our relationship," "I have been concerned about the little time we have spent together lately. I miss spending time with you," and "I think we should work together in sharing the household responsibilities given the pain I have."

Making a request or sharing a need means asking for something, using "I" statement stems such as "I would appreciate it if _____," "I really would like _____," and "It would mean a lot to me if _____."

Examples of requests include "I would appreciate it if you would take your plate up to the sink. It would really help me out" and "I would mean a lot to me if you would come to my next doctor's appointment. I am really nervous about seeing the doctor."

When patients share their feelings, they can use the following format: "I feel [emotion] _____ when _____ [a situation, thought, or behavior occurs]

The patient first identifies the emotion that he or she is feeling about a certain life event or situation—sad, glad, mad, scared, guilty, depressed, jealous, and so on. Then, the patient identifies the situation, personal thought, or behavior (self or other) that evokes that feeling. The words that follow "*when*" describe the situation and need to be as specific and concrete as possible to educate the recipient of the communication. Examples of "I feel" statements include "I feel depressed when you tell me my pain isn't real," "I feel scared when you are silent," "I feel guilty when I cannot complete household chores," "It hurts a great deal when I sweep the floors or make the bed."

Here is an example of a therapist–patient dialogue to illustrate the use of "I" statements.

Patient: Well, I hate to admit it, but sometimes I get so angry with Jonathan for not coming to my doctor's visits.

Therapist: How does this happen—that Jonathan doesn't come with you to the appointments?

Patient: Well, I tell him I have an appointment and he says something like, "Okay. Have a good time."

Therapist: So the situation is you have a doctor's appointment and Jonathan tells you "to have a good time." You begin to feel angry. What thoughts or images run through your mind?
Patient: He doesn't care about me.

Therapist: He doesn't care because . . .
Patient: He doesn't offer to accompany me to the doctor's office.

Therapist: How do you respond when he says this, "Have a good time"?
Patient: I usually walk away feeling frustrated and alone.

Therapist: Does he know you want him to come with you?
Patient: He should. [pause] He might not. I've only mentioned it once or twice.

Therapist: I want you to think about what you would like to share with Jonathan, specifically your thoughts and feelings about this issue. How would you complete this sentence: "I would appreciate it if . . ."
Patient: I would appreciate it if . . . [pause] I don't understand what I should say here.

Therapist: Think about what it is you want or need from Jonathan in this situation.
Patient: I would appreciate it if you would come to some of my doctor's appointments.

Therapist: Great! That is your main message.

Once patients learn the general format of assertive communications (listen, encourage, summarize, and share thoughts and feelings using "I" statements), then other rules of assertive communications can be discussed.

KEEP AN OPEN MIND: DON'T ASSUME OR JUDGE

To help patients listen more effectively, they need to keep an open mind and not assume they know the other person's experience or perspective. Patients can learn to listen to other people's feelings or points of view without judging or assuming. One way to do this is to focus on the content of the message and on the process (e.g., the other person's tone of voice, delivery of message) to ascertain what the person is trying to communicate. In other words, patients learn to focus on the person with whom they are communicating. When patients repeat or summarize what the person was saying, they do this to be sure that the other person feels heard and that they understand the other person's perspective correctly.

OWN YOUR THOUGHTS AND FEELINGS: AVOID "YOU" STATEMENTS AND USE "I" STATEMENTS

One form of blaming others is the use of "you" statements in communications. "You" statements foster defensiveness in the receiver of the communication because the focus of the communication is on the other person. Examples of "you" statements include "It's your fault. You are always pushing me," and "You don't care about my pain. You are selfish."

Patients can catch themselves using "you" statements and substitute "I" statements. "I" statements, which start with the word I, indicate one's interest and willingness to speak from one's own experiences. "I" statements also communicate a sense of ownership of one's thoughts or perceptions (e.g., "I have been thinking about what we discussed earlier, and I think we need to consider getting a wheelchair for me. I just can't get around anymore like I used to"), needs or requests (e.g., "I really would appreciate some time to talk about my condition"), and feelings without blaming others (e.g., "I feel depressed and down when my pain kicks in," "I feel lonely when we don't talk on a daily basis," and "I have been worried about my pain. How has this affected you?"). When patients own their thoughts and feelings, they are accepting responsibility for them.

COMMUNICATE IDEAS WITHOUT BLAME: AVOID "WHY" QUESTIONS

Blaming can also come in the form of "why" questions. "Why" questions are usually asked because the listener wants to understand the other person's motives for saying or doing something or for feeling a certain way. However, "why" questions tend to put people on the defensive, feeling as though they have to justify or explain their position. "Why" questions, no matter how they are delivered, tend to have a negative, judgmental quality. Examples of "why" questions include "Why aren't you more supportive?" "Why don't you come to my office visits with me?" "Why don't you care about my pain?" "Why are you like this?" and "Why are you so mean to me?"

In therapy, patients can be taught how to turn every "why" into a "what," "how," or "tell me more" type of communication, which will reduce defensiveness and increase open communication. "Why" questions can be turned into "I" statements, specifically focused on explaining one's wishes or desires in as much detail as possible (e.g., describing the behavior needed) without intending to "push other people's buttons." For example, if the original "why" question is "Why did you wreck the car and hurt yourself?" other alternatives are available that will communicate more openness and less blame. For example, a "what" question could be "What happened?" A "how" question could be "How did it happen?" "Tell me more" communications include "Tell me about the accident. Tell me about your injuries." An "I" statement might be "I am really concerned about you. Are you okay?" These alternative questions and statements typically request information or communicate care or concern. Below are the "why" questions mentioned earlier in this section along with alternative, more assertive comments or questions.

"Why" Questions	*Assertive Questions and Comments*
Why aren't you more supportive?	**I would really appreciate it if we could spend some time together.** I have been feeling lonely lately, and I miss doing things together.
Why don't you come to my office visits?	I realize that you have been busy lately. However, **I was wondering if you could come to my next office visit with me.** Sometimes, it's really hard to remember what the doctor is saying in there when we have such a brief office visit. **I could really use your support.**
Why don't you care about my pain?	**Lately, I have noticed that when I am talking about my pain, you tend to walk away from me.** I just want you to understand what I'm going through. But I also want to know how all of this is affecting you too. Could we set aside some time to talk about this?
Why are you like this?	**Help me understand what's going on.** (Tell me more.) I really want to know. **OR** **I feel hurt when you tell me I'm lazy.** I just want you to know that this pain really bothers me and I

am trying to do the best that I
can to return to work. **I don't
appreciate your assuming that I
am lazy.** I am in pain.

Why are you so mean to me?   **I've noticed that you have been
angry for the past week, especially
when you yell at me and tell me "I
am no good."** I don't want you to
yell at me or put me down. That
hurts my feelings. I do want to
know what is going on. Can we
talk about this? [pause for
response] If we can't talk with
each other, then I guess we need
more time. But I will not talk with
you if you start yelling or putting
me down.

The sentences in bold face are the key communications in each scenario, because the person is communicating feelings when something happens (without blame), the person is stating the behaviors or events that
are dissatisfying (sharing thoughts without blame), or the person is requesting something from the other person (without coercion).

GET TO THE MESSAGE OR KEY POINTS

What am I trying to communicate? What message am I trying to convey?
These questions direct patients to communicate their main points (getting to the heart of the matter) without cluttering it with other concerns.
     Therapists can help patients identify their main messages by using a
variety of strategies (e.g., questions, feedback, journaling, outlines, and
role-plays). For example, if a patient engages in a great deal of storytelling—sharing very specific, and often nonessential, details about life
events in session—the therapist can interrupt and ask the patient to summarize the important message he or she is trying to communicate in telling
this story.

Therapist: Let me interrupt you here for a moment. What were the main
     points that you were trying to communicate to me in telling this
     story?

Therapists also can provide feedback by sharing their own reactions to what their patients say. Here is an example.

Therapist: I think in your efforts to help me understand your experience of pain you may be providing more details than are necessary to get to the same point.
Patient: I never realized this before. That really takes me by surprise.

Therapist: Is this the first time you've received feedback like this?
Patient: Actually, come to think of it, it's not. Other people have told me that before. I guess it just never really sunk into my awareness until now.

Therapist: Well, maybe we could work on this to help you get your main points across to others.

Journal entries can help patients identify the main points or messages they want to convey. For example, patients could write down what they want to say to their physicians at the next office visit, including any questions they may have. Often patients do not feel they have enough time to talk with their physicians about their pain or other medical concerns.

Therapist: If you could ask your doctor one or two questions during your next appointment, what would those questions be?

Main ideas or points can also be written in outline form to help provide some structure. These outlines can serve as a guide when patients need to communicate their ideas or feelings with others. For example, patients may want to bring in a short list of questions they have for the prospective employer during a job interview. Or, if patients need to share some feelings with a family member, then a brief outline can help them stay focused on the main issues they want to communicate.

Role-plays can be used to help patients practice communicating their main points. This will be demonstrated later in this chapter.

WHEN GIVING FEEDBACK, BE SPECIFIC, AND CONCRETE

Part of communication involves not only sharing one's experiences but also providing feedback to others. As much as possible, it is important for patients to be specific and concrete in their feedback, addressing the behaviors or events that occurred.

For example, a patient may be inclined to give a negative label to himself or to others instead of giving specific feedback on inappropriate or upsetting behaviors. Examples of labels include "I'm stupid for thinking I can trust others." "My friend is a jerk for telling someone else about my problem." Examples of more specific, concrete feedback are "I wish you had not revealed my secret to someone else" and "I did not appreciate your breaking our promise, and it really hurt my feelings."

YOU HAVE RIGHTS, BUT SO DO OTHERS

Patients have the right to communicate with others as long as they do not infringe upon the rights of others. This means being a good listener, respecting people's physical and conversational space (give them room, not interrupting or talking over others), realizing that people have a right to disagree with one another, and not engaging in emotional (e.g., putting others down or yelling, manipulating), physical (e.g., throwing objects, hitting, punching), or sexual (e.g., unwanted exposure, fondling) means to control others. Patients need to remember that they have the same right as others to be treated respectfully.

PAY ATTENTION TO FREQUENCY AND TIMING OF COMMUNICATIONS

It's not just the words people use, or their "body language" (e.g., tone of voice, body posture) that is essential in effective communication; it's the frequency and timing—how often communications occur and when the other party is open to hearing the feedback or communication. For example, if patients are constantly talking about their pain with others, people may be turned off by their communications. On the other hand, if patients do not share their experiences at all, people will not understand their pain. Finding a balance in sharing experiences is key. It is also important to consider when people are open and receptive to certain communications. For example, if patients are trying to talk with their partners about something important when their partners are in the middle of watching a television show, they may not get the attention or the responsiveness they were anticipating. Finding an opportune time to talk is important. This may involve scheduling a special time to talk when both parties are available, receptive, and attentive.

ROLE-PLAYING ASSERTION SKILLS

Patients can learn these assertion skills by role-playing them in session. Usually the therapist starts out by demonstrating the skill, then lets the patient practice it in session. Next, conversation scenarios could be played out. In the first role-play scenario, the therapist will play the role of the patient, and the patient will play the role of someone in the patient's life with whom he or she wishes to communicate. This initial arrangement is helpful for several reasons. First, the therapists shows the patient how to put the communication skills in action in a regular conversation. Thus, the patient learns through this direct observation. Second, the therapist gains a better understanding of how other people relate or respond to the patient based on the patient's representation of a person's character in the role-play. Third, information from these first two steps can help with the transition when the patient and therapist switch roles (patient plays himself or herself, and therapist plays the role of the "other person"). Because the patient has had a chance to observe the therapist using the communication skills, the patient may experience more success in implementing them than if he or she did it from the beginning without this observation period. In addition, the therapist can play the role of the "other person" more accurately (based on the patient's interpretation) than before. This transition makes the conversational role-play feel more genuine and real for the patient. By acting out roles, therapists and patients can play out different conversations with important people in the patients' lives, with the goal of teaching patients how to be good listeners and good communicators.

The therapist–patient dialogue below is an example of how therapists can teach patients assertive communications in session. Kevin, a 65 year old gay man, has been feeling frustrated because his partner, Tom, does not understand his pain.

Patient: I just don't think anyone really understands what I am going through with this pain. I sure wish I had more support, particularly from Tom.

Therapist: The reality is that you know more about your experience of chronic pain than anyone else does—what it feels like and how it affects you. So, one way to feel more understood is to share your experiences with Tom.

Patient: I just feel like giving up. What's the use? I just feel so alone with this.

Therapist: What feelings do you get in touch with when these thoughts cross your mind?

Patient: So sad and hopeless.

Therapist: I am here to help you get more support from the people in your life, including your partner. Why don't we take a moment now, in session, for us to practice ways to do that?

Patient: I guess we could give it a try. I don't expect that it will make much of a difference.

Therapist: It might or it might not. Let's suspend our judgment on that thought and see what happens, okay? [Patient nods his head.] You mentioned wanting more support from Tom. Tell me what is going on.

Patient: Tom really does not understand what I'm going through. It's so upsetting to me. I think if I could tell him what I needed, then maybe I would feel better about our relationship and myself.

Therapist: Okay, in a moment, we are going to do a role-play of how you and Tom relate to one another. I need a better understanding of how Tom comes across to you, so, you will play the role of Tom first and I will pretend to be you. In my role, I will be showing you some ways to communicate your thoughts, feelings, and requests in an assertive way. Later, we will switch roles. To help us get started, think of a recent incident in which you felt that Tom didn't support you. Think about what he said or did that didn't feel supportive to you. This is where we will begin. When you are ready, you will go first as "Tom."

Patient: [playing the role of Tom] I really don't have time to talk with you about your pain now. I need to go mow the lawn.

Therapist: [playing the role of the patient] Before you go, could we set up a time to talk about this? It is really important to me.

Patient: I have got a lot of stuff to do right now. I don't have the time to talk.

Therapist: What I'm asking for is your support. Sometimes I just want to talk with you about my pain and what I'm going through. It really hurts me when you walk away, especially when I am reaching out to you.

Patient: Okay. I guess we could talk later today.

Therapist: Let's make it a date. What time would work for you?

Patient: How about 7 p.m.?

Therapist: Okay. Thanks, Tom. [Therapist steps out of the role.] Okay, let's stop the role-play for a moment. How did you feel about it?

Patient: I thought it went pretty good. I really tried to play Tom the best that I could. He gets so busy at times. He really doesn't want to talk about my pain much.

Therapist: How do you make sense of that?

Patient: Well, I told you earlier that I don't feel like he supports me.

But, after we did the role-play, I just realized that he might not know how to support me. He tends to shut down when I want to talk.

Therapist: Is that true about most topics, or just when it comes to your pain?

Patient: I think it's true of most topics, but I've noticed that Tom avoids my comments about my pain. Sometimes, I wonder if he thinks it is real or not.

Therapist: Well, certainly we could put that thought to the test later. Let's focus back on the role-play. What were the main points I was communicating when I was in your role?

Patient: I just want some time to talk and when can we do it. [pause] I think one of my problems is that I get into my "complaining mode" and whine about how no one cares. That seems to push him away more.

Therapist: What might keep him there in the same room? How could you communicate with him differently than before?

Patient: I think focusing on my message and not jumping to the conclusion that he doesn't care.

Therapist: Okay. Well, why don't we try that, then? Let's switch roles now. You are you, and I am Tom. Before we get started, tell me what your main messages are.

Patient: First of all, I love him. But I am also angry with him for not helping me out . . . for not listening to me. [Anger is escalating.]

Therapist: I can tell that you are feeling angry right now. What thoughts are running through your mind right now?

Patient: If he really cared about me, he would listen to me.

Therapist: Have you asked him to listen?

Patient: Well, sort of. I haven't been real direct about it.

Therapist: It is possible that you are assuming he can read your mind and know what you want and need.

Patient: Probably.

Therapist: Now, I want you to turn all of your angry "shoulds" into "wants." Instead of saying, "you should listen to me," you could say, "I really want you to listen to me." Do you see what I mean?

Patient: Okay, I would like for him to listen to me and to support me.

Therapist: Remember to be as specific and concrete about his behavior as possible. In other words, define "support" in more detail.

Patient: [pause] I would like for him to sit with me, listen to me, and help me with some of the things that I cannot do. Just taking some time with me would feel really supportive.

Therapist: Okay. That's great. Are you ready to begin the role-play? We've spent the last couple of minutes preparing you to share your main messages with Tom. Do you want to write them down as an outline before we start?

Patient: Sounds good. [Writes down: I want Tom to listen, to schedule some time to talk and to get his help with some of projects/chores]

Therapist: Okay, let's begin the role-play. Just as a reminder, I will not interrupt you during this role-play. I realize that Tom may do that at times. But I want you to have an opportunity to practice what you want to say to him first.

Patient: Okay. [playing the role of self.] I need to talk to you for a few minutes.

Therapist: [playing the role of Tom] I really don't have time to talk with you about your pain right now. I need to go mow the lawn.

Patient: Tom, I would like to find some time when we can talk today. I've been feeling very lonely. I want you to understand what I'm going through, with my pain and all. I really need your support.

Therapist: I have been supportive. I just need to mow the lawn.

Patient: When I try to tell you what I'm feeling or when I ask for your help, I notice that you tend to walk away or cut me off. It makes me wonder if you really care.

Therapist: [Steps out of the "Tom" role for a minute.] Tell me what you need from Tom as your partner.

Patient: I just want some time to talk with you about my pain—the doctor's visit, the evaluations, and the financial problems we are having. I want you to listen to me. I'm afraid that the wall is up and you don't want to talk, but it would really help me feel better if we did talk.

Therapist: Okay, how can I show you that I am invested in you—listening to you—supporting you? [asking the patient to be concrete and specific in his feedback to Tom]

Patient: I would appreciate it if you wouldn't talk down to me—like when you told me that this pain is all in my head. I wasn't sure if you were saying this just to get me mad or because you really believed it. I just can't handle hearing that message anymore, from anyone. I think that would be a beginning.

Therapist: Anything else?

Patient: I just want us to schedule times when we can talk without interruption. I know that you're busy, but I also need your support.

Therapist: Okay, let's stop the role-play and discuss how that went.

After the role-play, the therapist and patient discussed what he learned from this exercise. The patient learned to ask for support and to be more specific and concrete in defining what he meant by support. Timing was also an important consideration in the example above. It may not be realistic for the patient to request time to talk with his partner when he is heading out the door to mow the lawn. However, scheduling a later time to talk was more reasonable.

Just like any other skill, listening and sharing experiences takes practice. Patients need to realize that part of learning a skill is making mistakes. It takes a while to master a skill. As long as they can learn from the mistakes they have made and are patient and caring with themselves and others, they will make progress. Realistic expectations are key: to share one's thoughts and feelings and to understand other people's perspectives. Unrealistic expectations may relate to patients' need for control or power: to change someone else or their high need to master these skills right away.

PART VI

PHARMACOTHERAPY

17

Pharmacotherapy for Chronic Pain Patients

In medical school, students are often taught to treat surgery as an option only after medications have proven ineffective. The hope is that most of the time patients will heal without the need for major medical interventions such as back surgery. In some cases, medical interventions, including prescription drugs, can make disease states worse. Therefore, the best pharmacotherapy approach to acute and chronic pain management is no drug therapy at all. However, the option of not using medications is not practical. Medication management of pain has become an extremely important aspect of treatment, and it is important for therapists to understand how medication management varies based on the type of pain the patient has. It has been suggested that physicians may not be treating pain effectively due to fear of addiction to pain medications, societal and regulatory censure, and diversion of drugs to the street (Resnik, Rehm, & Minard, 2001; Sipkoff, 2001).

In this chapter, some of the myths related to the medication of pain will be mentioned and separated from the realities. Fortunately, treatment guidelines for managing pain are essentially similar, be it acute, chronic, cancer, or nonmalignant pain. The main differences lie in nociceptive versus neuropathic pain states, as these syndromes have different physical causes (i.e., pathophysiologic mechanisms).

For starters, medical professionals and therapists are encouraged to believe the patient's self-report of pain. An adequate assessment is the hallmark of coming up with a pain management plan. Oral analgesics (i.e., pain-relieving medications) are administered whenever possible, as this is the simplest way the patient can take medication. Ideally, potential side effects (e.g., constipation) should be treated before they occur. Medications generally are dosed around-the-clock rather than on an as-needed basis.

MEDICATION MANAGEMENT OF NOCIOCEPTIVE PAIN

It is important for medical professionals to identify and treat the underlying cause of pain (VonRoenn, Cleeland, Gonin, et al., 1993). Sometimes patients are diagnosed as having a so-called "chronic pain syndrome." However, pain is a symptom of disease, not a disease state in and of itself. There is always an illness causing pain. In order to adequately treat pain, medical professionals need to identify the cause of the pain and then come up with strategies to treat the underlying disease state. Assuming this is done, rational pharmacological treatments for pain can be implemented. The World Health Organization (WHO) established what is known as the Analgesic Pain Management Ladder, which has become the standard of medication management for cancer pain and has been extrapolated for use with noncancer, nocioceptive pain as well (see Figure 17.1). The goal is to achieve maximum benefit with the lowest drug dose and minimal side effects.

FIGURE 17.1 World Health Organization Analgesic Pain Management Ladder

Step 1	Nonopioid
	1. Acetaminophen
	2. NSAID (i.e. ibuprofen, naproxen sodium, indmethicin)
	  a. COX-2 inhibitors
	    (e.g., rofecoxib, celecoxib)

Step 2	Add opioid (i.e. oxycodone, morphine sulfate).
Step 3	Add adjuvant analgesics at any point during this process.
Step 4	For episodic pain, use short-acting opioids; for continuous pain, consider the use of long-acting opioids (e.g., controlled release morphine, controlled release oxycodone, controlled release fentanyl, or methadone). Be aware that although methadone has a long half-life, the analgesic effect wears off in approximately 6 hours. Also be aware that meperidine, (Demerol),

formerly the most commonly prescribed opioid in the United States, is potentially harmful. It metabolizes into meperidine which can cause seizures, psychosis and depression. It is therefore is a poor choice for analgesia. Propoxyphene, the ingredient in Darvocet and Darvon, also is problematic. It too metabolizes into an agent with many side effects. However, it is commonly used in the elderly, probably the worst population in terms of the development of side effects to this medication. In studies, propoxyphene was found to be no more effective than acetaminophen alone. It should also be noted that there is recent evidence suggesting that methadone may be a NMDA (N-methyl-D-aspartate) antagonist, which may make it one of the few opioids effective in neuropathic pain.

From "Pain Control and the World Health Organization Analgisic Ladder," by V. Ventufridda and J. Stjernsward, 1996, *Journal of the American Medical Association,* 275, p. 835–836. Copyright 1996 by World Health Organization. Reprinted with permission.

The progression of medication is based on the severity of pain. For mild to moderate pain, we begin by using nonopioids, for example, acetaminophen, or nonsteroidal anti-inflammatory drugs such as ibuprofen, or the new COX-2 (cyclooxygenase-2) inhibitors, celecoxb (Celebrex), rofecoxib (Vioxx), and valdecoxib (Bextra). The COX-2 inhibitors have a gastrointestinal-sparing effect. In other words, there is less risk of peptic ulcer disease as compared with conventional nonsteroidal anti-inflammatory (WSAID) drugs.

If the patient continues to experience pain, a nonopioid–opioid combination of medication is considered next. Compounded agents such as a combination of oxycodone and acetaminophen, the active ingredients in Percocet, are no longer used. Instead, it is now recommended to use each individual ingredient separately to allow greater flexibility in titration. For example, Percocet only allows us to dose 40 milligrams of oxycodone a day. Oxycodone is the opioid ingredient in Percocet. Going beyond this would result in acetaminophen toxicity. Cases of liver failure have been documented in patients who took massive doses of this agent on a daily basis. It is therefore much safer and makes more sense to separate out these ingredients, use them individually, and titrate them according to need. When the analgesic ladder was initially developed, it was recommended to begin with a low-potency opioid, or the so-called schedule 3 agents. (The lower the number on a schedule agent suggests higher potency as well as increased scrutiny by law enforcement and the Drug Enforcement Agency. For example, a schedule 2 agent is more potent and more closely scrutinized than a schedule 3. Agent.) It is now recommended to use a schedule 2 agent instead of a schedule 3 agent. This has the effect of getting patients comfortable immediately, therefore establishing better compliance and enhanced rapport with your patient.

Medical professionals used to start patients off on a schedule-3 or low-potency opioid because it was thought to reduce the potential risk for addiction. They did not understand the concept of addiction at that time. As an analogy, there was push, years ago, to develop low-dose nicotine cigarettes in the hope that smokers would cut down on the number of packs of cigarettes that they would smoke every day. The result was that smokers actually doubled the number of packs a day that they smoked.

In actuality, the potency (i.e., strength) of a narcotic medication (i.e., opioid) is not as important as it was once thought, because addiction is comprised of psychological dependence as well as a physiological process. It therefore makes sense to go right to a schedule 2 opioid and get the patient comfortable immediately. At this point, adjuvant medications can also be prescribed as well. An adjuvant medication is one that has approval from the U.S. Food and Drug Administration (FDA) for one area, but also has off-label uses in pain. For example, anticonvulsive agents are approved for treatment of seizures, but there are also data regarding their use in treating neuropathic pain. In addition, some antidepressants approved for the treatment of depression are also effective in treating neuropathic pain (based on pain research findings). As a result, much of what medical professionals do in medicating pain is off-label. In fact, off-label medication is also prescribed regularly in psychiatry. For example, Trazodone, a sedating antidepressant, has been used as a sleeping pill. The FDA has not approved it for this purpose, but we administer it for such purposes because we have empirical and clinical evidence to support its use. We also use hydroxyzine, an approved antihistamine, as an anxiolytic (i.e., antianxiety) medication because it has a sedative effect and does calm patients. It has become standard to use off-label or adjuvant medications in a variety of medical disease states and symptoms. This is particularly true in pain management.

Adjuvant medications are often used at any point in the analgesic ladder in order to enhance pain control. If the patient is suffering from moderate to severe pain, it is okay to go right to an opioid and then concurrently use the adjuvant medications. Nonopioid medications such as acetaminophen or the anti-inflammatory drugs are taken for granted because they are readily available over the counter without a prescription. People take these agents and often do not even tell their physicians they are taking these medications for pain relief. In reality, these agents can be quite dangerous if not monitored properly. It is not uncommon for people to overdose accidentally on acetaminophen or ibuprofen. Acetaminophen at high doses can cause liver toxicity. Anti-inflammatory drugs such as ibuprofen can cause kidney damage as well as peptic ulcer disease. In many respects, the opioid medications are actually safer than over-the-counter medications for pain or inflammation. There is no organ damage associated with opioids, and they are tightly controlled substances carefully monitored by the prescribing physician. The nonopioid medications also have a "ceiling" effect (American Pain Society, 1999). This is not the case for opioids. Opioid medications can be dosed as high as needed to achieve pain control. It is a myth that giving someone 10 milligrams of morphine will result in respiratory arrest. Pain is a very stimulating experience and actually stimulates the respiratory center of the brain. It is rare for chronic pain patients to become respiratorily depressed by opioid medications unless they are already respiratorily depressed, for example, a patient emerging from anesthesia postoperatively. We are therefore able to titrate opioids to the desired effect, and there is no ceiling dose.

A model for treating pain using the WHO analgesic ladder comes from the geriatric population (American Medical Directors Association, 1999). The general guidelines are as follows: Titrate to effect, starting with a short-acting opioid (e.g., oxycodone, codeine, or immediate release morphine) prescribed as needed for episodic pain; transition to equivalent doses of long-acting opioids (e.g., sustained release oxycodone [Oxycontin], sustained release morphine, fentanyl patch [Duragesic]) for continuous pain; then use fast-onset, short-acting opioids (hydrocodone, hydrocodeine, oxycodone, codeine, or immediate release morphine) for breakthrough pain; finally, use pain-modulating adjuvant agents (e.g., antidepressants or anticonvulsants) in combination with analgesic agents (e.g., opioids) to assist with baseline pain management and breakthrough pain. It is important to anticipate, prevent, and treat common side effects of these various medications such as sedation, nausea, itching, and constipation.

The WHO analgesic ladder was originally developed for treatment of cancer pain. However, patients suffering from noncancer pain, such as failed back surgery or advanced arthritis, feel that their pain is worse than that experienced by a patient who is terminally ill. Terminally ill patients know that there is an end to their suffering, whereas noncancer pain patients who are relatively healthy may be facing 30 or 40 years of agonizing pain. It is therefore crucial that pain be treated as aggressively as possible.

Although opioid therapy has been medically and ethically accepted for the management of malignant and acute pain, major controversies continue to surround the use of opioids for chronic, noncancer pain (Pappagallo, Heinberg, Semin, 1997). Why the controversy? Pain is very complex. The goals of therapy for chronic, noncancer pain involve a multitude of factors. Obviously, health care professionals want to control patients' pain, improve functioning, stabilize family relationships, return patients to an active lifestyle, and assist patients in achieving minimal reliance on the health care system.

Fears about addiction often prevent the use of opioids in the treatment of chronic, noncancer pain (Gruener, 2003). Patients themselves put up barriers. For example, most Americans would rather bear pain than take action to relieve it. According to one study, 92% believe pain is a fact of life, 82% believe it is too easy to become reliant on pain medication, 72% believe that medication will not be effective with continued use, and 46% avoid medication until pain becomes unbearable (Bostrom, 1997).

Health care professionals also put up barriers. Unfortunately, pain is viewed as a normal by-product of injury and disease, and, therefore, it is assumed not much can be done about it. Health care professionals may also see pain medication as addictive or believe that once patients start taking pain medication, there will be a vicious cycle, requiring the constant escalation (i.e., increasing) of the dose. There is a legitimate fear of scrutiny by regulatory agencies, something that has been worsening of late.

Pharmacists can also put up barriers. According to one survey, 33% of pharmacists believe that patients will become addicted if opioids are taken daily for a month; 42% reported addiction was the same as physical dependence, tolerance, and psychological dependence; and 47% thought the practice of prescribing opioids for several months for noncancer pain should be discouraged (Greenwald & Narcessian, 1999).

How do we overcome these barriers? It is important to conduct an addiction history assessment. We need to develop a controlled substance agreement for patients to sign. Our documentation needs to be excellent, and we should assess the patient at each visit for pain relief, improved functioning, side effects, and aberrant drug-related behaviors. In order to better understand the justification for using opioid medication in both cancer and noncancer pain states, the differences between addiction and legitimate use of these agents need to be examined. Part of the problem is that health care professionals do not understand the differences between tolerance, physical dependence, abuse, and addiction.

Tolerance involves the need to increase the dose of a medication periodically in order to achieve the same desired effect. Patients can develop tolerance to the cognitive side effects and the sedating properties of opioid analgesics, but generally not to the pain-relieving (analgesic) properties. This means that medical professionals have to periodically increase the dosages of opioid medications (to increase the pain-relieving properties of these medications) because progressive, chronic, debilitating diseases tend to get worse (e.g., become more painful) over time. For example, in treating diabetes, medical professionals often have to increase patients' insulin over time. It is not that the patient is becoming tolerant to insulin; rather, the pancreas continues to deteriorate. Therefore, the disease state is worsening, requiring an increase in insulin. If an arthritis patient's joints continue to deteriorate, it makes sense that his or her pain will increase and an increase in the dosage of medication is needed. So tolerance is merely an adaptation phenomenon.

Physical dependence is often erroneously equated with addiction. Physical dependence is defined as a predictable withdrawal syndrome following the abrupt withdrawal of a controlled substance. It is important to understand that if a patient is put on a controlled medication, he or she will develop physical dependence to it. There is nothing good or bad connoted by this; it is merely a cellular adaptation phenomenon. For example, some medical professionals may receive a referral letter like this: "I am sending you Mr. Smith, who is physically dependent on substance Y," as if to say that something aberrant is happening.

In the medical field, abuse is defined as the use of a legitimate medication outside the scope of medical practice (i.e., not taking medications as prescribed) or the use of an illicit substance. If a patient is told to take two time-release morphine pills every 12 hours by the clock and he or she is taking three or 4 every four hours without discussing it with his or her physician, then that it abuse. If a patient is smoking marijuana, using crack cocaine, and getting high, then that is also abuse. Abusers are not always addicted. They can be, but they do not have to be.

According to the *DSM-IV-TR* (American Psychiatric Association, 2000, p. 199), substance abuse refers to a maladaptive pattern of substance abuse that results in one or more of the following: failure to fulfill life roles, recurrent use when it is dangerous (e.g., drinking and driving), recurrent legal problems, and continued use despite social and interpersonal problems associated with the use. In other words, the consequences of using substances determine whether there is substance abuse or not.

Addiction involves psychological dependence on the medication or substance. Addicts are preoccupied with how they are going to get a substance. They may spend much of their time using the substance and recovering from its effects. They may take more of the substance than they had planned. They may desire to stop using or have tried to stop, but their efforts have not been successful. They may engage in harmful behaviors to get the drug, such as stealing from friends or relatives, breaking into pharmacies, breaking into liquor stores. They continue to use despite the potential harmful effects (e.g., physical, psychological) and consequences (e.g., going to jail, marriage/partnership problems, job loss). They tend to be in a state of denial as their lives go downhill.

Contrast this with legitimate pain patients. Their lives are improving as a result of taking the pain medications prescribed. Their relationships may be improving, and they may be less irritable because their pain is under better control. They may return to work. Their functioning may be improving.

Although health care professionals should assess for aberrant drug-taking behaviors, the majority of chronic pain patients are honest and legitimate users of prescription medications, not addicts. There are no studies demonstrating that pain patients abuse pain medications or illicit substances any more than the general population. In other words, pain itself is not a risk factor for substance abuse or addiction. According to the joint statement from 21 health care organizations and the Drug Enforcement Adminstration, "for many patients, opioid analgesics—when used as recomended by established pain management guidelines—are the most effect way to treat their pain, and often the only treatment option that provides significant relief (DEA, 2001). The medical professional can use the WHO analgesic ladder to treat noncancer pain, secure in the knowledge that most patients do not abuse medications.

Benzodiazepines, such as Diazepam (Valium), are used to treat anxiety and muscle spams associated with acute pain. These medications are not effective for other types of pain and should be used with caution because of the potential to abuse them (American Pain Society, 1999). Benzodiazepines are also harmful because they may dull cognition and memory, and, as a result, may actually interfere with progress in psychotherapy.

MEDICATION MANAGEMENT OF NEUROPATHIC PAIN

As mentioned in chapter 1, neuropathic pain has a different pathophysiologic mechanism than nocioceptive pain. Therefore, there are different treatment guidelines in terms of the medication management of this syndrome of illnesses. See Table 17.1 for a list of medications used in the management of neuropathic pain.

TABLE 17.1 Pharmacological Management of Neuropathic Pain

Medication Type	Examples
Antidepressants	amitriptyline (Elavil), nortriptyline (Pamelor), SSRIs: fluoxetine (Prozac), sertraline (Zoloft), paroxetine (Paxil); venlafaxine (Effexor)
Anticonvulsants	carbamazepine (Tegretol), oxcarbazepine (Trileptal), gabapentin (Neurontin), lamotrigine (Lamictal), topiramate (Topomax), tiagabine (Gabitril)
Antiarrhythmics	mexiletine, lidocaine
Topical formulations	capsaicin, lidocaine, aspirin
Analgesics	NSAID (Ibuprofen), COX-2 inhibitors (see text), tramadol (Ultram), opiates (oxycodone [Percocet], morphine, fentanyl [Duragesic patch])
Others	ketamine, dextromethorphan

NSAID = nonsteroidal anti-inflammatory drug
SSRI = Selective Serotomy Reuptake Inhilitor
Developed by Daniel Gruener, MD

The hallmark of treating neuropathic pain as opposed to nociceptive pain consists of antidepressants, particularly the tricyclics, as well as anticonvulsants. The use of antidepressants, for example, tricyclics, increase norepinephrine and serotonin levels in the brain, which inhibits descending pain messages (from the brain down the spinal cord), thus potentially dampening neuropathic pain. Tricyclic antidepressants such as amitriptyline (Elavil) and nortripyyline (Pamelor) have been shown to relieve the pain of diabetic neuropathy and postherpetic neuralgia (American Pain Society, 1999). Venlafaxine (Effexor) has been shown to produce pain relief in diabetic neuropathy in addition to its effects in alleviating depression (Kunz et al., 2000).

The newer so-called second generation anticonvulsants, for example, gabapentin (Neurontin), tiagabine (Gabitril), and oxcarbazepine (Trileptal), are often used off-label to treat the symptoms of neuropathic pain, because they have fewer side effects than their eralier counterparts, for example, carbamazepine (Tegretol). As mentioned earlier, gabapentin (Neurontin) is now FDA-approved for postherpetic neuralgia, which is a type of neuropathic pain. There is also a growing body of literature on anticonvulsant medications, and more studies are under way that may support the use of these agents in various pain syndromes.

In summary, the treatment of pain is relatively simple. We must determine if pain is nociceptive or neuropathic. If nociceptive, then we should utilize the WHO ladder, starting off with a nonopioid analgesic and progressing to an opioid if the pain is nonresponsive. If the pain is neuropathic, we should begin treatment with either an antidepressant or an anticonvulsant, combining these classes of agent if there are limited or no effects.

SUBSTANCE ABUSE IN CHRONIC PAIN PATIENTS

Although the majority of chronic pain patients will not have this problem, some chronic pain patients may be at risk for abusing substances, such as alcohol, illicit drugs, and prescription medication. The strongest risk factor of substance abuse issues in the chronic pain population is a history of substance abuse (Portenoy, 1990).

During the intake interview, as well as later in the therapy experience, therapists should assess patients' alcohol use, illicit drug use, and prescription medication use. Alcohol and illicit drug use can have a significant impact on the health of patients and may interfere with their physical progress and recovery. In addition, the abuse of alcohol, illicit drugs, and prescription medication can be potentially dangerous to the patients' health, especially if they are used in combination with one another. Physical and psychological difficulties can also occur if patients overuse certain prescribed or over-the-counter medications to cope with their pain, their sleeplessness, or their moods.

After therapists have obtained information about patients' use of these substances, they can have a better sense of direction with regard to the effects of substance use on the physical, psychological, and social problems of each patient. Unless therapists have specialized training in substance abuse treatment, it is recommended that they refer patients with substance abuse problems to qualified specialists (e.g., certified drug and alcohol counselors, medical specialists). Therapists who want to learn more about the cognitive therapy approach to helping patients with substance abuse can read the book *Cognitive Therapy of Substance Abuse* (Beck, Wright, Newman, & Liese, 1993).

TREATMENT ADHERENCE

One aspect of pain medication management is patients' adherence to pharmacotherapy treatment. Some patients may forget how much medicine they are supposed to take. This may be true of patients with cognitive impairments due to physical (e.g., head trauma) and/or psychological (e.g. severe depression) causes. Occasionally, patients may overuse medication.

It is recommended that therapists have an updated list of patients' medications, their dosage levels for each medication, the recommended administration times, and the purpose or function of each medication (i.e., inflammation, pain, sleep difficulties, or mood disturbances). If medical treatment adherance concerns arise, patients could be asked to keep track of their medications, dosage levels, and times of administration on a daily basis each week. This information could be provided to therapists to review to ensure that patients are taking their dosages on a time-contingent basis instead of an as-needed basis. The therapist can work with the patient, his or her physicians, and family members or close friends to ensure that the patient is taking the appropriate dosages of medication as recommneded and to identify potential barriers or pitfalls to appropriate medication use. If medications are overused or underused, then the reasons for these decisions, including the patient's beliefs about taking medication, should be explored.

PART VII

PREPARING FOR THE END
OF THERAPY AND BEYOND

18

Preparing for Termination and Relapse Prevention

As work draws to a close in therapy, it is a time for the therapist and patient to reflect on a number of issues, including what was learned in therapy, what was meaningful and helpful, what the patient plans to do in the future (i.e., self-help plan), and how effective therapy was for the patient. Developing a self-help plan and scheduling booster sessions are important components of relapse prevention.

PREPARING CHRONIC PAIN PATIENTS FOR THE END OF THERAPY

The therapist prepares the patient for the end of therapy from the very beginning, when goals are established. At different points during the therapeutic process, progress toward these goals should be reviewed. Once these goals are met, new goals are identified, or therapy is brought to a close.

As the therapist prepares the patient for the end of therapy, there are several important steps to follow: (1) encourage the patient to review his or her therapy notebooks, (2) review the key skills learned over the course of therapy, (3) discuss the skills that the patient plans to use in the future for each problem area (self-help plan), (4) schedule booster sessions as needed to prevent relapses, and (5) educate the patient that therapy services are available in the future as needed.

REVIEW THEIR THERAPY NOTEBOOK

Before the last session, the patient is asked to review all of the information sheets, therapy homework assignments, and notes that he or she has kept in their own folder or notebook. The therapy folder represents a summary of all the work done in therapy. It can include informational handouts on cognitive therapy, pain monitoring forms, Automatic Thought Records, activity monitoring/scheduling forms, advantages/disadvantages analysis forms, coping cards, core belief worksheets, cognitive conceptualization diagrams, problem-solving worksheets, relaxation handouts, relaxation tapes, and assertiveness training handouts, and medication logs. This process helps the patient reflect on what he or she has learned and accomplished in therapy. In fact, reviewing the therapy notebook on a regular basis after therapy has ended may be one component of the patient's self-help plan. In the following therapist–patient dialogue, the therapist asks the patient to review the therapy folder as a homework assignment. In the final session, this homework is discussed.

Therapist: Next week will be our last therapy session. As your last self-help homework assignment, I would like to suggest that you review all of your therapy handouts, and notes, and the worksheets, and coping cards we developed in therapy. As you review these materials, think about what you have learned and how you felt about the therapy experience, so we can discuss this next week. How does that sound to you?

[Next session]

Therapist: So, what was it like to review the materials in your therapy folder this past week?
Patient: It made me realize how much hard work we did! [laughs]

Therapist: We sure did! [laughs] Anything that stands out?
Patient: What stands out for me is that I do have less pain in my life than before, and I have some new ways to cope with my pain now.

Therapist: That's great. What do you think has helped to reduce your pain?
Patient: I think the relaxation techniques helped. Learning how to be more assertive with my doctor really helped us find the right medications for my pain. Thinking more realistically about my pain and my life has also had a big impact on me. I think I suffer less when I focus on what I can do and how I can cope.

REVIEW THE KEY SKILLS LEARNED OVER THE COURSE OF THERAPY

During the last therapy session, the therapist and patient can review and reflect on what was learned. The patient usually will be able to identify some new skills learned in therapy that helped him or her cope better with his or her pain, moods, relationships with others (including family, friends, physicians, and other treatment team members), and other areas of focus in therapy. Writing down these newly acquired skills in session will help create the patient's self-help plans for the future. Discussing pivotal moments or memories in the therapy experience will allow the patient to have some closure on the therapeutic relationship with the therapist.

In this part of the session, the therapist and patient discuss pivotal moments or memories.

Therapist: As you reflect back on your work in therapy, what stands out for you as some of the positive experiences?

Patient: Just knowing that you cared about me and my pain. I needed some space to talk about what I was going through. No one seemed to care then—at least, that was what I thought.

Therapist: I remember when you came into therapy. You were very distrustful and wanted to know what I was going to do for you. Do you remember that?

Patient: Yes, I was a tough cookie, wasn't I? [laughs]

Therapist: But somehow you learned to trust the therapy experience. You learned to trust me. What made the difference?

Patient: I remember in session you said that it was very natural for me to question what therapy was all about since I had never been in therapy before. And when you explained to me what I could expect, that made me feel better. But most importantly, you treated me like a person, not just another patient. I think I was sensitive to being moved around from one doctor's office to the next when I first started working with you.

Therapist: I'm glad you felt supported in here. What can you do in the future when you think professionals don't care about you or your pain, or when you think they can't be trusted?

Patient: I'll ask myself, "What's the evidence?" [laughs] I think I made some assumptions about professionals that may not be true. I'm sure that occasionally I may come across some professionals who don't care. In those cases, I can let them know I am concerned about their level of attention to my care, or I can find another professional to help me. I also have learned that doctors don't always have the answers or the "cure," and they don't have the time to talk like we do. I need to be more assertive with them in telling them about my experience of pain and how the treatments are working or are not working for me.

DEVELOPING A SELF-HELP PLAN FOR RELAPSE PREVENTION

After the patient and therapist have discussed what was learned in therapy, they can begin to explore what skills the patient plans to use in the future to cope with pain and his or her life. For example, developing a good relationship with the therapist may be viewed by some patients as one of the most important skills learned in therapy. If so, discussing what the patient learned in establishing this relationship will help him or her understand the skills he or she gained and can use in future relationships, particularly relationships with close friends and family, as well as other health care professionals, including physicians nurses and physical therapists.

The patient is then asked to anticipate potential problems or ongoing issues to work on in the future. These problems or issues should be written down along with a plan of action—identifying what skills will be used in the future to cope with each of them.

A self-help plan prepares the patient to handle problems on his or her own, without the therapist's help. Certainly, scheduling booster sessions or returning to therapy can be included as part of a self-help plan after patient has tried other prevention strategies.

In the following therapist–patient dialogue, a self-help plan for the patient is developed.

Therapist: Of all the skills you have learned in therapy, which ones do you think you are going to use in the future?

Patient: Definitely the relaxation techniques to reduce my pain. The Automatic Thought Record will help me catch my negative thoughts and evaluate them. Once I was able to look at my thoughts as possibilities instead of facts and reviewed all of the evidence, I realized that many of my thoughts and beliefs were not realistic. Life seems to be more manageable when I think more realistically about my pain. [pause] Reading the coping cards reminds me of the work we did in therapy and what I can do to cope, especially when I am in a lot of pain.

Therapist: Do you see yourself putting these skills into action in the future? Can you imagine it?

Patient: Definitely. I've practiced them so many times now that it almost feels automatic.

Therapist: Great! Do you foresee any difficulties in coping with your pain or other stresses in the future?

Patient: Sure. I may have periods when the pain is really intense, really severe. During those times, I plan to distract myself by playing the relaxation tapes. If I start to feel depressed, anxious, or angry about my pain, I can talk with my friends about it. I can also fill out my Automatic Thought Records to catch my negative thoughts and put them to the test when I am down or overwhelmed by the pain. This will help me think more realistically and focus on what I can do about the problems in my life.

Therapist: This sounds like a great plan. Let's write down some of these ideas.

Figure 18.1 is an example of a self-plan the therapist and patient developed during their last therapy session.

FIGURE 18.1 Self-Help Plan

Pain Management
When I am experiencing intense, severe pain, I need to remember to

1. Relax.
   - Practice my deep breathing exercises.
   - Use progressive muscle relaxation.
   - Use guided muscle relaxation.
   - Use guided imagery.

2. Catch my negative thoughts and evaluate them.
   - Use the Automatic Thought Record to write down the situation, my experience of pain, my emotions, and my automatic thoughts.
   - Remember that thoughts are not facts, but hypotheses or possibilities to test out.
   - Look for errors in my thinking.
   - Explore the evidence for and against my negative thoughts, especially the "hot" ones.
   - Come up with a realistic alternative explanation.
   - If my negative thoughts are true, move to problem solving (identify the problem, generate solutions, try one solution, and evaluate effectiveness).
   - Continue to review cognitive therapy self-help books, for example, *Mind over Mood: A Cognitive Therapy Treatment Manual for Clients* (1995) by Dennis Greenberger and Christine Padesky, and *The Feeling Good Handbook* (1989) by David Burns.

FIGURE 18.1 *(continued)*

3. Catch my negative images and stop them or change them in some way.
   - Stop/interrupt traumatic or distressing memories/images if they are bothering me.
   - Take images of pain beyond the worst.
   - Imagine coping in the image.
   - Become the director of my image and change it in some way.
   - Face my traumatic or distressing images when I am ready.

4. Be aware of my core beliefs that get activated when I am in pain.
   - When I think I'm inadequate or I'm unworthy of love and support, I will review my core belief worksheets.
   - I will continue to collect evidence for and against my beliefs and modify them.
   - I will fill out new core belief worksheets as needed.
   - Continue to review *Reinventing Your Life* (1994) by Jeffrey Young and Janet Klosko.

5. Take my medication as recommended by my physician.
   - Keep track of my medications, dosages, and frequency of use on a daily basis.
   - Don't underuse or overuse medications.
   - When I am concerned about increased pain or the reduced effectiveness of any medications, I will contact my physician and schedule an appointment.

6. Meet regularly with my physician to review my pain management plan.
   - Don't be afraid to ask questions. (I am the consumer of services. This is my body.)
   - Go in with specific, brief questions for my physician. (Write them down in outline form.)
   - Tell my physician what I am feeling when I am in pain. (Don't downplay or exaggerate it.)
   - Follow my physician recommendations or seek a second opinion.

7. Stay active to keep my body and mind healthy.
   - If my pain is really bothering me, try to distract myself and do something else if I can.
   - Continue exercising 3 to 4 days a week to condition my muscles and to combat stress. Adjust any exercise plans based on my physician's recommendations.
   - Don't sit or lie down for long periods (except at night when sleeping).
   - Put pleasurable activities into my daily life.

8. Seek support and be assertive.
   - Join support group in the community.
   - Review chronic pain self-help books. Examples include *Managing Pain before It Manages You: Revised Edition* (2000) by Margaret Caudill, *The Chronic Pain Control Workbook* (1996) by Ellen Catalano and Kimeron Hardin, and *Learning to Master Your Chronic Pain* (1996) by Robert Jamison.
   - Find other articles and book on my chronic pain condition and read them.
   - Keep in touch with my two best friends.
   - Tell people what I want using "I" statements.
   - Focus on listening first and summarize what I hear. Then state my own opinions or feelings without blame (no "you" statements or "why" questions).

9. Return to therapy for a booster session in 2 months.
   - Discuss my progress and focus on any potential problem areas.
   - If I need to return to therapy again, it is not a sign of weakness, but a sign of strength. We can identify new problems or issues to work on in therapy.

SCHEDULE BOOSTER COGNITIVE THERAPY SESSIONS AS NEEDED

Although the therapist and patient mutually agree to end therapy, the patient should be told that he or she may request a booster session. The booster session is often a "refresher" session to remind the patient of the skills that he or she learned in therapy and how these skills can be applied to a recent event or an upcoming stressor (e.g., surgery, ending a relationship). Usually, this session is focused on cognitive coping (e.g., identifying, evaluating, and modifying automatic thoughts/beliefs; use of imagery to cope) and problem-solving strategies (e.g., identify problem, generate solutions, and commit to trying out one solution; relaxation; distraction techniques, etc.). Some patients do not return for a follow-up, knowing that these booster sessions are available provides them with a great deal of security.

SEEK OUT FUTURE PSYCHOTHERAPY SERVICES AS NEEDED

Near the end of the last session, it is often helpful for the therapist to remind the patient that he or she can seek out psychotherapy services when needed. The patient has a right to find a therapist with whom he or she feels most comfortable. Providing the patient with the opportunity to return to work with the therapist as well as providing other referral resources will help guide the patient to a variety of professionals in the future. The patient also needs to understand that not all therapists use the same approach to therapy or have the same personalities. Each therapist is unique, so encouraging the patient to be a knowledgeable consumer of services will help to ensure positive experiences in therapy in the future.

In summary, cognitive therapy is an effective form of therapy with patients who have chronic pain. Cognitive therapy is not just a set of techniques or a theory for understanding pain and distress. This therapy approach embraces a supportive, compassionate and collaborative relationship between the therapist and the patient. Chronic pain patients have plenty of medical and health care consultants on their team who give them advice and provide brief interventions. These patients want a therapist who will give them the space to talk—a professional who won't interrupt them or rush them out the door. They need our attention, understanding, compassion, enthusiasm, and hopefulness as therapists. They want someone to validate their pain and their suffering. These patients can be difficult to work with due to the chronicity of their pain, psychosocial stressors, and/or personality problems. However, the commitment, optimism, and flexibility of the therapist are essential to promote positive changes in these patients' lives. It is very rewarding to work with these people. We hope this book will help you in enhancing the quality of these patients' lives, who in many cases, have come to us as a last resort.

Appendix

Patient's Name:_____

Date of Session:_____ Time Session Began_____AM/PM

Therapist's Name:_____

PART I. Please **circle** your response to each of the following:

1. Before you came in today, how much progress did you expect to make in dealing with your problems **in today's session?**
   MUCH   SOME   NO
   PROGRESS   PROGRESS   PROGRESS

2. **In today's session,** how much progress do you feel you actually made?
   MUCH   SOME   NO
   PROGRESS   PROGRESS   PROGRESS

3. **In future sessions,** how much progress do you think you will be able to make in dealing with your problems?
   MUCH   SOME   NO
   PROGRESS   PROGRESS   PROGRESS

4. How satisfied are you with **today's session?**
   VERY SATISFIED   SATISFIED   INDIFFERENT   DISSATISFIED

5. **In today's session,** how well do you think your therapist understood your problems?
   VERY WELL   FAIRLY WELL   POORLY

6. How well were you able to convey your concerns or problems **in this session?**
   VERY WELL   FAIRLY WELL   POORLY

7. **In today's session,** how much did you think you could trust (have confidence in) your therapist?
   VERY MUCH   SOME   NOT AT ALL

PART II. Please answer the following questions about **homework.**

1. Was homework assigned **last session?**

2. Did you discuss last week's homework **in today's session?**

3. How helpful was the homework and the discussion of it?
   VERY   SOME   NOT AT ALL   NOT APPLICABLE

4. How pleased are you with the homework that was assigned for **this coming week?**
   VERY   SOME   NOT AT ALL   NOT APPLICABLE

PART II. Rate the extent to which you believe you gained the following skills **in this therapy session.** Please refer only to **this session,** realizing that not all of these skills can be gained in any one session.

		VERY MUCH	SOME	NONE
1.	Better insight into and understanding of my psychological problems	2	1	0
2.	Methods or techniques for better ways of dealing with people (i.e., asserting myself)	2	1	0
3.	Techniques in defining and solving my everyday problems (i.e., home, work, school)	2	1	0
4.	Confidence in undertaking an activity to help myself	2	1	0
5.	Greater ability to cope with my moods	2	1	0
6.	Better control over my actions	2	1	0
7.	Greater ability to **recognize** my unreasonable **thoughts**	2	1	0
8.	Greater ability to **correct** my unreasonable **thoughts**	2	1	0
9.	Greater ability to **recognize** my self-defeating or erroneous **assumptions**	2	1	0
10.	Greater ability to **evaluate** my self-defeating or erroneous **assumptions**	2	1	0
11.	Better ways of scheduling my time	2	1	0

PART IV. Rate the extent to which your therapist was the following **in this session.**

	VERY MUCH	SOME	NONE
1. Sympathetic and caring	2	1	0
2. Competent (knew what he/she was doing)	2	1	0
3. Warm and friendly	2	1	0
4. Supportive and encouraging	2	1	0
5. Involved and interested	2	1	0

PART V. Please circle the response which applies to your reaction to **today's session.**

1. My therapist acted condescending (talked down to me).   YES   NO

2. My therapist was too quiet and passive.   YES   NO

3. My therapist talked too much.   YES   NO

4. My therapist was too bossy.   YES   NO

5. My therapist seemed to miss the point.   YES   NO

6. This therapy (cognitive therapy) does not seem to be   YES   NO
   suited to me and my problem.

PART VI. In the remaining space, please describe the most outstanding aspect of today's session.

References

Achterberg, J., McGraw, P., & Lawlis, G. (1981). Rheumatoid arthritis: A study of relaxation and temperature biofeedback training as an adjunctive therapy. *Biofeedback and Self Regulation, 6,* 207–223.

ADA (1990). *The Americans with Disabilities Act.*

AGS Panel on Persistent Pain in Older Persons. (2002). Management of persistent pain in older persons. *Journal of the American Geriatrics Society, 60,* 205–224.

al Absi, M., & Rokke, P. (1991). Can anxiety help us tolerate pain? *Pain, 46,* 43–51.

American Pain Society. (1999). *Principles of analgesic use in the treatment of acute pain and cancer pain* (4th ed.). Glenview, IL: Author.

American Psychiatric Association. (2000). *Diagnostic and statistical manual of mental disorders* (4th ed., text rev.). Washington, DC: Author.

Appelbaum, K. (1991). The role of regular home practice in the relaxation treatment of tension headache. *Journal of Consulting and Clinical Psychology, 59,* 467–470.

Arntz, A., Dreessen, L., & De Jong, P. (1994). The influence of anxiety on pain: Attentional and attributional mediators. *Pain, 56,* 307–314.

Attanasio, V., Andrasik, F., & Blanchard, E. (1987). Cognitive therapy and relaxation training in muscle contraction headache: Efficacy and cost-effectiveness. *Headache, 27,* 254–260.

Banks, S., Jacobs, D., Gevirtz, R., & Hubbard, D. (1998). Effects of autogenic relaxation training on electromyographic activity in active myofascial trigger points. *Journal of Musculoskeletal Pain, 6*(4), 23–32.

Banks, S., & Kerns, R. (1996). Explaining high rates of depression in chronic pain: A diathesis-stress framework. *Psychological Bulletin, 119,* 95–110.

Basler, H., Jakle, C., & Kroner-Herwig, B. (1997). Incorporation of cognitive-behavioral treatment into the medical care of chronic low back pain patients: A controlled randomized study in German pain treatment centers. *Patient Education and Counseling, 31,* 113–124.

Basler, H., & Rehfisch, H. (1990). Follow-up results of a cognitive-behavioural treatment for chronic pain in a primary care setting. *Psychology and Health, 4,* 293–304.

Beck, A., Emery, G., & Greenberg, R. (1985). *Anxiety disorder and phobias: A cognitive perspective.* New York: Basic Books.

Beck, A., Epstein, N., Brown, G., & Steer, R. (1988). An inventory for measuring clinical anxiety: Psychometric properties. *Journal of Consulting and Clinical Psychology, 56,* 893–897.

Beck, A., Rush, J., Shaw, B., & Emery, G. (1979). *Cognitive therapy of depression.* New York: Guilford Press.

Beck, A., & Steer, R. (1988). *Beck Hopelessness Scale: Manual.* San Antonio, TX: The Psychological Corp.

Beck, A., Steer, R., & Brown, G. (1996). *The Beck Depression Inventory.* San Antonio, TX: The Psychological Corp.

Beck, A., Wright, F., Newman, C., & Liese, B. (1993). *Cognitive therapy of substance abuse.* New York: Guilford Press.

Beck, J. (1995). *Cognitive therapy: Basics and beyond.* New York: Guilford Press.

Bennett, G. (1994). Neuropathic pain. In R. Wall & R. Melzack (Eds.), *Textbook of pain* (pp. 201–224). New York: Churchill Livingstone.

Blanchard, E. (1992). Psychological treatment of benign headache disorders. *Journal of Consulting and Clinical Psychology, 60,* 537–551.

Bonica, J. (1990). *The management of pain.* Philadelphia: Lea & Pebiger.

Boothby, J., Thorn, B., Stroud, M., & Jensen, M. (1999). Copying with pain. In R. Gatchel & D. Tark (Eds.), *Psychosocial factors in pain critical perspectives* (pp. 343–359). New York: The Guilford Press.

Bostrum, M. (1997). Summary of the Mayday Fund Survey: Public attitudes about pain and analgesics. *Journal of Pain Symptom Management, 13,* 166–168.

Bradley, L., Young, L., Anderson, K., McDaniel, L., Turner, R., & Agudelo, C. (1984). Psychological approaches to the management of arthritis pain. *Social Science Medicine, 19*(12), 1353–1369.

Braha, R., & Catchlove, R. (1986–1987). Pain and anger: Inadequate expression in chronic pain patients. *Pain Clinic, 1,* 125–129.

Brescia, F., Porteroy, R., Ryan, M., Krdsnoff, L., & Gray, G. (1992). Pain, opioid use, and survival in hospitalized patients with advanced cancer. *Journal of Clinical Oncology, 10,* 149–155.

Brown, G., Nicassio, P., & Wallston, K. (1989). Pain coping strategies and depression in rheumatoid arthritis. *Journal of Consulting and Clinical Psychology, 57*(5), 652–657.

Burns, D. (1989). *The feeling good handbook.* New York: Penguin.

Burns, J., Johnson, B., Mahoney, N., Devine, J., & Pawl, R. (1996). Anger management style, hostility and spouse responses: Gender differences in predictors of adjustment among chronic pain patients. *Pain, 64,* 445–453.

Butcher, I., Dahlstrom, W., Graham, J., Tellegen, A., & Kaemmer, B. (1989). *Manual for administration and scoring. MMPI-2.* Minneapolis: University of Minnesota Press.

Cardona, L. (1994). Behavioral approaches to pain and anxiety in the pediatric patient. *Child and Adolescent Psychiatric Clinics of North America, 3*(3), 449–464.

Catalano, E., & Hardin, K. (1996). *The chronic pain control workbook: A step-by-step guide for coping with and overcoming pain.* Oakland, CA: New Harbinger Publications.

Caudill, M. (2000). *Managing pain before it manages you: Revised edition.* New York: Guilford Press.

Corne, S., Wilson, K., Pontefract, A., & deLaplante, L. (2000). Cognitive behavioral treatment of insomnia secondary to chronic pain. *Journal of Consulting and Clinical Psychology, 68,* 407–416.

Cutler, R., Fishbain, D., Rosomoff, H., Abdel-Moty, E., Khalil, T., & Rosomoff, R. (1994). Does nonsurgical pain center treatment of chronic pain return patients to work? A review and meta-analysis of the literature. *Spine, 19,* 643–652.

Dahl, J., & Faellstroem, C. (1989). Effects of behavioral group therapy on chronic pain. *Scandinavian Journal of Behaviour Therapy, 18,* 137–143.

DEA (2001). Drug Enforcement Administration, 21 health groups call for balanced policy on prescription pain medications like OxyContin. http://www. usdoj.gov/dea/pubs/pressrel/pr102301.html. Accessed May 5, 2003.

Deardoff, W. (2000). The MMPI-2 and chronic pain. In R. Gatchel & J. Weisberg (Eds.), *Personality characteristics of patients with pain* (pp. 109–128). Washington, D.C.: American Psychological Association.

Emmelkamp, P., & van Oppen, P. (1993). Cognitive interventions in behavioral medicine. *Psychotherapy Psychosomatics, 59,* 116–130.

Engstrom, D. (1983). Cognitive behavioral therapy methods in chronic pain treatment. In J. J. Bonica (Ed.), *Advances in pain research and therapy* (pp. 829–838). New York: Raven Press.

Erdal, K. J., & Zautra, A. J. (1995). Psychological impact of illness downturns: A comparison of new and chronic conditions. *Psychology and Aging, 10,* 570–577.

Faucett, J., & Levine, J. (1991). The contributions of interpersonal conflict to chronic pain in the presence or absence of organic pathology. *Pain, 44,* 35–43.

Feldman, S., Downey, G., & Schaffer-Neitz, R. (1999). Pain, negative mood, and perceived support in chronic pain patients: A daily diary study of people with Reflex Sympathetic Dystrophy Syndrome. *Journal of Consulting and Clinical Psychology, 67,* 776–785.

Feverstein, M., Bürrell, L., Miller, V., Lincoln, A., Huang, G., & Berger, R. (1999). Clinical Management of Carpaltunnel Syndrome: A 12-year review of outcomes. *American Journal of Industrial Medicine, 35,* 232–245.

Flor, H., Fydrich, T., & Turk, D. (1992). Efficacy of multidisciplinary pain treatment centers: A meta-analytic review. *Pain, 49,* 221–230.

Fordyce, W. (1976). *Behavioral methods for chronic pain and illness.* St. Louis: C. V. Mosby.

Fordyce, W., Brockway, J., Bergman, J., & Spengler, D. (1986). Acute back pain: A control-group comparison of behavioral vs. traditional management methods. *Journal of Behavioral Medicine, 9*(2), 127–140.

Fordyce, W., Fowler, R., & DeLateur, B. (1968). An application of behavior modification technique to a problem of chronic pain. *Behaviour Research and Therapy, 6,* 105–107.

Gaskin, M., Greene, A., Robinson, M., & Geisser, M. (1992). Negative affect and the experience of chronic pain. *Journal of Psychosomatic Research, 36,* 707–713.

Gatchel, R., & Weisberg, J. (Eds.). (2000). *Personality characteristics of patients with pain.* Washington, DC: American Psychological Association.

Grant, L., & Haverkamp, B. (1995). A cognitive-behavioral approach to chronic pain management. *Journal of Counseling and Development, 74,* 25–31.

Greene, B., & Blanchard, E. (1994). Cognitive therapy for irritable bowel syndrome. *Journal of Consulting and Clinical Psychology, 62*(3), 576–582.

Greenberger, D., & Padesky, C. (1995). *Mind over mood: A cognitive therapy treatment manual for clients.* New York: Guilford Press.

Greenwald, B., & Narcessian, E. (1999). Opioids for managing patients with chronic pain: Community pharmacists' perspectives and concerns. *Journal of Pain Symptom Management, 17,* 369–375.

Gruener, D. (2003). Opioid analgesics. In D. Gruener & S. Lande (Eds.), *Pain control in the hospital.* Philadelphia: Greater Philadelphia Pain Society.

Gupta, M. (1986). Is chronic pain a variant of depressive illness? A critical review. *Canadian Journal of Psychiatry, 31,* 241–248.

Gutkin, A., Holborn, S., Walker, J., & Anderson, B. (1992). Treatment integrity of relaxation training for tension headaches. *Journal of Behavioral Therapy and Experimental Psychiatry, 23,* 191–198.

Hasenbring, M., Ulrich, H., Hartmann, M., & Soyka, D. (1999). The efficacy of a risk factor-based cognitive behavioral intervention and electromyographic biofeedback in patients with acute sciatic pain. An attempt to prevent chronicity. *Spine, 24,* 2525–2535.

Holroyd, K., & Andrasik, F. (1982). Do the effects of cognitive therapy endure? A two-year follow-up of tension headache sufferers treated with cognitive therapy or biofeedback. *Cognitive Therapy and Research, 6,* 325–334.

Holroyd, K., Holm, J., Hursey, K., Penzien, D., Cordingley, G., Theofanous, A., Richardson, S., & Tobin, D. (1988). Recurrent vascular headache: Home-based behavioral treatment versus abortive pharmacological treatment. *Journal of Consulting and Clinical Psychology, 56,* 218–223.

Hyman, S., & Cassen, N. (1996). Pain. In *Scientific American Medicine, 3.*

Jacobson, E. (1938). *Progressive relaxation* (2nd ed.). Chicago: University of Chicago Press.

James, L., Thorn, B., & Williams, D. (1993). Goal specification in cognitive-behavioral therapy for chronic headache pain. *Behavior Therapy, 24,* 305–320.

Jamison, R. (1996). *Learning to master your chronic pain.* Sarasota: Professional Resource Exchange, Inc.

Jamison, R., & Virts, K. (1990). The influence of family support on chronic pain. *Behaviour Research and Therapy, 28,* 283–287.

Jensen, M., Karoly, P., & Huger, R. (1987). The development and preliminary validation of an instrument to assess patients' attitudes toward pain. *Journal of Psychosomatic Research, 31,* 393–400.

Jensen, M., Romano, J., Turner, J., Good, A., & Wald, L. (1999). Patient beliefs predict patient functioning: Future support for a cognitive-behavioural model of chronic pain. *Pain, 81,* 95–104.

Kaivanto, K., Estlander, A., Moneta, G., & Vanharanta, H. (1995). Isokinetic performance in low back pain patients: The predictive power of the Self-Efficacy Scale. *Journal of Occupational Rehabilitation, 5,* 87–99.

Kanazi, G., Johnson, R., & Dworkin, R. (2000). Treatment of postherpetic neuralgia: An update. *Drugs, 59,* 1113–1126.

Keefe, F., Caldwell, D., Williams, D., Gil, K., Mitchell, D., Robertson, C., Martinez, S., Nunley, J., Beckham, J., Crisson, J., & Helms, M. (1990). Pain coping skills training in the management of osteoarthritic knee pain: A comparative study. *Behavior Therapy, 21,* 49–62.

Keefe, F., & Van Horn, Y. (1993). Cognitive-behavioral treatment of rheumatoid arthritis pain. *Arthritis Care and Research, 6,* 213–222.

Keefe, F., Williams, D., & Smith, S. (2001). Assessment of pain behaviors. In R. Gatchel & J. Weisberg (Eds.), *Personality characteristics of patients with pain* (pp. 109–128). Washington, DC: American Psychological Association.

Keel, P., Bodoky, C., Gerhard, U., & Muller, W. (1998). Comparison of integrated group therapy and group relaxation training for fibromyalgia. *Clinical Journal of Pain, 14,* 232–238.

Kerns, R., Haythornthwaite, J., Southwick, S., & Giller, E. (1990). The role of marital interaction in chronic pain and depressive symptom severity. *Journal of Psychosomatic Research, 34,* 401–408.

Kerns, R., Turk, D., Holzman, A., & Rudy, T. (1986). Comparison of cognitive behavioral and behavioral approaches to the outpatient treatment of chronic pain, *Clinical Journal of Pain, 1,* 195–203.

Kole-Snijders, A., Vlaeyen, J., Goossens, M., Rutten-van Moelken, M., Heuts, P., van Breukelen, G., & von Eek, H. (1999). Chronic low-back pain: What does cognitive coping skills training add to operant behavioral treatment? Results of a randomized clinical trial. *Journal of Consulting and Clinical Psychology, 67,* 931–944.

Kunz, N., Goli, V., Entsuah, A. et al. (2000, October). *Venlafaxine in painful diabetic neuropathy.* Abstract presented at the annual meeting of the American Diabetes Association, Denver.

Labus, J., Keefe, F., & Jensen, M. (2003). Self-reports of pain intensity and direct observations of pain behavior: When are they correlated? *Pain, 102,* 109–124.

Lackner, J., Carosella, A., & Feuerstein, M. (1996). Pain expectancies, pain, and functional self-efficacy expectancies as determinants of disability in patients with chronic low back disorders. *Journal of Consulting and Clinical Psychology, 64*(1), 212–220.

Larsson, B., & Melin, L. (1989). Follow-up on behavioral treatment of recurrent headache in adolescents. *Headache, 29,* 249–253.

Lefebvre, M. (1981). Cognitive distortion and cognitive errors in depressed psychiatric and low back pain patients. *Journal of Consulting and Clinical Psychology, 49,* 517–525.

Linton, S. (1979). Behavioral approaches to low back pain. *Scandinavian Journal of Behaviour Therapy, 8,* 121–132.

Linton, S., & Andersson, T. (2000). Can chronic disability be prevented? A randomized trial of a cognitive-behavior intervention and two forms of information for patients with spinal pain. *Pain, 25,* 2825–2831.

Linton, S., Bradley, L., Jensen, I., Spangfort, E., & Sundell, L. (1989). The secondary prevention of low back pain: A controlled study with follow-up. *Pain, 36,* 197–207.

Lisspers, J., & Ost, L. (1990). Long-term follow-up of migraine treatment: Do the effects remain up to six years? *Behaviour Research and Therapy, 28,* 313–322.

Magni, G., Caldieron, C., Rigatti-Luchini, S., & Merskey, H. (1990). Chronic musculoskeletal pain and depressive symptoms in the general population: An analysis of the 1st National Health and Nutrition Examination Survey data. *Pain, 43,* 299–307.

Marcus, D. (2003). Tips for managing pain. Implementing the latest guidelines. *Postgraduate Medicine, 113,* 49–50, 55–56, 59–60.

McCracken, L., Zayfert, C., & Gross, R. (1992). The Pain Anxiety Symptom Scale: Development and validation of a scale to measure fear of pain. *Pain, 50,* 67–73.

Melzack, R. (1975). The McGill pain questionnaire: Major properties and scoring methods. *Pain, 1,* 277–299.

Melzack, R. (1987). The short-form McGill pain questionnaire. *Pain, 30,* 191–197.

Merskey, H., & Bogduk, N. (Eds.). (1994). *Classification of chronic pain: Description of chronic pain syndromes and definition of pain terms.* Seattle; IASP Press.

Miller, L. (1993). Psychotherapeutic approaches to chronic pain. *Psychotherapy, 30(1),* 115–124.

Mims, B. C. (1989). Sociologic and cultural aspects of pain. In C. D. Tollison (Ed.), *The handbook of chronic pain management* (pp. 17–25). Baltimore: Williams & Wilkins.

Morley, S., Eccleston, C., & Williams, A. (1999). Systematic review and meta-analysis of randomized controlled trials of cognitive behaviour therapy and behaviour therapy for chronic pain in adults, excluding headache. *Pain, 80,* 1–13.

Morrison, J. (1996). *The first interview.* New York: Guilford Press.

Murphy, A., Lehrer, P., & Jurish, S. (1990). Cognitive coping skills training and relaxation training as treatments for tension headaches. *Behavior Therapy, 21,* 89–98.

Newton-John, T., Spence, S., & Schotte, D. (1995). Cognitive-behavioural therapy versus EMG biofeedback in the treatment of chronic low back pain. *Behaviour Research and Therapy, 33,* 691–697.

Nicholas, M., Wilson, P., & Goyen, J. (1992). Comparison of cognitive-behavioral group treatment and an alternative non-psychological treatment for chronic low back pain. *Pain, 48,* 339–347.

Nicholson, N., & Blanchard, E. (1993). A controlled evaluation of behavioral treatment of chronic headache in the elderly. *Behavior Therapy, 24,* 395–408.

Ollat, H., & Cesaro, P. (1995). Pharmacology of neuropathic pain. *Clinical Neuropharmacology, 18,* 391–404.

Padesky, C., & Greenberger, D. (1995). *Clinician's guide to mind over mood.* New York: Guilford Press.

Parker, J., Frank, R., Beck, N., Smarr, K., Buescher, K., Phillips, L., Smith, E., Anderson, S., & Walker, S. (1988). Pain management in rheumatoid arthritis patients: A cognitive-behavioral approach. *Arthritis and Rheumatism, 31,* 593–601.

Parker, J., Iverson, G., Smarr, K., & Stucky-Ropp, R. (1993). Cognitive-behavioral approaches to pain management in rheumatoid arthritis. *Arthritis Care and Research, 6,* 207–212.

Paulsen, J., & Altmaier, E. (1995). The effects of perceived versus enacted social support on the discriminative cue function of spouses for pain behaviors. *Pain, 60,* 103–110.

Payne, R., & Dale, D. (1996). Pain. In *Scientific American Medicine, 3,* p. 3.

Pearce, S., & Erskine, A. (1993). Evaluation of the long-term benefits of a cognitive-behavioural out-patient programme for chronic pain. In M. Hodes & S. Moorey (Eds.), *Psychological treatment in disease and illness* (pp. 140–150).

Murray, L., et al. (Eds.). (2003). *Physicians desk reference* (57th ed.). Montvale, NJ: Thompson, PDR.

Pilowsky, I., & Spence, N. (1976). Illness behavior syndromes associated with intractable pain. *Pain, 2,* 61–71.

Pilowsky, I., Spence, N., Rounsefell, B., Forsten, C., & Soda, J. (1995). Out-patient cognitive-behavioural therapy with amitriptyline for chronic non-malignant pain: A comparative study with 6-month follow-up. *Pain, 60,* 49–54.

Portenoy, R. (1990). Chronic opioid therapy in nonmalignant pain. *Journal of Pain and Symptom Management, 5*(1), 46–62.

Reese, L. (1983). Coping with pain: The role of perceived self-efficacy. *Disertations Abstracts International, 44*(5-B), 1641.

Resnik, D., Rehm, M., & Minard, R. (2001). The undertreatment of pain: Scientific, clinical, cultural, and philosophical factors. *Medicine Health Care, and Philosophy, 4,* 277–288.

Romano, J., Jensen, M., Turner, J., Good, A., & Hops, H. (2000). Chronic pain patient-partner interactions: Further support for a behavioral model of chronic pain. *Behavior Therapy, 31,* 415–440.

Romano, J., & Turner, J. (1985). Chronic pain and depression: Does the evidence support a relationship? *Psychological Bulletin, 97,* 18–34.

Romano, J., Turner, J., Jensen, M., Friedman, L., Bulcroft, R., Hops, H., & Wright, S. (1995). Chronic pain patient–spouse behavioral interactions predict patient disability. *Pain, 63,* 353–360.

Rosenstiel, A., & Keefe, F. (1983). The use of coping strategies in chronic low back pain patients: Relationship to patient characteristics and current adjustment. *Pain, 17,* 33–44.

Ross, M. J., & Berger, R. S. (1996). Effects of stress inoculation training on athletes' postsurgical pain and rehabilitation after orthopedic injury. *Journal of Consulting and Clinical Psychology, 64*(2), 406–410.

Ruksznis, E. (1996). Consensus on pain and insomnia. *APS Observer, 9*(1).

Saarijarvi, S., Rytokoski, U., & Karppi, S. (1990). Marital satisfaction and distress in chronic low-back pain patients and their spouses. *Clinical Journal of Pain, 6,* 148–152.

Schwartz, L., Slater, M., & Birchler, G. (1996). The role of pain behaviors in the modulation of marital conflict in chronic pain couples. *Pain, 65,* 227–233.

Schwarz, S., Taylor, A., Scharff, L, & Blanchard, E. (1990). Behaviorally treated irritable bowel syndrome patients: A four-year follow-up. *Behavioral Research and Therapy, 29*(4), 331–335.

Seaburn, D. B., Lorenz, A., & Kaplan, D. (1992). The transgenerational development of chronic illness meanings. *Family Systems Medicine, 10*(4), 385–394.

Severeijns, R., Vlaeyen, J., van den Hout, M., & Weber, W. (2001). Pain catastrophizing predicts pain intensity, disability, and psychological distress independent of the level of physical impairment. *Clinical Journal of Pain, 17,* 165–172.

Spikoff, M. (2001). Regulatory attitudes improve, but fear of opioid use continues. http://www.mdoptions.com/cgi-bin/article.cgi?article_id=928, accessed April 10, 2003.

Söderlond, A., & Lindberg, P. (2001). An integrated physiotherapy/cognitive-behavioral approach to the analysis and treatment of chronic whiplash associated disorders. *Disability and Rehabilitation, 23,* 436–437.

Sorbi, M., Tellegen, B., & du-Long, A. (1989). Long-term effects of training in relaxation and stress-coping in patients with migraine: A 3-year follow-up. *Headache, 29,* 111–121.

Spence, S. (1998). Cognitive-behavior therapy in the management of upper extremity cumulative trauma disorder. *Journal of Occupational Rehabilitation, 8,* 27–45.

Spence, S., Sharpe, L., Newton-John, T., & Champion, D. (1995). Effect of EMG biofeedback compared to applied relaxation training with chronic, upper extremity cumulative trauma disorder. *Pain, 63,* 199–206.

Spielberger, C. (1999). The State-Trait Anger Expression Inventory-2: Professional manual. Odessa, FL: Psychological Assessment Resources.

Stanton-Hicks, M., Baron, R., Boas, R., Gordh, T., Harden, N., Hendler, N., Koltzenburg, M., Raj, P., & Wilder, R. (1998). Complex regional pain syndromes: Guidelines for therapy. *Clinical Journal of Pain, 14,* 155–166.

Stroud, M., Thorn, B., Jensen, M., & Boothby, J. (2000). The relation between pain beliefs, negative thoughts, and psychosocial functioning in chronic pain patients. *Pain, 84,* 347–352.

Stucky, C., Gold, M., & Zhang, X. (2001). Mechanisms of pain. *Proceedings of the National Academy of Sciences of the United States of America, 98,* 11845–11846.

Sullivan, M., Reesor, K., Mikail, S., & Fisher, R. (1992). The treatment of depression in chronic low back pain: Review and recommendations. *Pain, 50,* 5–13.

Sullivan, M., Thorn, B., Haythornthwait, J., Keefe, F., Martin, M., Bradley, L., et al. (2001). Theoretical perspectives on the relation between catastrophizing and pain. *Clinical Journal of Pain, 17,* 52–64.

Summers, J., Rapoff, M., Varghese, G., Porter, K., & Palmer, R. (1991). Psychosocial factors in chronic spinal cord injury pain. *Pain, 47,* 183–189.

Tearnan, B., & Lewandowski, M. (1992). The Behavioral Assessment of Pain Questionnaire: The development and validation of a comprehensive self-report instrument. *American Journal of Pain Management, 2,* 181–191.

Tobin, D., Holroyd, K., Baker, A., Reynolds, R., & Holm, J. (1988). Development and clinical trial of a minimal contact, cognitive-behavioral treatment of tension headache. *Cognitive Therapy and Research, 12,* 325–339.

Tollison, C. (1993). The magnitude of the pain problem: The problem in perspective. In R. Weiner (Ed.), *Innovations in pain management: A practical guide for clinicians* (vol. 1, pp. 3–9). Orlando, FL: Paul M. Deutsch Press.

Tollison, C. & Hinnant, D. (1996). Psychological testing in the evaluation of the patient in pain. In S. Waldman & A. Winnie (Eds.), *Interventional pain management* (pp. 119–128). Philadelphia: W. B. Saunders.

Toner, B., Segal, Z., Emmott, S., Myran, D., Ali, A., DiGasbarro, I., & Stuckless, N. (1998). Cognitive-behavioral group therapy for patients with irritable bowel syndrome. *International Journal of Group Psychotherapy, 48,* 215–243.

Tota-Faucette, M., Gil, K., Williams, D., Keefe, F., & Goli, V. (1993). Predictors of response to pain management treatment: The role of family environment and changes in cognitive processes. *Clinical Journal of Pain, 9,* 115–123.

Trief, P. M., Elliott, D. J., Stein, N., & Frederickson, B. B. (1987). Functional vs. organic pain: A meaningful distinction? *Journal of Clinical Psychology, 43*(2), 219–226.

Turk, D., Kerns, R., & Rosenberg, R. (1992). Effects of marital interaction on chronic pain and disability: Examining the down side of social support. *Rehabilitation Psychology, 37,* 259–274.

Turk, D., Meichenbaum, D., & Genest, M. (1993). *Pain and behavioral medicine: A cognitive-behavioral perspective.* New York, NY: Guilford Press.

Turk, D., & Melzack, R. (2001). *Handbook of pain assessment* (2nd ed.). New York: Guilford Press.

Turk, D., Rudy, T., & Steig, R. (1987). Chronic pain and depression. *Pain Management, 7,* 141–149.

Turkat, I., & Pettegrew, L. (1983). Development and validation of the Illness Behavior Inventory. *Journal of Behavioral Assessment, 5,* 35–47.

Turner, J. (1982). Comparison of group progressive-relaxation training and cognitive-behavioral group therapy for chronic low back pain. *Journal of Consulting and Clinical Psychology, 50*(5), 757–765.

Turner, J., & Clancy, S. (1988). Comparison of operant behavioral and cognitive-behavioral group treatment for chronic low back pain. *Journal of Consulting and Clinical Psychology, 56*(2), 261–266.

Van Peski-Oosterbaan, A., Spinhoven, P., van Rood, Y., van der Does, J., Bruschke, A., & Rooijmans, H. (1999). Cognitive-behavioral therapy for noncardiac chest pain: A randomized trial. *American Journal of Medicine, 106,* 424–429.

van Tulder, M., Ostelo, R., Vlaeyen, J., Linton, S., Morley, S., & Assendelft, W. (2000). Behavioral treatment for chronic low back pain. *Spine, 26,* 270–281.

Varni, J. (1981). Self-regulation techniques in the management of chronic arthritic pain in hemophilia. *Behavior Therapy, 12,* 185–194.

Varni, J., & Gilbert, A. (1982). Self-regulation of chronic arthritic pain and long-term analgesic dependence in a hemophiliac. *Rheumatology and Rehabilitation, 22,* 171–174.

Varni, J., Gilbert, A., & Dietrich, S. (1981). Behavioral medicine in pain and analgesia management for the hemophilic child with factor VIII inhibitor. *Pain, 11,* 121–126.

Ventafridda, V., & Stjernsward, J. (1996). Pain control and the World Health Organization analgesic ladder. *Journal of the American Medical Association, 275,* 835–836.

Vlaeyen, J., Haazen, I., Schuerman, J., & Kole-Snijders, A., & van Eek, H. (1995). Behavioural rehabilitation of chronic low back pain: Comparison of an operant treatment, an operant-cognitive treatment and an operant respondent treatment. *British Journal of Clinical Psychology, 34,* 95–118.

Vollmer, A., & Blanchard, E. (1998). Controlled comparison of individual versus group cognitive therapy for irritable bowel syndrome. *Behavior Therapy, 29,* 19–33.

Waldrop, D., Lightsey, O., Jr., Ethington, C., Woemmel, C., & Coke, A. (2001). Self-efficacy, optimism, health competence, and recovery from orthopedic surgery. *Journal of Counseling Psychology, 48*(2), 233–238.

Weisberg, J., & Keefe, F. (1999). Personality, individual differences, and psychopathology in chronic pain. In R. Gatchel & D. Turk (Eds.), *Psychosocial factors in pain: Critical perspectives* (pp. 56–73). New York: Cuilford Press.

Woolf, G., & Mannion, R. (1999). Neuropathic pain: Etiology, symptoms, mechanisms and management. *Lancet, 353,* 1959–1964.

Weiner, R.S. (Ed.), (1993). *Innovations in Pain Management: A Practical Guide for Clinicians,* Volume I, Chapter 1.

Williams, A., Richardson, P., Nicholas, M., Pither, C., Harding, V., Ridout, K., Ralphs, J., Richardson, I., Justins, D., & Chamberlain, J. (1996). Inpatient vs. outpatient pain management: Results of a randomized controlled trial. *Pain, 66*, 13–22.

World Health Organization. (1995). The WHO analgesic ladder for cancer pain management: Stepping up the quality of its evaluation. *Journal of the American Medical Association, 274*, 1870–1873.

Young, J. (1999). *Cognitive therapy for personality disorders: A schema-focused approach* (3rd. ed.). Sarasota, FL: Professional Resource Press.

Young, J., & Klosko, J. (1994). *Reinventing your life.* New York: Plume Books.

Index

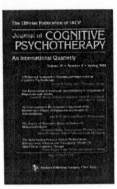

$ *Springer Publishing Company*

Clinical Advances in Cognitive Psychotherapy

Theory and Application

Robert L. Leahy, PhD, and
E. Thomas Dowd, PhD, ABPP, Editors

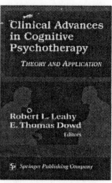

A virtual Who's Who in the field of cognitive psychotherapy! Briefly tracing the history and derivation of cognitive psychotherapy, the authors discuss its recent developments as an evolving and integrative therapy. Several of the chapters illustrate the applications of cognitive psychotherapy to treat such disorders as anxiety, depression, and social phobia. Other chapters discuss integration with therapy models such as schema-focused and constructivism. New empirically-based research is cited for treating the HIV-positive depressed client, the anorexic or bulimic sufferer, as well as applying cognitive therapy to family and group issues.

Partial Contents:

2002   464pp   0-8261-2306-6   hard

536 Broadway, New York, NY 10012 • Fax: 212-941-7842
Order Toll-Free: 877-687-7476 • Order On-line: www.springerpub.com